Health Disparities in Allergic Diseases

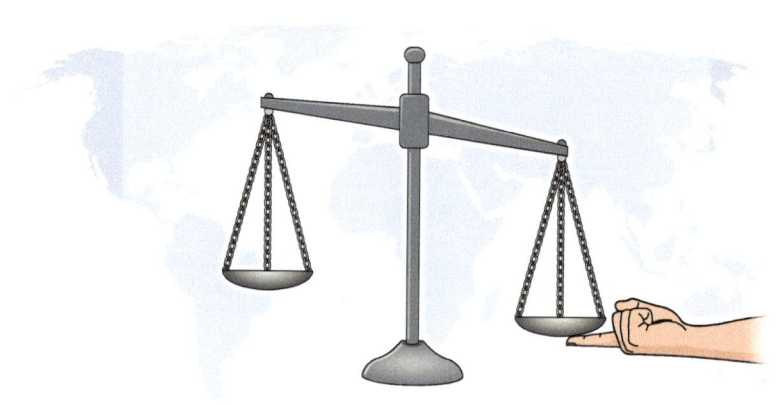

Mahboobeh Mahdavinia

Editor

Health Disparities in Allergic Diseases

An Evidence-Based Look at Causes, Conditions, and Outcomes

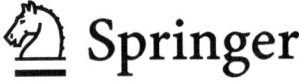 Springer

Editor
Mahboobeh Mahdavinia
Rush University
Chicago, IL
USA

ISBN 978-3-030-31221-3   ISBN 978-3-030-31222-0   (eBook)
https://doi.org/10.1007/978-3-030-31222-0

This Springer imprint is published by the registered company Springer Nature Switzerland AG
The registered company address is: Gewerbestrasse 11, 6330 Cham, Switzerland

Preface

On a daily basis, I take care of patients with severe allergies, people from all walks of life, different age groups, races, and genders and varied resources in life. An observation obvious from first days of training as a physician occupied my mind and later drove my research toward the field of disparity. I often take care of children with severe asthma in the hospital who have been intubated for asthma attacks and spend 1–2 days per months in average in the emergency department. These children can hardly keep up with their school work or even run for a fun play. Sometimes, we never hear of these children again, even after calling the number in the file multiple times to follow up on them or reschedule an appointment. I also take care of children, adolescents, and adults with the same type of asthma who run marathons, are part of the hockey or soccer teams, and do greatly at school and work. Allergies are chronic conditions and in most cases are carried throughout life. These conditions need to be properly managed and followed. Certain time points in life are key in their management and prevention of adverse outcomes.

Access to health care is a right to everyone in the society. As physicians, we are under the oath to provide care, not harm. It is extremely painful to see how incapacitated we are in delivering this oath sometimes, due to the existing health-care inequities, when we are unable to prescribe the medication of choice and do the proper testing, or when our patients are lost to follow up as they cannot afford to come back. This has been a drive for multiple epidemiologists and physicians around the globe to develop alternative methods to bridge the gaps in health care. However, despite these efforts, today, we still witness a great deal of preventable poor outcomes and damages that are certainly more common in minorities and socioeconomically deprived communities.

Health disparity is defined as health difference that is linked to social or economic disadvantage. These disparities adversely affect groups of people who have experienced greater social or economic obstacles to health based on race, socioeconomic status, gender, geographic location, or other characteristics that are historically linked to discrimination or exclusion. The extent of the problem is beyond a specific part of the globe. Most parts of the world including developed and developing countries witness such disparities at a great extent. Health disparities significantly affect patients with allergic diseases. In some allergic conditions, such as asthma or food allergy, these disparities can result in higher preventable mortality, while disparities result in higher morbidities in all allergic conditions such as eczema or rhinitis.

Addressing disparities in allergic diseases requires a multifactorial approach at the levels of public health policy, health-care providers, and individuals. Systematic interventions should be aimed at decreasing risk factors that disproportionally affect racial and ethnic minorities and impoverished populations. These include campaigns to reduce air pollution in inner city areas, control indoor allergen exposure, promote smoking cessation, and prevent violence in neighborhoods.

As individuals involved in health care, we can all play our part. Extra efforts to remove barriers to care such as taking the patient's language fluency and health literacy into account or spending more time to reassure proper rapport can go a long way. As health-care providers, we can sense and inquire about possible cultural beliefs and fears related to management, such as concerns about the use of controller inhalers for asthma which has been shown to be a major barrier to adherence to these lifesaving medications. Proper discussion and providing evidence can help them overcome these fears. If patients and their families feel that we truly care and are available if they need us, they will reach out on time and follow our recommendations. These efforts can increase adherence to medications and increase the outpatient follow-up that is necessary for reassessment and reinforcement of treatments.

In this book, we provide evidence and discuss studies from both developed and developing countries that witness health disparities in allergic disease. We tell stories of our patients with allergic diseases who had very poor preventable outcomes due to their lack of access and inadequate care. While it might be late for some of our patients, it is still time for a lot more children and adults suffering from allergic diseases. In the last chapters, we provide examples of programs and strategies that can help prevent or at least decrease such stories.

Chicago, IL, USA   Mahboobeh Mahdavinia, MD, PhD

Contents

Part III   Providing Solutions

Contributors

Hassan A. Ahmad Rush University Medical Center, Department of Internal Medicine, Division of Allergy/Immunology, Chicago, IL, USA

Sindhura Bandi, MD Allergy and Immunology, Rush University Medical Center, Chicago, IL, USA

Arnaldo Capriles-Hulett, MD Hospital San Juan de Dios, Caracas, Venezuela
Centro Medico de Caracas, Centro Medico Docente La Trinidad, Caracas, Venezuela

Christopher D. Codispoti, MD, PhD Department of Internal Medicine, Rush University Medical Center, Chicago, IL, USA

Brandon E. Cohen, MD Dermatology, University of Southern California, Los Angeles, CA, USA

Fernando De Maio, PhD Department of Sociology and Center for Community Health Equity, DePaul University, Chicago, IL, USA

Anne Marie Ditto Department of Medicine, Division of Allergy-Immunology, Northwestern University Feinberg School of Medicine, Chicago, IL, USA

Sareh Eghtesad, MS, RD Liver and Pancreatobiliary Diseases Research Center, Digestive Diseases Research Institute, Tehran University of Medical Sciences, Tehran, Iran

Nada Elbuluk, MD, MSC Dermatology, University of Southern California, Los Angeles, CA, USA

Roselyn M. Hicks, MD Satcher Health Leadership Institute, Division of Health Policy, Morehouse School of Medicine, Atlanta, GA, USA

Kylie N. Jungles Department of Allergy and Immunology, Rush University Medical Center, Chicago, IL, USA

Anjeni Keswani, MD, MSCI GW School of Medicine & Health Sciences, Washington, DC, USA

Jonatan Konfino, MD, MSc Centro de Estudios de Estado y Sociedad (CEDES), Buenos Aires, Argentina

Molly A. Martin, MD, MAPP Department of Pediatrics, University of Illinois at Chicago, Chicago, IL, USA

Leena Padhye Rush University Medical Center, Department of Internal Medicine, Division of Allergy/Immunology, Chicago, IL, USA

Andrea A. Pappalardo, MD Department of Pediatrics, University of Illinois at Chicago, Chicago, IL, USA

Department of Medicine, University of Illinois at Chicago, Chicago, IL, USA

Nima Parvaneh, MD Division of Allergy and Clinical Immunology, Department of Pediatrics, Tehran University of Medical Sciences, Tehran, Iran

Research Center for Immunodeficiencies, Children's Medical Center, Tehran University of Medical Sciences, Tehran, Iran

Mario Sánchez-Borges, MD Allergy and Clinical Immunology Department Centro Medico Docente La Trinidad, Caracas, Venezuela

Clinica El Avila, Caracas, Venezuela

Hendrik Sy Department for Infectious Diseases and Pulmonary Medicine, Charité – University Medicine Berlin, Berlin, Germany

Mary C. Tobin, MD Rush University Medical Center, Department of Internal Medicine, Division of Allergy/Immunology, Chicago, IL, USA

Ulyana Trytko Rush University Medical Center, Department of Internal Medicine, Division of Allergy/Immunology, Chicago, IL, USA

Alicia T. Widge, MD, MS National Institutes of Health, National Institute of Allergy and Infectious Diseases, Bethesda, MD, USA

Part I
Introductory Chapters

Chapter 1
Global Health: Reimagining Perspectives

Fernando De Maio and Jonatan Konfino

Introduction

Global health offers a particularly valuable lens to view the world. On the one hand, global health offers an image of development and overall improvements, with progression from the "age of pestilence and famine" to a newer age where more and more populations live longer and longer. This is supported by a number of indicators showing widespread (aggregate) improvements in critical epidemiological indicators, including life expectancy and infant mortality, over the past 50 years [1]. Yet, on the other hand, global health offers an image of great heartbreak and disappointment – with millions suffering from the burdens of neglected diseases and coping with morbidity and mortality from preventable causes associated with chronic non-communicable diseases [2–5]. This is supported by the brute facts indicative of broad inequity: life expectancy varies from 50 years to over 80 years in different countries, and diarrhoea remains a leading cause of death for children aged 5 and younger [1]. The toll of tuberculosis – despite the development of effective medications more than 40 years ago – is still unacceptably high [1, 5]. And when we go beyond national averages to look at within-country inequities, we recognize that the national pictures are misleading, hiding the very real and substantial inequities that exist in rich and poor countries alike [6]. Understanding the complexities of global health requires us to grapple with the world as deeply unequal and unjust [7]. Disparities in management and hence outcomes of non-communicable diseases such as asthma and allergies are examples of these inequities. Inequities are observed

F. De Maio (✉)
Department of Sociology and Center for Community Health Equity, DePaul University, Chicago, IL, USA
e-mail: fdemaio@depaul.edu

J. Konfino
Centro de Estudios de Estado y Sociedad (CEDES), Buenos Aires, Argentina

© Springer Nature Switzerland AG 2020
M. Mahdavinia (ed.), *Health Disparities in Allergic Diseases*,
https://doi.org/10.1007/978-3-030-31222-0_1

not only between populations in different countries but also within the same populations living in one city in countries with overall good levels of population health [8].

We can discern different ways of conceptualizing global health [2, 3, 9]. One tradition, the "statist" tradition, frames global health primarily as a question of security; it sees disease as a *threat* to be defeated [10, 11]. It invokes the state's obligation to defend its borders from external threats. In doing so, this type of thinking pathologizes the suffering of poor people, seeing their existence as a threat that must be contained [10]. In this light, Ebola matters to rich countries because it strikes fear, and "vulnerability" is generalized to everyone [11]. National policies based on this perspective actively screen out "sick" immigrants, erecting barriers (in the case of the United States under the Trump administration, calling for a physical wall on the southern border with Mexico). Under the statist perspective, migration itself becomes a danger to rich countries [4, 12, 13]. Under the statist perspective, global health takes place "out there", in so-called developing countries [14], and interventions often take the guise of charity [5] – a type of intervention that sidesteps the underlying questions of social justice [15].

The alternative way of understanding global health is from the perspective of human rights. This "globalist" tradition offers a rebuke to the statist tradition – from this perspective, we are interested in global health not because global patterns of disease are necessarily a *threat* but because we recognize the interconnectedness of all populations and the right of every individual on the planet to benefit from advances in medical care [5]. From this perspective, global health is not just about what happens *out there*. Instead, global health is concerned with how health/disease is shaped by global economic, political and cultural forces that transcend national boundaries. When our health is influenced by international food processing regulations, we witness global health in practice. When we work with or for companies with a global presence, we are part of a chain of events connected to global health; health "there" is influenced by actions here. For Koplan et al., global health:

> refers to any health issue that concerns many countries or is affected by transnational determinants, such as climate change or urbanisation, or solutions, such as polio eradication. Epidemic infectious diseases such as dengue, influenza A (H5N1), and HIV infection are clearly global. But global health should also address tobacco control, micronutrient deficiencies, obesity, injury prevention, migrant-worker health, and migration of health workers. *The global in global health refers to the scope of the problems, not their location* (emphasis added). [14]

Seeing global health from the globalist tradition shifts our intervention efforts from charity towards something far more structural – towards what the WHO has named the "uneven distribution of power, money, and resources" [16].

In this chapter, we explore the statist and globalist traditions in global health through an analysis of an important theoretical framework: epidemiologic transition. We identify the broad contours of the model and discuss some of its main critiques, before moving to a discussion of the United Nations' Sustainable Development Goals (SDGs). Our analysis identifies challenges and opportunities for adopting an equity-based perspective that would call out and challenge the root causes of avoidable and unnecessary morbidity and mortality in the world today.

Theorizing Global Health

One of the most influential (and debated) models in global health is Abdel Omran's theory of epidemiologic transition. His theory describes changes in a country's leading causes of death from infectious (or communicable) to chronic (or non-communicable) diseases [2, 17, 18]. The classic formulation of this model posits that the transition is primarily associated with a country's economic development. It describes how countries transition over time from an "era of pestilence and famine," characterized by brutally low life expectancies and outbreaks of infectious pathogens, to an era of "receding pandemics" and finally to an era of "man-made and degenerative" diseases, where life expectancy is high and mortality relatively predictable from 1 year to the next. Omran's model certainly describes the experience of the rich industrialized countries of the world – but the extent to which it applies to countries of the global south today is much debated.

As a theoretical framework, the epidemiologic transition is often implicit in global health thinking. It is often taken for granted that the model works and that it describes with some degree of precision the development of global health over time. Indeed, we have seen shifts in the leading causes of death towards chronic non-communicable diseases [19]. Yet researchers have also paused to unpack the model, sometimes developing ways of extending the theory to better fit contemporary epidemiological profiles in specific countries and regions [20–26] and sometimes criticizing it and calling for its abandonment altogether [27–29].

The most recent research in this area has questioned the assumptions of epidemiologic transition theory, and empirical findings show that many countries of the global south experience a persistent "dual burden" of disease, something that the original theory did not foresee in its stages of transition. Omran's model was very optimistic about the shift in population health profiles from infectious to non-communicable diseases. The coexistence of chronic diseases such as cancer, cardiovascular disease, adult-onset diabetes and arthritis with infectious diseases such as tuberculosis and malaria presents formidable challenges to fragmented and under-funded healthcare systems. Understanding epidemiologic transition, or what we might instead see as epidemiologic *overlap*, is therefore critical to gauging the pressures on healthcare systems in the global south, as well as to thinking about strengthening those healthcare systems.

Omran's theory, like all theories, was a product of its time – steeped in modernization theory and lacking the nuanced critiques raised by dependency theory and, later, world-systems approaches [2]. Omran saw development naturally occurring over time, though the pacing of that development could vary from place to place. But the notion of progress, of development through stages, was nevertheless fundamental to Omran's theory – from his theory, we have an image of the world *developing* towards higher and higher levels of population health, with longer life expectancies. And on this issue, epidemiologic transition is incompatible with more critical approaches to understand the world today [28, 30]. Martínez and Leal argue, for example, that the model is grossly *optimistic*, assuming that epidemiologic and economic improvement will naturally occur over time, ultimately labelling it an *illusion* [27]. Critics argue that Omran's model was naïve about economic development (which dependency and world-systems theories argue are not inevitable) and about infectious diseases (with HIV/AIDS being the clearest rebuke to the idea that infectious diseases could no longer threaten "post-transition" populations). Omran's theory also had very little, if anything, to say about global health inequities – which the WHO CSDH has poignantly framed as the critical social justice question of our time [2, 7, 16].

Global health discussions have turned from the passive perspective of Omran's epidemiologic transition theory to the far more active "structural determinants of health" model advocated by the WHO *Commission on the Social Determinants of Health*. The WHO Commission shifted the focus of the work from economic development to health equity, ultimately concluding that "reducing health inequalities is an ethical imperative. Social injustice is killing people on a grand scale" [16]. The CSDH took an openly progressive political stance, emphasizing that "it does not have to be this way and it is not right that it should be like this. Where systematic differences in health are judged to be avoidable by reasonable action they are, quite simply, unfair. Putting right these inequities – the huge and remediable differences in health between and within countries – is a matter of social justice" [16]. The CSDH openly questioned the benefits of globalization for the world's poor, observing that increasingly transnational risks are borne by low- and middle-income countries, while the financial benefits of new global trade agreements are unequally distributed in favour of high-income regions [2].

Overall, the WHO CSDH proposed 12 objectives categorized into three broad principles:

1. Improve daily living conditions

    • A more equitable start in life
    • A flourishing living environment
    • Fair employment and decent work
    • Universal social protection
    • Universal healthcare

2. Tackle the inequitable distribution of power, money and resources

    • Coherent approach to health equity
    • Fair financing
    • Market responsibility
    • Improving gender equity for health
    • Fairness in voice and inclusion
    • Good global governance

3. Measure and understand the problem and assess the impact of action

    • Enhanced capacity for monitoring, research and intervention [16]

The report emphasized the need for the pragmatic improvement of day-to-day living conditions for the world's poor. Building on a large literature on the health effects of childhood deprivation, the CSDH took a life course perspective and called for a major emphasis on early child development and education. At the same time, it called for strengthened social policies and legislation for working age populations, emphasizing the need to "improve the working conditions for all workers to reduce their exposure to material hazards, work-related stress, and health-damaging behaviours" [16]. Moreover, the CSDH called for living wage legislation and emphasized the need to "establish and strengthen universal comprehensive social protection policies that support a level of income sufficient for healthy living for all" [16]. The WHO CSDH advocated for a clear focus on the structural and social determinants of health.

The Commission described the 40-year gap in life expectancy from the poorest to the richest as four decades that are "denied" [16]. At the same time, it documented *within*-country inequities based on a variety of factors – economic, political and gender-based. The Commission calls for a refocusing of much of the global discourse on health, away from development towards equity, towards social justice.

We argue that responding to the WHO Commission's call will require global health researchers to name and challenge the status quo, to name and challenge our roles and our institutions' roles in the maintenance of an unequal system. At the core of this work is the concept of structural violence, defined by Paul Farmer et al. as "social arrangements that put individuals and populations in harm's way... The arrangements are *structural* because they are embedded in the political and economic organization of our social world; they are *violent* because they cause injury to people". It is structural violence that maintains the patterns of global health inequities that we see in the world today [31].

Selected Global Health Targets

Much of the contemporary global health discourse revolves around the United Nations' Sustainable Development Goals (SDGs), which build upon the previous Millennium Development Goals (MDGs) [32–34]. There are 17 SDGs:

1. No Poverty
2. Zero Hunger
3. Good Health and Well-Being
4. Quality Education
5. Gender Equality
6. Clean Water and Sanitation
7. Affordable and Clean Energy
8. Decent Work and Economic Growth
9. Industry, Innovation and Infrastructure
10. Reduced Inequality
11. Sustainable Cities and Communities
12. Responsible Consumption and Production
13. Climate Action
14. Life Below Water
15. Life on Land

16. Peace and Justice Strong Institutions
17. Partnerships to Achieve the Goal

While SDG 3 is the only one explicitly framed in the language of health, all of the other SDGs connect to health outcomes (perhaps, most clearly SDG 1, dealing with poverty; SDG 2, dealing with hunger; and SDG 10, dealing with inequality). SDG 3 is then organized into 13 targets, as shown in Table 1.1.

Table 1.1 Targets associated with SDG 3 "General Health and Well-Being". (Source: https://www.who.int/sdg/targets/en/)

By 2030, reduce the global maternal mortality ratio to less than 70 per 100,000 live births	Achieve *universal health coverage*, including financial risk protection, *access to quality essential health-care services and access to safe, effective, quality and affordable essential medicines and vaccines for all*
By 2030, end preventable deaths of newborns and children under 5 years of age, with all countries aiming to reduce neonatal mortality to at least as low as 12 per 1,000 live births and under-5 mortality to at least as low as 25 per 1,000 live births	By 2030, substantially reduce the number of deaths and illnesses from hazardous chemicals and air, water and soil pollution and contamination
By 2030, end the epidemics of AIDS, tuberculosis, malaria and neglected tropical diseases and combat hepatitis, water-borne diseases and other communicable diseases	Strengthen the implementation of the World Health Organization Framework Convention on Tobacco Control in all countries, as appropriate
By 2030, reduce by one third premature mortality from non-communicable diseases through prevention and treatment and promote mental health and well-being	Support the research and development of vaccines and medicines for the communicable and noncommunicable diseases that primarily affect developing countries, provide access to affordable essential medicines and vaccines, in accordance with the Doha Declaration on the TRIPS Agreement and Public Health, which affirms the right of developing countries to use to the full the provisions in the Agreement on Trade Related Aspects of Intellectual Property Rights regarding flexibilities to protect public health, and, in particular, provide access to medicines for all
Strengthen the prevention and treatment of substance abuse, including narcotic drug abuse and harmful use of alcohol	Substantially increase health financing and the recruitment, development, training and retention of the health workforce in developing countries, especially in least developed countries and small island developing States
By 2020, halve the number of global deaths and injuries from road traffic accidents	Strengthen the capacity of all countries, in particular developing countries, for early warning, risk reduction and management of national and global health risks
By 2030, ensure *universal access to sexual and reproductive health-care services*, including for family planning, information and education, and the integration of reproductive health into national strategies and programmes	

Several of the targets aim at big mortality indicators – with explicit targets associated with reductions in maternal mortality and child mortality by 2030. The epidemics of AIDS, tuberculosis, malaria and neglected tropical diseases are also called out for particular attention, as is the burden of chronic non-communicable diseases – the latter building on a great deal of advocacy lead by the WHO in the past 20 years [19, 35, 36]. Morbidity indicators take a backseat, and allergic diseases (the focus of this book) are problematically not highlighted as priorities.

Challenges and Opportunities

The WHO CSDH and the new SGD framework offer important opportunities for global health research and advocacy. The WHO CSDH, in particular, has attempted to shift attention towards structural and social determinants of health, framing global health inequities in the language of social justice. And the SDGs, much like the previous MDGs, attempt to set quantitative benchmarks to track progress and galvanize attention. However, as well intentioned as these works may be, we face an unequal playing field, and the fundamental question of how to nurture health equity in an increasingly unequal world is unaddressed. We live in a world that contains more scientific, technological and medical power than ever before. Yet what Paul Farmer describes as the "fault lines of inequality" are also more pronounced than ever [37].

The charitable sector is one of the fastest-growing industries in the global economy. This deluge of philanthropy has helped create a world where billionaires wield more power over education policy, global agriculture and global health than ever before [38]. Yet, the charitable model has failed to address the root causes of inequality. As Farmer notes:

> Those who believe that charity is the answer to the world's problems often have a tendency – sometimes striking, sometimes subtle, and surely lurking in all of us – to regard those needing charity as intrinsically inferior. This is different from regarding the poor as powerless or impoverished because of historical processes and events…. There is an enormous difference between seeing people as the victims of innate shortcomings and seeing them as the victims of structural violence. [5]

In place of charity, Farmer would have us adopt a social justice lens – one with a clear eye focus on structural violence as a driver of health and economic inequities despite overall economic growth (whose benefits do not "trickle down" to the poor).

One of the most promising developments in global health – a development with the real potential to change "business as usual" towards a more progressive system guided by equity – is the global revival in "social medicine". The term social medicine has deep roots – associated in Europe with Rudolph Virchow and in Latin America with a long-standing tradition symbolized perhaps most clearly by Argentina's Ramon Carrillo [39] and Chile's Salvador Allende [40, 41]. Most recently, it has been taken up by the "Social Medicine Consortium" (see http://www.socialmedicineconsortium.org/), who declares itself: "rooted in the belief that inequity kills, and that together we can achieve health equity by constructing systems that demand justice, recognize our global interconnectedness, and enable the next generation of health professionals". Groups like the Social Medicine Consortium actively develop local and global discussions focused on the structural roots of illness, guided by the conviction that health systems can and must address inequities in health in far deeper ways than are allowed by the traditional biomedical perspective.

Other groups, including the "People's Health Movement" (https://phmovement. org/), visualize a world in which equity between and within countries is achieved and health for all is a reality. They "demand that governments, international financial institutions and the United Nations agencies including the WHO be accountable to people, not to transnational corporations and their agents". They base their analysis on politics and economics, seeing those parts of life as integral to the delivery of healthcare; their analysis is rooted in Carillo and Allende's social medicine and echoes in the work of the WHO CDSH:

> High income countries, working closely with transnational corporations, are promoting neo-liberal policies to manage the contemporary crisis of globalized capitalism in the interests of the transnational capitalist class. With help from a network of one-sided 'trade and investment' agreements, these policies are either being accepted by or being forced on the governments of low and middle income countries. The resulting national policies are having far reaching consequences for the social conditions that shape people's health, and also for the approach and funding of comprehensive health care. Such policies are worsening the fundamental determinants of health, and progressively crippling healthcare infrastructure and delivery of services. Such policies are encouraging national governments to abdicate their responsibilities to public health... [42]

Groups like the Social Medicine Consortium and the People's Health Movement call the "decolonizing" of global health, prioritizing, instead, collaborations and partnerships that do not impose agendas onto poor people in the global south. To be clear, the default setting – the charity model – is rooted in unequal power relations, implying that the global north has answers for problems in the global south. What we require – if the promise of the WHO CSDH is to be followed through – is a new type of global health research, one based on science but also cognizant of politics and history. This reimagined global health must acknowledge and respect the great resources that exist in the global south and must look for insights from low-income countries that may actually be transferable to wealthier (but still unequal) contexts [43]. A great example of this is the critical role that community health workers may play in improving health outcomes in a range of settings [44–46].

Conclusion

Global health is at a crossroad. There are more funds available for global health research and advocacy than ever before. There are important global agenda-setting documents, including the WHO CSDH and the United Nations' SDGs, that frame global health in innovative new ways, bringing focus to the structural and social determinants of health. And we have better epidemiological data than ever before. Yet, do we have the political will to prioritize global health? Or will global health matter first and foremost when it becomes a security threat (the statist perspective), perhaps calling for more and more well-intentioned but ultimately ineffective charity? Our challenge is to reimagine global health – acknowledging that the overall improvements we have seen in aggregate-level indicators have not been equally shared, acknowledging the persistent and growing inequities that exist despite unprecedented global economic growth. This reimagined global health may conceptualize health inequities as a manifestation of structural violence, calling for the structural solutions identified by social medicine.

From this broad-ranging review of global health thinking, we now turn our attention to allergic diseases in the global south, an important but neglected issue in global health.

References

1. WHO. World health statistics 2018. Geneva: World Health Organization; 2018.
2. De Maio F. Global health inequities: a sociological perspective. Basingstoke: Palgrave Macmillan; 2014.
3. Cockerham GB, Cockerham WC. Health and globalization. Cambridge: Polity Press; 2010.
4. Farmer P. Infections and inequalities: the modern plagues. Berkeley: University of California Press; 1999.
5. Farmer P. Pathologies of power: health, human rights, and the new war on the poor. Berkeley: University of California Press; 2003.
6. De Maio FG. Understanding chronic non-communicable diseases in Latin America: towards an equity-based research agenda. Glob Health. 2011;7:36.
7. Muntaner C, Sridharan S, Solar O, Benach J. Against unjust global distribution of power and money: the report of the WHO commission on the social determinants of health: global inequality and the future of public health policy. J Public Health Policy. 2009;30(2):163–75.
8. De Maio F, Shah RC, Mazzeo J, Ansell D. Community health equity: a Chicago reader. Chicago: University of Chicago Press; 2019.
9. Kim JY, Millen JV, Irwin A, Gershman J, editors. Dying for growth: global inequality and the health of the poor. Monroe: Common Courage Press; 2000.
10. Davies SE. Global politics of health. Cambridge: Polity Press; 2010.
11. Brown T. 'Vulnerability is universal': considering the place of 'security' and 'vulnerability' within contemporary global health discourse. Soc Sci Med. 2011;72(3):319–26.
12. Hotez PJ, Dumonteil E, Woc-Colburn L, Serpa JA, Bezek S, Edwards MS, et al. Chagas disease: "the new HIV/AIDS of the Americas". PLoS Negl Trop Dis. 2012;6(5):e1498.
13. De Maio FG, Llovet I, Dinardi G. Chagas disease in non-endemic countries: 'sick immigrant' phobia or a public health concern? Crit Public Health. 2014;24(3):372–80.
14. Koplan JP, Bond TC, Merson MH, Reddy KS, Rodriguez MH, Sewankambo NK, et al. Towards a common definition of global health. Lancet. 2009;373(9679):1993–5.
15. Guzmán RG. Latin American social medicine and the report of the WHO Commission on Social Determinants of Health. Soc Med. 2009;4(2):113–20.
16. WHO. Closing the gap in a generation: health equity through action on the social determinants of health. Geneva: World Health Organization; 2008.

17. Omran AR. The epidemiologic transition. A theory of the epidemiology of population change. Milbank Mem Fund Q. 1971;49(4):509–38.
18. Omran AR. The epidemiologic transition theory. A preliminary update. J Trop Pediatr. 1983;29(6).305–16.
19. WHO. Preventing chronic diseases: a vital investment. Geneva: World Health Organization; 2005.
20. Cook IG, Dummer TJ. Changing health in China: re-evaluating the epidemiological transition model. Health Policy. 2004;67(3):329–43.
21. Gaylin DS, Kates J. Refocusing the lens: epidemiologic transition theory, mortality differentials, and the AIDS pandemic. Soc Sci Med. 1997;44(5):609–21.
22. Heuveline P, Guillot M, Gwatkin DR. The uneven tides of the health transition. Soc Sci Med. 2002;55(2):313–22.
23. Waters WF. Globalization and local response to epidemiological overlap in 21st century Ecuador. Glob Health. 2006;2:8.
24. Frenk J, Bobadilla JL, Sepúlveda J, Cervantes ML. Health transition in middle-income countries: new challenges for health care. Health Policy Plan. 1989;4(1):29.
25. Olshansky SJ, Ault AB. The fourth stage of the epidemiologic transition: the age of delayed degenerative diseases. Milbank Mem Fund Q. 1986;64(3):355–91.
26. Salomon JA, Murray CJL. The epidemiologic transition revisited: compositional models for causes of death by age and sex. Popul Dev Rev. 2002;28(2):205.
27. Martínez CS, Leal FG. Epidemiological transition: model or illusion? A look at the problem of health in Mexico. Soc Sci Med. 2003;57(3):539–50.
28. Avilés LA. Epidemiology as discourse: the politics of development institutions in the Epidemiological Profile of El Salvador. J Epidemiol Community Health. 2001;55(3):164–71.
29. Barreto ML. The globalization of epidemiology: critical thoughts from Latin America. Int J Epidemiol. 2004;33(5):1132–7.
30. Barreto ML, De Almeida-Filho N, Breilh J. Epidemiology is more than discourse: critical thoughts from Latin America. J Epidemiol Community Health. 2001;55(3):158–9.
31. De Maio F, Ansell D. "as natural as the air around us": on the origin and development of the concept of structural violence in health research. Int J Health Serv. 2018;48(4):749–59.
32. Zamora G, Koller TS, Thomas R, Manandhar M, Lustigova E, Diop A, et al. Tools and approaches to operationalize the commitment to equity, gender and human rights: towards leaving no one behind in the Sustainable Development Goals. Glob Health Action. 2018;11(sup1):1463657.
33. Urbina-Fuentes M, Jasso-Gutierrez L, Schiavon-Ermani R, Lozano R, Finkelman J. Transition from Millennium Development Goals to Sustainable Development Goals from the perspective of the social determinants of health and health equity. Gac Med Mex. 2017;153(6):697–730.
34. Marmot M, Bell R. The sustainable development goals and health equity. Epidemiology. 2018;29(1):5–7.
35. Beaglehole R, Ebrahim S, Reddy S, Voute J, Leeder S. Prevention of chronic diseases: a call to action. Lancet. 2007;370(9605):2152–7.
36. Beaglehole R, Yach D. Globalisation and the prevention and control of non-communicable disease: the neglected chronic diseases of adults. Lancet. 2003;362(9387):903–8.
37. De Maio F. Paul Farmer: structural violence and the embodiment of inequality. In: Collyer F, editor. Handbook of social theory for health and medicine. Basingstoke: Palgrave Macmillan; 2015. p. 675–90.
38. McGovey L. No such thing as a free gift: the gates foundation and the price of philanthropy. London: Verso; 2016.
39. Lerace V. Ramon Carrillo, actualidad y vigencia de su pensamiento sanitario. Revista Mestiza. 2016.
40. Waitzkin H, Iriart C, Estrada A, Lamadrid S. Social medicine then and now: lessons from Latin America. Am J Public Health. 2001;91(10):1592–601.
41. De Maio F. Health & Social Theory. Basingstoke: Palgrave Macmillan; 2010.

42. Peoples' Health Movement. The struggle for health is the struggle for a more equitable, just and caring world. Declaration of the Fourth People's Health Assembly – PHA4 Savar, Bangladesh. 2018.
43. Binagwaho A, Nutt CT, Mutabazi V, Karema C, Nsanzimana S, Gasana M, et al. Shared learning in an interconnected world: innovations to advance global health equity. Glob Health. 2013;9:37.
44. O'Donovan J, Verkerk M, Winters N, Chadha S, Bhutta MF. The role of community health workers in addressing the global burden of ear disease and hearing loss: a systematic scoping review of the literature. BMJ Glob Health. 2019;4(2):e001141.
45. Inobaya MT, Chau TN, Ng SK, MacDougall C, Olveda RM, Tallo VL, et al. Mass drug administration and the sustainable control of schistosomiasis: community health workers are vital for global elimination efforts. Int J Infect Dis. 2018;66:14–21.
46. Schneider H, Okello D, Lehmann U. The global pendulum swing towards community health workers in low- and middle-income countries: a scoping review of trends, geographical distribution and programmatic orientations, 2005 to 2014. Hum Resour Health. 2016;14(1):65.

Chapter 2
Allergic Diseases in the Developing World: An Emerging Problem or an Overseen Issue?

Sareh Eghtesad

Allergic diseases are defined as a hypersensitivity or overreaction of the immune system to seemingly harmless substances in the environment. While being impacted by the environment, they are also closely linked to the genetic background of the individuals affected. A number of allergic conditions can be observed as a result of this altered immune response, such as atopic dermatitis, asthma, allergic rhinitis, and food sensitivity/allergy. Although allergens are different throughout the world and in different environments, some are more commonly known to cause an allergic response in many populations; these include pollens, dust mites, animal dander, insect bites, and certain foods such as nuts and seafood.

Historically, allergic diseases were seen more commonly in industrialized populations and more so in urban areas compared to rural regions. However, in the past few decades, a changing trend has been witnessed, and higher incidence of allergic diseases is observed in developing countries as well. This rise has been attributed to the effects of modernization, industrialization, and improved sanitation in those countries, as well as greater access to various foods. Modern life changes such as overcleaning, access to filtered and sanitized water, use of pesticides, detergents and cleaners, as well as food storage and transportation have decreased exposure to many antigens that individuals would previously be in contact with on a daily basis. But how does this affect allergic diseases? The answer is described by the "hygiene hypothesis," which is, perhaps, the most credible explanation for the observed change caused by modernization [1, 2]. The hygiene hypothesis states that decreased exposure to bacteria early on in life inhibits full immune system development, making individuals prone to allergic diseases [1]. Therefore, the more sterile the living environment in early life, the higher the incidence of allergic diseases. The hygiene hypothesis is supported by migration studies where individuals from developing countries with low incidence of allergic and autoimmune diseases who migrated to

S. Eghtesad (✉)
Liver and Pancreatobiliary Diseases Research Center, Digestive Diseases Research Institute, Tehran University of Medical Sciences, Tehran, Iran

© Springer Nature Switzerland AG 2020
M. Mahdavinia (ed.), *Health Disparities in Allergic Diseases*,
https://doi.org/10.1007/978-3-030-31222-0_2

developed countries with high incidence of these diseases acquired these conditions at rates similar to that of natives of the developed country, emphasizing the role of modern lifestyles and the environment in the development of these conditions [3]. With that said, two important factors influencing this observation are the length of stay of migrants and their age at the time of migration. This reinforces the idea that the lack of exposure to bacteria in *early childhood* is what leads to the exacerbated immune response.

Some of the consequences of this altered immune function have a greater impact on individuals' lives than others. Asthma, for example, characterized by inflammation and narrowing of the airways, affected 339 million people worldwide in 2018. Although its exact cause is not known, there is strong evidence linking atopy and asthma to the hygiene hypothesis [4]. However, most observations of asthma as an allergic disease come predominantly from high-income, developed countries, and the association of the two is weaker in low- and middle-income or developing countries. Could this be a truly weak association though? Or is it simply because data are lacking from developing countries?

Although it is speculated that the prevalence of allergic diseases in developing countries is growing, data is lacking on the exact rates of these conditions in various parts of the world. What is certain, however, is that prevalence rates are still lower than those observed in developed countries. With that said, because of poorer economic conditions and lack of access to appropriate medical care, the health and economic impact of these diseases appear to be higher in developing and underprivileged countries [5].

In the following sections, we will first review the available data on the prevalence of allergic diseases in developing countries and discuss trends and patterns seen over the past few decades, and then, we will discuss the overall risk factors and common allergens, followed by the burden caused by allergic diseases in these countries.

Prevalence of Allergic Diseases: An Overview

The International Study of Asthma and Allergies in Childhood (ISAAC) is the largest worldwide collaborative epidemiological research project investigating asthma, rhinitis, and eczema, including data from over 100 countries. The study started in 1991 and has had several phases carried out thus far. Early data from the study reported an astounding 20-fold to 60-fold difference in asthma, allergic rhinoconjunctivitis, and atopic dermatitis (eczema) among children in different parts of the world [6]. As expected, these diseases were highest in developed countries, such as the United Kingdom, Australia, New Zealand, and Ireland, and lowest in developing countries, such as Indonesia, China, Taiwan, Uzbekistan, India, and Ethiopia [7]. But prevalence rates increased throughout the world from Phase I to Phase III studies, with 6- to 7-year-old children of Jodhpur, India, experiencing the lowest rates (2.4%) and those in Costa Rica experiencing the highest (37.6%).

Asthma trends: The rates of asthma are markedly varied across the globe. Adolescents (13–14 years of age) in Tibet and New Zealand experienced the lowest and highest rates of asthma, respectively (0.8% vs. 32.6%) [5]. The countries experiencing the highest rates of asthma most often had higher rates of allergic rhinoconjunctivitis as well.

Atopic dermatitis followed different patterns, with African countries being among those with higher prevalence rates. Studies on atopic dermatitis revealed rates as low as <2% in Iran to over 16% in Japan and Sweden in 6–7 year olds. The rates were also varied in older children in different parts of the world with rates of <1% in Albania and over 17% in Nigeria in 13- to 14-year-old children [7]. Phase III data from ISAAC in 2008 showed the increasing trend in atopic dermatitis with the highest rates being in Asia and Latin America. In children 13–14 years of age, atopic dermatitis ranged from 0.2% in China to 24.6% in Columbia with the highest rates again in Africa and Latin America [8].

Food allergies are another major category of allergic diseases, and although there is a lack of high-quality studies using gold standard techniques of diagnosing food allergies, the available data still shows an increasing trend in developed and developing countries, with some developing countries showing rates as high as developed countries [9, 10]. Genome–environment interactions are evidenced by studies investigating food allergies in migrants or descendants of low- and middle-income countries growing up in developed countries. These studies have shown that the rates of food allergies in these immigrant populations are even higher than that observed in natives of those developed countries [10].

One very important factor when comparing prevalence rates among different countries is having the same diagnostic criteria for a disease, as different criteria in the same population can give varying results, let alone in different populations around the world. And while not all studies published in the past few decades use the same diagnostic criteria, many are either part of the ISAAC project or have adopted its protocols and questionnaires, performing the same study in 6-to 7-year-old and 13- to 14-year-old children, making their results ideal for comparison. Although all relevant studies have been included in the sections presented in this chapter, for the sake of convenience, studies using ISAAC guidelines are marked in the tables associated with each section.

Prevalence and Trends of Allergic Diseases: Africa

The prevalence of allergic diseases varies widely between African countries and even within different regions of one country. Data from selected countries are presented in Table 2.1. The lowest rates of asthma are reported in children from a low socioeconomic region of Nigeria (0.9%), while highest rates are observed in South Africa and Congo (20.3% and 19.9%, respectively) [11, 12]. Allergic rhinitis rates as high as 38.5% and 61.7% have been reported in the general population of South Africa and Benin, respectively [13, 14]. Data from African countries is very limited,

Table 2.1 African countries

Region	Countries n = 27	Prevalence rates before 1999	Prevalence rates 2000–2009	Prevalence rates 2010–2019	Risk factors/common allergens reported	References
Africa	Algeria	Asthma: 1.2–1.34% (GP) 1.6% (<5Y) 3.4–4.1% (5–25Y)	Asthma: 3.45% (GP)			[52, 196, 197]
	Angola			Asthma: 15.8% (6–7Y)[ISAAC] 13.4% (13–14Y)[ISAAC, a] Allergic rhinitis: 19% (6–7Y)[ISAAC] 27% (13–14Y)[ISAAC, a] Eczema/atopic dermatitis: 22% (6–7Y)[ISAAC] 20% (13–14Y)[ISAAC, a]		[6, 198]
	Benin			Allergic rhinitis 35.7% (6–65Y) Allergic rhinoconjunctivitis: 61.7% (6–65Y)	Indoor allergens: house dust, pets (dogs and cats) Outdoor allergens: air pollution	[13]
	Botswana			Asthma: 15.9% (6–7Y)[ISAAC, a] 16.3% (13–14Y)[ISAAC, a]		[59]

Country				Reference
Burkina Faso	Asthma: 9.6% (15–64Y)			[199]
Cameroon	Current wheeze: 0.8–5.4% (5–15Y) 1.3–2.5% (>15Y)	Asthma: 2.7% (A) Current wheeze: 2.9% (A) Allergic rhinitis: 10.4% (A) 24.5% (A) Allergic rhinoconjunctivitis: 5.4% (A)	Indoor allergens: mites Food allergens: wheat	[200–202]
Congo (Democratic Republic of)	Asthma: 19.9% (GP)	Current wheeze: 15.4% (5–83Y) Allergic rhinitis: 30.8% (5–83Y) Allergic rhinoconjunctivitis: 24.4% (5–83Y)	Indoor allergens: cockroach, D. pteronyssinus	[107]
Egypt	Asthma: 9.4% (11–15Y)ISAAC Current wheeze: 14.7% (11–15Y)ISAAC Allergic rhinoconjunctivitis: 15.3% (11–15Y)ISAAC			[54]

(continued)

Table 2.1 (continued)

Region	Countries n = 27	Prevalence rates before 1999	Prevalence rates 2000–2009	Prevalence rates 2010–2019	Risk factors/common allergens reported	References
	Ethiopia	Asthma: 2.8% (13–14Y)ISAAC Current wheeze: 18.2% (13–14Y)ISAAC	Current wheeze: 16.2% (13–14Y)ISAAC Allergic rhinoconjunctivitis: 14.5% (13–14Y)ISAAC Eczema/atopic dermatitis: 1.2% (GP) 10.9% (13–14Y)ISAAC	Current wheeze: 11.5% (1Y) Eczema/atopic dermatitis: 8.6% (1Y)	Indoor/housing allergens: residence in brick houses, wooden walls and floors, place of sleeping (floor vs. bed/platform) Outdoor allergens: pollen	[53, 56, 203–205]
	Ghana			Allergic rhinoconjunctivitis: 39.9% (C–T) Eczema/atopic dermatitis: 1.5–1.6% (C–T)ISAAC	Indoor allergens: mite, cockroach Other allergens: inner-city residence	[58, 206]
	Guinea		Asthma: 18.6% (GP)			[11]
	Ivory coast	Asthma: 10.8% (C) Current wheeze: 19.8% (C)	Asthma: 19.3% (GP)			[207]

Kenya	Asthma: 6.6% (13–14Y)^{ISAAC} Current wheeze: 21.2% (13–14Y)^{ISAAC} Allergic rhinitis: 14.9% (13–14Y)^{ISAAC} Eczema/atopic dermatitis: 13.9% (13–14Y)^{ISAAC}	Asthma: 12.6% (13–14Y)^{ISAAC} 18.0% (GP) Current wheeze: 23.6% (13–14Y)^{ISAAC} Allergic rhinitis: 38.6% (13–14Y)^{ISAAC} Eczema/atopic dermatitis: 28.5% (13–14Y)^{ISAAC}	[15]
Madagascar		Current wheeze: 25.2% (7–14Y)^{ISAAC}	[208]
Mongolia	Asthma: 1.1%–2.4 (10–60Y) Allergic rhinoconjunctivitis: 9.3–18.4% (10–60Y)		[106]

(continued)

Table 2.1 (continued)

Region	Countries $n = 27$	Prevalence rates before 1999	Prevalence rates 2000–2009	Prevalence rates 2010–2019	Risk factors/common allergens reported	References
	Morocco		Asthma: 3.89% (GP) Current wheeze: 6.4–16.2% (13–14Y)[ISAAC] Allergic rhinitis: 37.8% (<10–49Y)[ISAAC] Allergic rhinoconjunctivitis: 8.8–28% (13–14Y)[ISAAC] Eczema/atopic dermatitis: 13.3–20.2% (13–14Y)[ISAAC]			[90, 196, 209]
	Mozambique		Asthma: 11.9% (13–14Y)[ISAAC]			[210]

				Indoor allergens	
Nigeria	Asthma: 18.4% (C)^{ISAAC} Current wheeze: 10.7–16.4% (C)^{ISAAC} Allergic rhinitis: 45.2–54.1% (C)^{ISAAC} Eczema/atopic dermatitis: 22.4–26.1% (C)^{ISAAC}	Asthma: 14.7% (18–45Y) Current wheeze: 4.8–5.5% (6–7Y)^{ISAAC} 7.2% (6–7Y)^{ISAAC} 10.7–13.0% (13–14Y)^{ISAAC} Allergic rhinitis: 11.3% (6–7Y)^{ISAAC} 29.6% (18–45Y) Eczema/atopic dermatitis: 10.1% (6–7Y)^{ISAAC}	Asthma: 0.9% (7–14Y)^{ISAAC} Current wheeze: 5.4% (7–14Y)^{ISAAC} Allergic rhinitis: 19.2% (7–14Y)^{ISAAC}	Indoor allergens: house dust mites, mold	[12, 55, 211–213]
Reunion island		Asthma: 21.5% (GP)			[11]
Senegal			Asthma: 3% (C)^{ISAAC} 12.8% (<15Y)^{ISAAC} Current wheeze: 9% (C)^{ISAAC} Allergic rhinoconjunctivitis: 12.5% (<15Y)^{ISAAC} Eczema/atopic dermatitis: 12.2% (<15Y)^{ISAAC}		[214, 215]

(continued)

Table 2.1 (continued)

Region	Countries n = 27	Prevalence rates before 1999	Prevalence rates 2000–2009	Prevalence rates 2010–2019	Risk factors/common allergens reported	References
	South Africa	Asthma: 13.1% (13–14Y)[ISAAC] Current wheeze: 16% (13–14Y)[ISAAC] Allergic rhinitis: 30.4% (13–14Y)[ISAAC] Allergic rhinoconjunctivitis: 17.6% (13–14Y)[ISAAC] Eczema/atopic dermatitis: 11.8% (13–14Y)[ISAAC]	Asthma: 14.4% (13–14Y)[ISAAC] 18.0–20.3% (GP) Current wheeze: 20.3% (13–14Y)[ISAAC] Allergic rhinitis: 38.5% (13–14Y)[ISAAC] Allergic rhinoconjunctivitis: 24.3% (13–14Y)[ISAAC] Eczema/atopic dermatitis: 19.4% (13–14Y)[ISAAC]	Asthma 3.4% (9–11Y)[ISAAC, a] Current wheeze: 12.9% (9–11Y)[ISAAC, a] Food allergy (peanuts) 15–38% (C) 40% (C)	Indoor allergens: visible mold growth, dampness, paraffin use for cooking Food allergens: peanuts	[14, 19, 216]
	Tanzania		Current wheeze: 1.9–5.2% (5–15Y) 2.2–5.0% (>15Y)	Asthma (self-reported): 6.4–17.6% (17Y)[ISAAC] Current wheeze 12.1–23.1% (17Y)[ISAAC]		[108, 202]
	Togo			Eczema/atopic dermatitis: 31.3% (0–15Y)		[217]

Country				References
Tunisia	Asthma: 3.53% (GP) Current wheeze: 13.2% (13–14Y)[ISAAC] Allergic rhinoconjunctivitis: 29.7% (13–14Y)[ISAAC] Eczema/atopic dermatitis: 8.3% (13–14Y)[ISAAC]	Asthma: 6.5% (2–52Y)[ISAAC] Allergic rhinitis: 11.7% (<15Y)[ISAAC] 13.4% (>15Y)[ISAAC]		[196, 218, 219]
Uganda		Asthma: 6.8 (>35Y) Allergic rhinitis: 11.9% (>35Y) Eczema/atopic dermatitis: 8.2% (>35Y)	Indoor allergens: use of gas for cooking	[109, 220]

The superscript [ISAAC] indicates studies that have used ISAAC protocol/questionnaires

A adults, C children, E elderly, GP general population, T teens, Y years

[a]Results from multicenter studies

and it is hard to pinpoint exact high and low regions, but even with the scarce amount of data available, the increasing trend in allergic diseases over the past few decades is evident. The same survey repeated 6 years apart in Kenyan adolescents showed significant changes over time. The rate of asthma increased from 6.6% to 12.6%, while allergic rhinitis increased from 14.9% to 38.6% and atopic dermatitis increased from 13.9% to 28.5% [15]. South Africa also showed similar trends with a 1–8.5% increase in different allergic diseases over a 7-year period [14].

Food allergies also appear to be on the rise in African countries with highest rates reported in Zimbabwe (10%) and Morocco (9.5%) [16]. Self-reported food reactions are as high as 28% in Nigeria [17]. Forty percent of children with atopic dermatitis in South Africa have a peanut allergy, one of the most common allergens [18, 19]. Other foods known to cause allergic reactions in various African countries include apples, tomatoes, soy, crab, egg whites, and milk. Sea food allergy is also high in certain regions of South Africa [20].

Prevalence and Trends of Allergic Diseases: Middle East

Most data in the Middle East come from studies performed in Turkey followed by Iran and Saudi Arabia. Before talking about individual countries, however, it would be best to get an overall picture of asthma status in that region by noting the meta-analysis performed in 2018 in the Eastern Mediterranean Region countries (Afghanistan, Bahrain, Djibouti, Egypt, Iran, Iraq, Jordan, Kuwait, Lebanon, Libya, Morocco, Oman, Pakistan, Palestine, Qatar, Saudi Arabia, Somalia, Sudan, Syria, Tunisia, United Arab Emirates (UAE), Yemen, and Cyprus). Using the World Health Organization definition of asthma, Masjedi et al. reported a pooled asthma prevalence of 9.38% (confidence interval: 9.20–9.55) [21]. While not all countries had the same amount of data to be reflected in this analysis equally, the highest prevalence rate was observed in Kuwait and the lowest in Syria. Another systematic review from the Arabian Peninsula including seven countries (Kuwait, UAE, Bahrain, Qatar, Oman, Kingdom of Saudi Arabia, and Yemen) reported a prevalence range of 8–23%, while the SNAPSHOT program reported lower prevalence rates of 3.6%, 6.4%, and 6.4% in Egypt, Turkey, and the Gulf Cluster (Kuwait, Saudi Arabia, and the UAE) [22, 23].

Selected data from different countries in addition to time trends are shown in Table 2.2. Based on these data, the highest reported prevalence of asthma in the years 2010–2019 was 35.4% in children (Iran—single-center study) and 15% in adults (Kuwait—national survey) [24, 25]. The lowest rates reported in children and adults were 8.9% (Turkey) and 1.9% (Kazakhstan), respectively [26, 27]. Given that allergic diseases are predominantly diagnosed for the first time in childhood, the majority of studies in the Middle East have focused on children, using ISAAC guidelines. While the rates of allergic diseases vary among different countries, they do show an anticipated rise in allergic diseases. In Turkey, the same survey repeated in 1994, 2004, and 2014 shows this trend well. The rate of allergic rhinitis, asthma,

Table 2.2 Middle eastern countries

Region	Countries n = 18	Prevalence rates before 1999	Prevalence rates 2000–2009	Prevalence rates 2010–2019	Risk factors/common allergens reported	References
Middle East	Afghanistan			Asthma: 12.5% (6–7Y)[ISAAC] 17.3% (13–14Y)[ISAAC]		[221]
	Azerbaijan			Asthma: 2.68% (≥18Y) Current wheeze: 12.3% (≥18Y)		[26]
	Iran	Asthma: 0.71% (6–11Y) Current wheeze: 3.9% (6–11Y)	Asthma: 3.9% (6–12Y)[a] 13.14% (C)[a] 2.7–35.4% (C)[ISAAC]	Asthma: 12.2% (5–6Y) 9.4% (6–7Y)[ISAAC] 3.9% (6–12Y)[a] 7.5% (6–14Y)[ISAAC] 12.4% (T)[ISAAC] 7.6% (18–45Y) 8.9% (20–44Y)[b] 7.8% (20–60Y) 7.95% (GP)[a]	Indoor allergens: house dust mites, feathers, cockroach, pets Outdoor allergens: pollen, grass, willow, insect stings, weeds, Russian thistle Food allergens: cow's milk, eggs (yolk and whites), wheat, honey, walnuts, hazelnuts, tomatoes, sesame, fish, shrimp, pepper, curry	[24, 28, 30, 65, 118, 222–233]
				Current wheeze: 23.3% (T)[ISAAC] Allergic rhinitis: 28.5% (5–6Y) 40.8% (6–7Y)[ISAAC] 28.3% (18–45Y) 26.7% (A)	Fungal allergens: Aspergillus, Alternaria, Cladosporium, Penicillium Other allergens: nickel, chromium, cobalt	

(continued)

S. Eghtesad

Table 2.2 (continued)

Region	Countries n = 18	Prevalence rates before 1999	Prevalence rates 2000–2009	Prevalence rates 2010–2019	Risk factors/common allergens reported	References
				Allergic rhinoconjunctivitis: 15.9% (18–45Y) Eczema/atopic dermatitis: 15% (5–6Y) 3.9% (18–45Y)		
	Israel		Asthma: 4.5% (17Y)		Other allergens: nickel sulfate, potassium dichromate, fragrance mix	[234, 235]
	Jordan		Asthma: 8.8–9.5% (6–14Y)[ISAAC]	Asthma: 6.2% (T)[ISAAC] Current wheeze: 11.7% (T)[ISAAC]		[236]
	Kazakhstan			Asthma: 1.9% (≥18Y) Current wheeze: 25.5% (≥18Y)		[26]
	Kuwait	Current wheeze: 16.1% (13–14Y)[ISAAC]	Asthma: 15.6% (13–14Y)[ISAAC] 16.8% (13–14)[ISAAC]	Asthma: 18% (C)[b] 11.9% (18–26Y) 15% (A)[c] Allergic rhinitis: 20.4% (18–26Y)	Outdoor allergens: pollen (especially in high humidity), environmental tobacco smoke	[25, 33, 223, 237–244]

Lebanon	Allergic rhinitis: 25.5% (13–14Y)ISAAC	Current wheeze: 7.6% (13–14Y)ISAAC 16.1% (13–14Y)ISAAC Allergic rhinitis: 22.2% (13–14Y)ISAAC 17.1% (13–14Y)ISAAC Eczema/atopic dermatitis: 12.8% (13–14Y)ISAAC 11.3% (13–14Y)ISAAC	Eczema/atopic dermatitis: 14.9% (T)ISAAC 9.2% (18–26Y) Food allergy (perceived, probable): 12.02%, 5.4% (C-T)	Food allergens: cow's milk, peanut, fish, sesame, egg, wheat, shellfish Other allergens: nickel	[245–247]
	Allergic rhinoconjunctivitis: 15.9% (13–4Y)ISAAC Eczema/atopic dermatitis: 11% (13–14Y)ISAAC	Asthma: 8.3% (13–14Y)ISAAC Allergic rhinitis: 45.2% (13–14Y)ISAAC Eczema/atopic dermatitis: 12.8% (13–14Y)ISAAC	Food allergy: 4.1% (C) 3.2% (A)	Indoor allergens: humidity on bedroom walls, spongy pillow, pets, noncotton mattress	

(continued)

Table 2.2 (continued)

Region	Countries n = 18	Prevalence rates before 1999	Prevalence rates 2000–2009	Prevalence rates 2010–2019	Risk factors/common allergens reported	References
	Oman	Asthma: 13.8% (6–7Y)[ISAAC] Current wheeze: 8.7% (6–7Y)[ISAAC]	Asthma: 17.8% (6–7Y)[ISAAC] 10.5% (6–7Y)[ISAAC] 15.4% (10Y)[ISAAC] 20.7% (13–14Y)[ISAAC]			[248–250]
			Current wheeze: 13.8% (6–7Y)[ISAAC] Allergic rhinitis: 7.4% (6–7Y)[ISAAC] 10.5% (13–14Y)[ISAAC]			
			Eczema/atopic dermatitis: 7.5% (6–7Y)[ISAAC] 14.4% (13–14Y)[ISAAC]			
	Pakistan		Asthma: 15.8% (3–16Y)[ISAAC] 9.4% (11–15Y) 10.6% (A)	Asthma (self-reported): 10.2% (3–17Y)[ISAAC] 1.8% (A)	Indoor allergens: house dust mite, Dermatophagoides farina, D. pteronyssinus, ill-ventilated kitchens	[63, 119, 251–253]

		Outdoor allergens: pollen Food allergens: wheat, egg, milk, shite lentils, corn, rice, soya, peanut		
	Current wheeze: 14.7% (11–15Y) Allergic rhinitis: 28.5% (3–16Y)[ISAAC]			
	Allergic rhinoconjunctivitis: 15.3% (11–15Y)			
Palestine	Asthma: 8.4% (5–8Y)[ISAAC] 9.4% (6–12Y) 5.9% (12–15Y)[ISAAC]		[254, 255]	
	Current wheeze: 9.6% (5–8Y)[ISAAC] 8.8% (6–12Y) 7.2% (12–15Y)[ISAAC]			
Qatar	Asthma: 19.8% (6–14Y)[ISAAC] Allergic rhinitis: 30.5% (6–14Y)[ISAAC]		[31]	
	Eczema/atopic dermatitis: 22.5% (6–14Y)[ISAAC]			

(continued)

Table 2.2 (continued)

Region	Countries n = 18	Prevalence rates before 1999	Prevalence rates 2000–2009	Prevalence rates 2010–2019	Risk factors/common allergens reported	References
	Saudi Arabia	Asthma: 6.8% (7–12Y) 8–23% (C)[ISAAC]	Asthma: 6.01% (C)[ISAAC]	Asthma: 23.6% (6–8Y)[ISAAC] 27.5% (C) 14.3% (<16Y)[ISAAC, a] 4.05% (>15Y)[b] 19.6% (16–18Y)[ISAAC] 11.4% (16–18Y)[ISAAC] 11.3% (22–40Y)	Indoor allergens: pets (dogs, dog hair), using wood as cooking fuel	[32, 117, 141, 256–264]
		Allergic rhinitis: 17.9% (7–12Y) 12–17% (7–12Y) 20–25% (C)[ISAAC]	Allergic rhinitis: 26.51% (C)[ISAAC]	Current wheeze: 18.2% (22–40Y) Allergic rhinitis: 24.2% (6–8Y)[ISAAC] 6.3% (C) 21.4% (<16Y)[ISAAC, a] 38.6% (16–18Y)[ISAAC]	Outdoor allergens: distance from brick factories, exposure to dense truck traffic, pigweed, Bermuda grass	
		Eczema/atopic dermatitis: 10.8% (7–12Y) 12–13% (C)[ISAAC]		Eczema/atopic dermatitis: 10.3% (6–8Y)[ISAAC] 12.5% (C)	Food allergens: eggs, vegetables Fungal allergens: cladosporium	

| Turkey | Asthma:
5% (6–14Y)ISAAC
16.8%–17.4%
(6–13)
5.2–5.8%
(7–12Y)
16.4% (7–12)
8.1% (7–14Y)

Allergic rhinitis:
18.7–28% (6–13)
8.8%
(6–14Y)ISAAC
12.3% (7–12) | Asthma:
4.6%
(6–14Y)ISAAC
12.9%
(13–14Y)ISAAC
8.6–12.1%
(7–12Y)
3.1–5.3% (A)
4.5% (A)

Current wheeze:
13.4%
(13–14Y)ISAAC
Allergic rhinitis:
11.4%
(6–14Y)ISAAC
4.3–7%
(13–14Y)ISAAC | Asthma:
27.3% (5–6Y)
8.9% (6–14Y)ISAAC
11.9% (C)ISAAC
3.6% (30–49Y)
4.4% (A)

Current wheeze:
33.3% (5–6Y)
15.8%
(9–11Y)ISAAC, c
12.0% (30–49Y)
Allergic rhinitis:
8.9% (C)ISAAC
13.4% (5–6Y)
8.1% (6–7Y)
15.6%
(6–14Y)ISAAC
14.5% (12–15Y)
4.5%
(13–14Y)ISAAC
16.5% (30–49Y)
6.4% (A)
31.0% (9–11Y) | Indoor allergens: living in apartments, more rooms in house (crowding), housing condition (living in shanty-type houses), molds at home, use of wood or biomass for heating or cooking, pets (cats)

Outdoor allergens: air pollution, bee stings, living at altitude below 1000 m, pollen | [23, 34, 61, 66, 116, 136, 142, 147, 153, 158, 265–278] |

(continued)

Table 2.2 (continued)

Region	Countries n = 18	Prevalence rates before 1999	Prevalence rates 2000–2009	Prevalence rates 2010–2019	Risk factors/common allergens reported	References
		Eczema/atopic dermatitis: 6.1–6.5% (6–13) 5% (6–14Y)[ISAAC] 2.2% (7–12)	Eczema/atopic dermatitis 9.9% (6–14Y)[ISAAC] Food allergy 0.3% (GP)	Allergic rhinoconjunctivitis: 23.5% (9–11Y)[ISAAC, c] 27.3% (C)[ISAAC]	Food allergens: fish, sea food, fermented drinks made from millets and various seeds, animal fats and butter, kiwi, peach, tomatoes, melon and watermelon, cow's milk, eggs, chicken meat, bananas	
				Eczema/atopic dermatitis: 4.3% (1Y) 8.3% (5–6Y) 3.6% (C)[ISAAC] 8.1% (9–11Y)[ISAAC, c] 8.1% (10–11Y)[ISAAC, c] 7% (6–14Y)[ISAAC] 9.6% (30–49Y) Food allergy: 6.5% (C)[ISAAC]	Other allergens: metal dust, volatile fumes, wood/coal smoke, paper dust	

The superscript [ISAAC] indicates studies that have used ISAAC protocol/questionnaires

A adults, C children, E elderly, GP general population, T teens, Y years

[a]Results from systematic review/meta-analysis

[b]Results from national surveys

[c]Results from multicenter studies

and atopic dermatitis increased from 8.8% to 15.6%, 5% to 8.9%, and 5% to 7%, respectively [27]. Other similar trends are seen in Oman, Iran, Saudi Arabia, and Lebanon (Table 2.2).

Of the different allergic diseases, the highest rates in all Middle Eastern countries belong to allergic rhinitis. In Iran, about 40% of children and 26–28% of adults experience allergic rhinitis independent from or along with asthma [28–30]. Rates as high as 20%, 30%, and 38% have also been reported in Kuwait, Qatar, and Saudi Arabia, respectively [31–33]. Data on food allergy prevalence is lacking in the Middle East; however, the available data show an increase in this category of allergic diseases as well. In Turkey, seafood, fermented drinks made with millets, and animal fats are among common food allergens reported [34]. Peanuts were the most common food allergen in Saudi Arabia, and in Israel, egg, cow's milk, and sesame caused the most number of allergic reactions [35, 36].

Prevalence and Trends of Allergic Diseases: Asia

In general, asthma prevalence is lower in Asian developing countries compared to those in other regions of the world. A range of 1.1–11.0% was found in a systematic review of 74 studies in various regions of China, with the lowest prevalence being observed in Tibet and highest in Hong Kong [37]. Most studies performed in mainland China have used Chinese diagnostic guidelines, yielding a lower prevalence of 3% [37]. Crude prevalence of asthma in India, Sri Lanka, Bangladesh, Nepal, and Pakistan were found to be 6.3%, 5.3%, 5.2%, 4.2%, and 3.7%, respectively [38]. The highest rate of allergic rhinitis was reported for adults in Thailand (37.7%), followed by those in Vietnam (29.6%) [39, 40]. Food allergy prevalence appears to be comparable to prevalence rates observed in Europe and the West, even though the types of foods consumed vary widely [41, 42]. Various seafood are major allergens in the adult population, while eggs and milk commonly affect children. In India, beef and wheat allergies are reported as well. Table 2.3 summarizes results of selected studies performed throughout Asia. Similar to many other developing countries, data from most countries are insufficient, especially in the adult population.

Prevalence and Trends of Allergic Diseases: Latin America

Based on the data available, the highest rate of asthma in adults and children living in Latin American countries is 9.5% (Argentina) and 28.6% (Brazil), respectively, while the lowest rates reported are 4.4% (Brazil) and 6.1% (Mexico) [43–46]. The same increasing trend observed in other developing countries is reported in Latin America as well, although data from most countries excluding Mexico and Brazil are scarce. Selected data from these countries are shown in Table 2.4. As with other

Table 2.3 East Asian countries

Region	Countries n = 13	Prevalence rates before 1999	Prevalence rates 2000–2009	Prevalence rates 2010–2019	Risk factors/common allergens reported	References
Asia	Bangladesh	Asthma: 7.3% (5–14Y) 5.3% (15–44Y)				[68]
	China	Asthma: 0.91% (0–14Y) 2.1% (3–7Y) 3.9% (13–14Y)[ISAAC] 1.8% (>6Y)	Asthma: 1.5% (0–14Y) 1.97% (0–14Y)[c] 1.59% (0–14Y)[a] 0.8% (9–20Y) 4.6–6.9% (13–14Y)[ISAAC]	Asthma: 4% (0–8Y) 2.09–7.45% (0–14Y) 3.3% (6–13Y)[ISAAC, a] 2.36% (0–14Y) 2.32% (0–14Y) 3.69% (0–14Y)[ISAAC] 1.12% (0–14Y) 4.56% (0–14Y) 4.13% (0–14Y) 5.92% (3–6Y) 10.2% (3–7Y) 2.11% (0–14Y)[a] 3.45% (C) 2.9% (C) 1.8% (>6Y) 2.46% (A) 1.25% (≥18)[c]	Indoor allergens: mites, house dust mites, cockroach, pets (dog, cat), pests and visible mold, *D. pteronyssinus*, *D. farina*, cooking with gas, foam pillows, damp housing	[75–78, 85, 86, 101, 146, 148, 154, 15c, 279–30c]

Current wheeze: 3.4% (13–14Y)[ISAAC] Food allergy: 3.5% (0–2Y)	Current wheeze: 3.4–5.8% (C) 9.3% (2–6Y) 1–7.2% (13–14Y)[ISAAC] 4.8–6.1% (13–14Y)[ISAAC] Allergic rhinitis: 10.8% (3–6Y) 8–21.4% (GP) 1.1–6.3% (13–14Y)[ISAAC] Food allergy: 7.7% (0–2Y)	Allergic rhinitis: 9% (0–8Y) 7.83%–20.42% (0–14Y) 9.8% (6–13Y)[ISAAC, a] 15.79% (C)[a] Eczema/atopic dermatitis: 39% (0–8Y) 12.94% (1–7Y) 7.22%–20.64% (0–14Y) 5.5% (6–13Y)[ISAAC, a] 4.6–10.2% (3–6Y) Food allergy: 3.8% (0–1Y) 5.5–7.3% (0–2Y) 0.3–0.5% (0–14Y)	Outdoor allergens: pollen, weed pollens, house adjacent to traffic or near pollution source, damaged water source, living near major roads Food allergens: egg, cow's milk, wheat, peanut, crab, shellfish, fish, shrimp, oranges, mango

(continued)

Table 2.3 (continued)

Region	Countries n = 13	Prevalence rates before 1999	Prevalence rates 2000–2009	Prevalence rates 2010–2019	Risk factors/common allergens reported	References
	China	Asthma: 0.91% (0–14Y) 2.1% (3–7Y) 3.9% (13–14Y)[ISAAC] 1.8% (>6Y)	Asthma: 1.5% (0–14Y) 1.97% (0–14Y)[c] 1.59% (0–14Y)[a] 0.8% (9–20Y) 4.6–6.9% (13–14Y)[ISAAC]	Asthma: 4% (0–8Y) 2.09–7.45% (0–14Y) 3.3% (6–13Y)[ISAAC, a] 2.36% (0–14Y) 2.32% (0–14Y) 3.69% (0–14Y)[ISAAC] 1.12% (0–14Y) 4.56% (0–14Y) 4.13% (0–14Y) 5.92% (3–6Y) 10.2% (3–7Y) 2.11% (0–14Y)[a] 3.45% (C) 2.9% (C) 1.8% (>6Y) 2.46% (A) 1.25% (≥18Y)[c]	Indoor allergens: mites, house dust mites, cockroach, pets (dog, cat), pests and visible mold, *D. pteronyssinus*, *D. farina*, cooking with gas, foam pillows, damp housing	[75–78, 85, 86, 101, 146, 148, 154, 159, 279–304]
		Current wheeze: 3.4% (13–14Y)[ISAAC] Food allergy: 3.5% (0–2Y)	Current wheeze: 3.4–5.8% (C) 9.3% (2–6Y) 1–7.2% (13–14Y)[ISAAC] 4.8–6.1% (13–14Y)[ISAAC]	Allergic rhinitis: 9% (0–8Y) 7.83%–20.42% (0–14Y) 9.8% (6–13Y)[ISAAC, a] 15.79% (C)[a]	Outdoor allergens: pollen, weed pollens, house adjacent to traffic or near pollution source, damaged water source, living near major roads	

	Asthma: 15.7% (4–17Y) Current wheeze: 20.8% (4–17Y)	Allergic rhinitis: 10.8% (3–6Y) 8–21.4% (GP) 1.1–6.3% (13–14Y)ISAAC Food allergy: 7.7% (0–2Y)	Eczema/atopic dermatitis: 39% (0–8Y) 12.94% (1–7Y) 7.22%–20.64% (0–14Y) 5.5% (6–13Y)ISAAC, a 4.6–10.2% (3–6Y) Food allergy: 3.8% (0–1Y) 5.5–7.3% (0–2Y) 0.3–0.5% (0–14Y)	Food allergens: egg, cow's milk, wheat, peanut, crab, shellfish, fish, shrimp, oranges, mango	
Hong Kong		Current wheeze: 9.6% (2–6Y)ISAAC			[301]
India		Asthma: 2.3% (6–7Y)ISAAC 3.3% (13–14Y)ISAAC 10.7% (C)ISAAC, a 2.38%a 4.19% (GP)	Asthma: 1.7% (A) 12.1% (6–15Y) 4.9% (C) 5.49% (GP) 5.35% (6–7Y)ISAAC 6.05% (13–14Y)ISAAC 1.8–1.9% (20–49Y)	Indoor allergens: house dust mite, D. pteronyssinus, D. farina, mite antigens, use of biomass, solid fuels and smoke-v-producing fuels at home, pets, absence of smoke outlets	[71, 96, 121–123, 126, 127, 131, 134, 305–313]

(continued)

Table 2.3 (continued)

Region	Countries n = 13	Prevalence rates before 1999	Prevalence rates 2000–2009	Prevalence rates 2010–2019	Risk factors/common allergens reported	References
			Current wheeze: 6.2% (6–7Y)[ISAAC] 7.8% (13–14Y)[ISAAC] 7.3% (7–8)[ISAAC]		Outdoor allergens: pollen Food allergens: cow milk, beef–mutton, eggs, banana, brinjal, wheat Chemical allergens: nickel sulfate, *Parthenium hysterophorus*	
	Laos		Allergic rhinoconjunctivitis: 23.7% (13–14Y)[ISAAC] Eczema/atopic dermatitis: 7.1 (13–14Y)[ISAAC]			[314]
	Malaysia	Current wheeze: 5.4% (6–7Y)[ISAAC] 6% (5–14Y) 6.8% (13–14Y)[ISAAC] Allergic rhinitis: 27% (5–14Y)	Asthma: 7.1% (1–5Y) 134% (GP) Current wheeze: 6.2% (1–5Y) 4.3% (6–7Y)[ISAAC] 5.7% (13–14Y)[ISAAC]		Indoor allergens: house dust mites Outdoor allergens: acacia and Bermuda grass pollens	[120, 145, 315–317]
		Allergic rhinoconjunctivitis: 4.6% (6–7Y)[ISAAC] 11% (13–14Y)[ISAAC] Eczema/atopic dermatitis: 13.7% (5–7Y)[ISAAC] 9.9% (12–14)[ISAAC]	Allergic rhinoconjunctivitis: 5% (6–7Y)[ISAAC] 15% (13–14Y)[ISAAC]		Food allergens: eggs, cow's milk	

Country					
Mongolia			Asthma: 4.7% (>20Y) 20.9% (6–7Y)[ISAAC] Current wheeze: 15.7% (>20Y) Allergic rhinoconjunctivitis: 14.6% (>20Y)		[150, 318]
Philippines			Food allergy: 0.33–0.43% (14–16Y)	Food allergens: shellfish	[319, 320]
Singapore			Food allergy: 0.28–0.64% (4–6Y) 0.3–0.47% (14–16)	Food allergens: peanuts, tree nuts, shellfish	[319, 320]
Sri Lanka			Asthma: 17% (5–17Y) Current wheeze: 21.3% (3–5Y)	Indoor allergens: combined kitchen/living area, inadequate ventilation in sleeping area	[321–323]
			Allergic rhinitis: 21.4% (5–17Y) Eczema/atopic dermatitis: 5% (5–17Y)	Food allergens: wheat	

(continued)

Table 2.3 (continued)

Region	Countries n = 13	Prevalence rates before 1999	Prevalence rates 2000–2009	Prevalence rates 2010–2019	Risk factors/common allergens reported	References
	Thailand	Asthma: 18.3% (6–7Y)[ISAAC] 12.7% (13–14Y)[ISAAC] Allergic rhinitis: 44.2% (6–7Y)[ISAAC] 38.7% (13–14Y)[ISAAC]	Asthma: 8.8 (16–31Y) 9.8% (17–53Y) Current wheeze: 14.3% (6–7Y)[ISAAC] 9.8% (13–14Y)[ISAAC] 10.1% (16–31Y) 12.1% (17–53Y)	Asthma: 16% (20–66Y)	Indoor allergens: house dust mites, cockroaches	[40, 69, 70, 139, 301, 324–327]
		Eczema/atopic dermatitis: 15.4% (6–7Y)[ISAAC] 14% (13–14Y)[ISAAC]	Allergic rhinitis: 42.6% (6–7Y)[ISAAC] 33.3% (13–14Y)[ISAAC] 26.3% (16–31Y) 57.4% (17–53Y)	Allergic rhinitis: 37.7% (20–66Y) Food allergy: 9.3% (3–7Y)	Food allergens: shrimp, cow's milk, fish, chicken eggs, ant eggs Chemical allergens: potassium dichromate, nickel sulfate, cobalt chloride, fragrance mix	
			Eczema/atopic dermatitis: 13.5% (6–7Y)[ISAAC] 11.2% (13–14Y)[ISAAC] 9.4% (16–31Y) 15% (17–53Y) Food allergy: 9.3% (0–3Y)			
	Tibet		Asthma: 1.1% (13–14Y)[ISAAC] Current wheeze: 0.8% (13–14Y)[ISAAC]			[91]

	Allergic rhinoconjunctivitis: 5.2% (13–14Y)[ISAAC] Eczema/atopic dermatitis: 0.4% (13–14Y)[ISAAC]			
Vietnam	Asthma: 2.4% (A)	Asthma: 3.9–5.6% (21–70Y) 5.1% (6Y) Allergic rhinitis: 10–29.6% (21–70Y)	Indoor allergens: house mites, storage mites, cockroaches Food allergens: crustaceans, fish, mollusk beef, milk, egg	[183, 308, 328–331]
		Allergic rhinoconjunctivitis: 11.5% (6Y) Eczema/atopic dermatitis: 6.7% (6Y) Food allergy: 5.7% (A) 5–8.4% (C)		

The superscript [ISAAC] indicates studies that have used ISAAC protocol/questionnaires
A adults, *C* children, *E* elderly, *GP* general population, *T* teens, *Y* years
[a]Results from multicenter studies
[c]Results from national surveys

Table 2.4 Latin American countries

Region	Countries n = 13	Prevalence rates before 1999	Prevalence rates 2000–2009	Prevalence rates 2010–2019	Risk factors/common allergens reported	References
Latin America	Argentina			Asthma: 9.5% (A) Current wheeze: 13.9% (A) Food allergy (cow milk): 0.8% (C)	Indoor allergens: carpeted rooms Outdoor allergens: living <300 m from an industry Other allergens: wearing synthetic clothes	[43, 5_]
	Brazil	Asthma: 4.9–7.3% (6–7Y)^{ISAAC} 9.8–10.2% (13–14Y)^{ISAAC}	Asthma: 20.4% (6–7Y)^{ISAAC} 19.7% (13–14)^{ISAAC} 26.5% (6–14Y) 18.4% (4Y) 23.8% (13–14Y)^{ISAAC} 12.8% (C) 24.3% (6–7Y)^{ISAAC} 19% (13–14Y)^{ISAAC} 16.5–31.2% (6–7Y)^{ISAAC} 11.8–30.5% (13.14Y)^{ISAAC} 15.3% (13–14Y)^{ISAAC}	Asthma: 11.8% (C)[a] 11.6% (13–14Y)^{ISAAC} 13.3% (T) 25.2% (C) 15.9% (T) 22% (6–7Y)^{ISAAC} 8.5% (10Y)[c] 22.6% (13–14Y)^{ISAAC} 15.3% (13–14Y)^{ISAAC} 7% (5–17Y) 19.1% (13–14Y)^{ISAAC} 9.1% (C) 29.7% (T) 12.4% (T) 25.8% (C) 4.4% (A) 12.8% (13–14Y)^{ISAAC} 28.6% (8–16Y) 20.4% (13–14Y)^{ISAAC}	Indoor/housing allergens: moisture, pets (cats/dog), mold, more number of rooms, *D. pteronyssinus*, *Dermatophagoides farina*, *Blomia tropicalis*	[44, 4_7, 83, 87, 88, 12_8, 140, 155, 157, 332–352]

				Allergens	Refs
Current wheeze: 6% (13–14Y)[ISAAC]	Current wheeze: 21.1% (4Y) 12.5% (0.5–5Y) 15.8% (13–14Y)[ISAAC] 15–19% (13–14Y)[ISAAC] 11.7% (C) 31.2% (6–7Y)[ISAAC] Allergic rhinitis: 28.8% (6–7Y)[ISAAC] 31.7% (13–14Y)[ISAAC] 26.6% (6–7Y)[ISAAC] 34.2% (13–14Y)[ISAAC] 12.2% (13–14Y)[ISAAC] 40.7% (13–14Y)[ISAAC] 36.6% (13–14Y)[ISAAC] Allergic rhinoconjunctivitis: 12.6% (6–7Y)[ISAAC] 10.3–17.4% (6–7Y)[ISAAC] 14.6% (13–14Y)[ISAAC] 8.9–28.5%(13–14Y)[ISAAC] Eczema/atopic dermatitis: 13.6% (13–14Y)[ISAAC] 8.2% (6–7Y)[ISAAC] 5% (13–14Y)[ISAAC]	Current wheeze: 44.1% (13–14Y)[ISAAC] 6% (20–69Y) Allergic rhinitis: 27.3% (6–7Y)[ISAAC] 43.2% (13–14Y)[ISAAC] 36.6% (13–14Y)[ISAAC] 28.1% (6–7Y)[ISAAC] 18.5% (13–14Y)[ISAAC] Allergic rhinoconjunctivitis: 12.7% (6–7Y)[ISAAC] 18.7% (13–14Y)[ISAAC] 15.4% (6–7Y)[ISAAC] Eczema/atopic dermatitis: 9.6% (6–7Y)[ISAAC] 11.3% (6–7Y)[ISAAC] Food allergy: 0.61% (0.5–5Y)	Outdoor allergens: insects, grasses Food allergens: processed foods, cow's milk	
Chile	Asthma: 9.7–16.5% (6–7Y)[ISAAC] 7.3–12.4% (13–14Y)[ISAAC] Current wheeze: 16.5–20% (6–7Y)[ISAAC] 6.8–11.7% (13–14Y)[ISAAC]	Food allergy: 6% (C)	Indoor allergens: mold or dampness in the house Outdoor allergens: farm animal contact	[353, 354]

(continued)

Table 2.4 (continued)

Region	Countries n = 13	Prevalence rates before 1999	Prevalence rates 2000–2009	Prevalence rates 2010–2019	Risk factors/common allergens reported	References
	Colombia	Asthma: 12.2% (GP)	Food allergy: 14.9% (1–83Y)	Asthma: 9.0% (adults) Current wheeze: 11.9% (adults) Allergic rhinitis: 30.8% (6–7Y)[ISAAC] 36.6% (13–14Y)[ISAAC]	Indoor allergens: cats	[49, 69, 355–358]
				Allergic rhinoconjunctivitis: 17.2% (6–7Y)[ISAAC] 24.9% (13–14Y)[ISAAC]	Food/drug allergens: acetaminophen, cereals, eggs, milk, antibiotics in first year of life	
	Costa Rica	Asthma: 23.4% (children) 23.0–27.7% (6–7)[ISAAC]	Asthma: 27.1% (10Y) 23.4% (5–17Y)	Asthma: 21.9% (6–13Y)[ISAAC] Allergic rhinitis: 42.6% (6–13Y)[ISAAC] 27% (6–14)	Indoor allergens: dust, mold, dust mites, cockroach	[48, 79, 129, 137, 359, 360]
				Eczema/atopic dermatitis: 19.2% (6–13Y)[ISAAC]	Outdoor allergens: tree pollen	
	Ecuador			Asthma: 10.1% (GP) Current wheeze: 9.4–10.3% (C)		[361, 362]
	El Salvador			Food allergy: 5.7% (C)	Food allergens: milk, shrimp, chili, chocolate, nuts	[50]
	Grenada			Current wheeze: 30.5% (6–7Y)[ISAAC]		[363]
	Honduras			Eczema/atopic dermatitis: 28.2% (1Y)		[364]

Jamaica			Asthma: 16.7% (2–17Y)[ISAAC] Current wheeze: 19.6% (2–17Y)[ISAAC] Allergic rhinitis: 24.5% (2–17Y)[ISAAC] Eczema/atopic dermatitis: 17.3% (2–17Y)[ISAAC]	Indoor allergens: mold, pets (cats and dogs)	[365]
Mexico	Asthma: 8.7% (6–12Y) 34% (6–12Y) 21.8% (6–14Y)[ISAAC] 5.8% (6–14Y)[ISAAC] Current wheeze: 5.8% (6–14Y)[ISAAC]	Asthma: 18% (2–5Y) 4.5% (6–7Y)[ISAAC] 9.9% (6–7Y)[ISAAC] 9.1% (6–14Y) 9.5% (9.1Y) 31.8–33.6% (C) 7.4% (C) 8% (13–14Y)[ISAAC] 7.8% (T) Current wheeze: 6.8% (6–7Y)[ISAAC] 9.9% (13–14Y)[ISAAC] 7.3% (T)	Asthma: 11.9% (C) 6.1% (C) 7.8% (15–16Y) 12.7% (T) 6.8% (A) 10% (E) Current wheeze: 10.3% (T) Allergic rhinitis: 11.9% (3–15Y) 5.5% (6–12Y) 15% (C) 5.4% (C) 9% (T) 6.9% (A) 60% (E)	Indoor allergens: pets, indoor plants stuffed toys, dust, dust mites, wall saltpeter, dampness (mold growth) Outdoor allergens: contact with farm animals, living close to cement factory, tree pollen	[46, 151, 360, 366–383]

(continued)

Table 2.4 (continued)

Region	Countries n = 13	Prevalence rates before 1999	Prevalence rates 2000–2009	Prevalence rates 2010–2019	Risk factors/common allergens reported	References
		Allergic rhinitis: 4.9% (6–14Y)[ISAAC] Eczema/atopic dermatitis: 4.1% (6–14Y)[ISAAC]	Allergic rhinitis: 44% (2–5Y) 4.5% (T) 7.6% (GP) Eczema/atopic dermatitis: 10.1% (6–10Y) 5.4% (11–16Y) 3.8% (T)	Eczema/atopic dermatitis: 3.4% (C) 3% (12Y) 5.2% (T) 3.8% (A) Food allergy: 4.9% (C)	Food allergens: early consumption of cow's milk, early introduction of cereals, egg, beef, pulses, pecans, peanuts, sesame, sea food (shellfish, mollusk, fish, shrimp, and crustaceans), strawberries, chocolate, soy, oranges, onion, beans, tomato, lettuce	[98, 334, 385]
Peru				Asthma: 16.7% (6–18Y) Allergic rhinitis: 18% (13–15Y)	Chemical allergens: Nickel sulfate, palladium chloride, cobalt chloride, potassium dichromate	
Trinidad and Tobago			Asthma: 12.8–13.5% (11–19Y)[ISAAC] Current wheeze: 13.1–13.4% (11–19Y)[ISAAC]			[386]

The superscript [ISAAC] indicates studies that have used ISAAC protocol/questionnaires
A adults, C children, E elderly, GP general population, T teens, Y years
[a]Results from multicenter studies
[c]Results from national surveys

countries, allergic rhinitis is the most common allergic disease with rates as high as 43.2%, 42.6%, and 36.6% reported in Brazilian, Costa Rican, and Colombian youth [47–49]. Given the tropical climate of many Latin American countries, dampness, mold, and different fungi commonly trigger allergic reactions. Food allergies range from 0.8% in Argentina to 5.7% in El Salvador, where milk, shrimp, chili, chocolate, and nuts were the most common allergens [50, 51].

Risk Factors and Common Allergens in Developing Countries

So there is evidently an increasing trend in allergic diseases in developing countries, and while risk factors such as gender, age, family history of atopic diseases, and socioeconomic status affect the development of allergic diseases [14, 19, 29, 33, 34, 52–83], these factors have been present at times of lower prevalence rates as well and do not contribute much to the increasing rates over the past few decades. What risk factors do affect allergic diseases then? Probably, those that have changed as a result of urbanization and modernization. Examples of these are increase in caesarian section rates, smoking, obesity, and exposure to air pollutants.

Mode of delivery Birth delivery mode has been shown to affect the rate of allergic diseases [49, 72, 73, 84–88]. More caesarian sections are being performed now compared to past decades, since it seems to be the "modern" way of delivering a child in many countries where it is performed without adequate indication. In 2010, the World Health Organization reported over 6.2 million unnecessary caesarian sections being performed worldwide, 50% of which belonged to China and Brazil [89].

Obesity Greater consumption of high-fat foods and lower physical activity leading to overweight and obesity are also common trends in urbanized societies. Fast food consumption, weight gain, and higher body mass index have been reported to be risk factors of asthma and its related symptoms as well [26, 65, 75, 78, 90–105].

Smoking Most studies in different developing countries have reported higher rates of allergic diseases in urban vs. rural areas [62, 101, 106–115]. Furthermore, many reports have indicated that exposure to tobacco smoking is an important risk factor for asthma [55, 62, 73–75, 77, 78, 81, 90, 92, 93, 95, 96, 116–135]. One interesting observation made in several studies is the effects of maternal smoking on increased allergic diseases in children [72, 73, 88, 121, 136–140]. One possible explanation for this observation is that in many societies, female smoking was previously regarded as a taboo, but it appears that cultures have overcome this taboo and female smoking has become more common in developing countries. The effects of smoking during pregnancy and low-birth-weight children have been extensively studied and proven before, and now higher rates of allergic diseases are observed in children born underweight and to mothers who smoke.

Pet allergy Many of the allergens reported in various countries also reflect modernization features. Pets are a common allergen in many developing countries, as having a pet inside the home (dogs and cats) is more common now [13, 34, 77, 92, 104, 116–118, 121, 127, 132, 134, 140–148]. This can contribute to the increased rate of pet allergy.

Industrial sites and pollution Other allergens of urbanized living reported include living in close proximity of different industries such as cement or brick factories, air pollution, and chemical compounds and volatile fuel that individuals were less commonly exposed to prior to the increase in allergic diseases [13, 79, 82, 148–152]. Living conditions often experienced in urban societies such as apartment living, more crowding in small areas, and crowded day-care attendance have been shown to be associated with higher asthma and its related symptoms as well [56, 61, 68, 76, 151, 153–158].

Now not all modern techniques adversely affect allergic diseases. For example, use of electricity as a cooking method was shown to be a protective factor compared to wood, coal, and other smoke-producing biomass that were previously used for indoor cooking and heating [39, 126, 127, 134, 159].

The High Burden of Allergic Diseases in Developing Countries

As mentioned in the previous sections, the impact of allergic diseases appears to be higher in developing countries in comparison to developed countries, despite of their lower prevalence rates. But why so? There are several reasons for this phenomenon. Lack of knowledge by patients, caregivers, and most importantly physicians is one critical, influential, and preventable factor. Many studies evaluating physicians' ability to identify and manage allergic diseases have reported poor and insufficient knowledge about asthma, its pathophysiology and related symptoms [160–166], delayed or inaccurate diagnosis [167, 168], lack of knowledge about standard medications and guidelines [160, 165, 168–170], and general mismanagement [160, 163–165, 171–175]. In one study evaluating the quality of asthma management, 40% of individuals diagnosed were not informed about their disease, and those who were informed were not given any educational materials [176]. Of course, these extreme cases are uncommon; however, poor physician–patient interactions further affect disease management. Given that the majority of allergic symptoms first develop in childhood, parental knowledge about these diseases and their management is critical, yet in many instances, missing [177–181]. In one study in Africa, parents perceived asthma to be contagious and transmitted from one person to another, while others believed it was transmitted through contaminated food [182]. In Brazil, some parents believed rescue medications may cause their children harm [44]. Research regarding psychosocial factors affecting asthma management in nine Arab countries has also shown parental knowledge to be generally insufficient [179]. Many parents perceive that their children cannot lead normal lives [175] and these misconceptions adversely affect their children's quality of life as they are often passed down to them, making them believe that they cannot overcome and control their medical condition. Besides social pressures, lack of knowledge in patients leads to noncompliance with therapy [177, 178, 183, 184], exacerbating disease status.

Even when knowledge is adequate, however, other obstacles such as limited resources hinder better care in developing countries. Many times, the most appropriate medications and therapies are not readily available [168, 185], and even when they are, individuals from lower socioeconomic levels are not able to afford them. The economic burden of allergic diseases is a great concern for many countries. The highest costs in various countries are attributed to inpatient and emergency room visits as well as medications [186–188]. In Iran and India, where health care is mostly self-funded, the annual cost per child is very high compared to the average family incomes, draining on family resources [187, 189].

There is a low level of asthma control reported by many developing countries, even those with larger, more rapidly growing economies [184, 186, 187, 190–193]. In China, physicians reported 75% of patients to be well-controlled, while according to Global Initiative for Asthma (GINA) criteria, less than 15% of them were well-controlled [194].

In Qatar, a country with the highest gross domestic product per capita in the world and high health expenditure per capita, 31% and 26% of patients had uncontrolled and partly controlled asthma, respectively, most of which stemmed from incorrect use of inhalers and misunderstanding the role of reliever and controller medications, signifying that the effects of insufficient knowledge on asthma control are greater than the effects economic limitations may have [190]. Allergic diseases in general, but more so uncontrolled asthma, affect individuals' quality of life and cause behavioral and emotional problems in children [44, 167, 179]. They cause school and work absences in 52% of children and 30% of adults in Oman, respectively, and similar patterns are observed in other countries as well [44, 179, 186, 191, 195]. Work productivity, daily activities, and sleep quality are also reported to be low by asthma patients in different developing countries. Although decreased quality of life does pertain not only to developing countries but also to anyone with uncontrolled asthma all over the world, the impact is more significant in low-income developing countries because of the higher rate of uncontrolled asthma observed in these populations.

Allergic Diseases: An Emerging Problem or an Overseen Issue?

So are allergic diseases an emerging problem in low-income and developing countries? Or are they an overseen issue in these populations? The answer appears to be both. Allergic diseases are an emerging problem because of changes in disease patterns and rates over the past few decades, caused by multiple risk factors mainly linked to modernization. The majority of the available data is very recent or only partial, indicating that the issue had been overlooked before and not anticipated in many populations. On the other hand, while there is still a substantial amount of work to be done, most developing countries are now aware of the increasing rate of allergic diseases and are trying to do something about it. For so many years, the greatest health obstacle in developing countries was controlling communicable diseases (still the greatest obstacle in underdeveloped countries), as they caused the highest rates of morbidity and mortality. However, with the global disease trends seen over the past decades, changing from high rates of communicable disease to high noncommunicable diseases, there is a need for change in public health policies in order to better control the burden associated with noncommunicable diseases, including allergic diseases. This change has not yet occurred in many developing countries. Medical and political authorities must get engaged in order to develop adequate resources to manage these problems. As with most things, education definitely plays a major role. Turkey has been a pioneer is conducting different educational workshops targeting different levels of care, from formal educational workshop for physicians to allergy camps for children, all of which have been found to be significantly effective and a great first step for combating the burden of allergic diseases in this country. Similar approaches for the development of infrastructures of education, research, and management are needed throughout the world. These programs need to be culturally sensitive and specific to each population in order to precisely address the needs of each group of people and impact their audience.

References

1. Bach J-F. The hygiene hypothesis in autoimmunity: the role of pathogens and commensals. Nat Rev Immunol. 2017;18:105.
2. Strachan DP. Hay fever, hygiene, and household size. BMJ. 1989;299(6710):1259–60.
3. Okada H, Kuhn C, Feillet H, Bach JF. The 'hygiene hypothesis' for autoimmune and allergic diseases: an update. Clin Exp Immunol. 2010;160(1):1–9.
4. The Global Asthma Report 2018. Auckland: Global Asthma Network; 2018.
5. Lai CK, Beasley R, Crane J, Foliaki S, Shah J, Weiland S. Global variation in the prevalence and severity of asthma symptoms: phase three of the International Study of Asthma and Allergies in Childhood (ISAAC). Thorax. 2009;64(6):476–83.
6. Worldwide variation in prevalence of symptoms of asthma, allergic rhinoconjunctivitis, and atopic eczema: ISAAC. The International Study of Asthma and Allergies in Childhood (ISAAC) Steering Committee. Lancet. 1998;351(9111):1225–32.
7. Williams H, Robertson C, Stewart A, Ait-Khaled N, Anabwani G, Anderson R, et al. Worldwide variations in the prevalence of symptoms of atopic eczema in the International Study of Asthma and Allergies in Childhood. J Allergy Clin Immunol. 1999;103(1 Pt 1):125–38.
8. Odhiambo JA, Williams HC, Clayton TO, Robertson CF, Asher MI. Global variations in prevalence of eczema symptoms in children from ISAAC Phase Three. J Allergy Clin Immunol. 2009;124(6):1251–8.e23.
9. Prescott SL, Pawankar R, Allen KJ, Campbell DE, Sinn J, Fiocchi A, et al. A global survey of changing patterns of food allergy burden in children. World Allergy Organ J. 2013;6(1):21.

10. Loh W, Tang MLK. The epidemiology of food allergy in the global context. Int J Environ Res Public Health. 2018;15(9):E2043.
11. Ait-Khaled N, Odhiambo J, Pearce N, Adjoh KS, Maesano IA, Benhabyles B, et al. Prevalence of symptoms of asthma, rhinitis and eczema in 13- to 14-year-old children in Africa: the International Study of Asthma and Allergies in Childhood Phase III. Allergy. 2007;62(3):247–58.
12. Adetoun Mustapha B, Briggs DJ, Hansell AL. Prevalence of asthma and respiratory symptoms in children in a low socio-economic status area of Nigeria. Int J Tuberc Lung Dis. 2013;17(7):982–8.
13. Flatin MC, Ade S, Hounkpatin SH, Ametonou B, Vodouhe UB, Adjibabi W. Symptoms of allergic rhinitis in Parakou, Benin: prevalence, severity and associated factors. Eur Ann Otorhinolaryngol Head Neck Dis. 2018;135(1):33–6.
14. Zar HJ, Ehrlich RI, Workman L, Weinberg EG. The changing prevalence of asthma, allergic rhinitis and atopic eczema in African adolescents from 1995 to 2002. Pediatr Allergy Immunol. 2007;18(7):560–5.
15. Esamai F, Ayaya S, Nyandiko W. Prevalence of asthma, allergic rhinitis and dermatitis in primary school children in Uasin Gishu district, Kenya. East Afr Med J. 2002;79(10): 514–8.
16. Boye JI. Food allergies in developing and emerging economies: need for comprehensive data on prevalence rates. Clin Transl Allergy. 2012;2(1):25.
17. Achinewu SC. Food allergy and its clinical symptoms in Nigeria. Food and Nutrition Bulletin. 1983;5(3):18–19.
18. Frank L, Marian A, Visser M, Weinberg E, Potter PC. Exposure to peanuts in utero and in infancy and the development of sensitization to peanut allergens in young children. Pediatr Allergy Immunol. 1999;10(1):27–32.
19. Gray CL, Levin ME, du Toit G. Ethnic differences in peanut allergy patterns in South African children with atopic dermatitis. Pediatr Allergy Immunol. 2015;26(8):721–30.
20. Zinn C, Lopata A, Visser M, Potter PC. The spectrum of allergy to South African bony fish (Teleosti). Evaluation by double-blind, placebo-controlled challenge. S Afr Med J. 1997;87(2):146–52.
21. Masjedi M, Ainy E, Zayeri F, Paydar R. Assessing the prevalence and incidence of asthma and chronic obstructive pulmonary disease in the Eastern Mediterranean Region. Turk Thorac J. 2018;19(2):56–60.
22. Al-Herz W. A systematic review of the prevalence of atopic diseases in children on the Arabian Peninsula. Med Princ Pract. 2018;27(5):436–42.
23. Al-Digheari A, Mahboub B, Tarraf H, Yucel T, Annesi-Maesano I, Doble A, et al. The clinical burden of allergic rhinitis in five Middle Eastern countries: results of the SNAPSHOT program. Allergy Asthma Clin Immunol. 2018;14:63.
24. Entezari A, Mehrabi Y, Varesvazirian M, Pourpak Z, Moin M. A systematic review of recent asthma symptom surveys in Iranian children. Chron Respir Dis. 2009;6(2): 109–14.
25. Khadadah M. The cost of asthma in Kuwait. Med Princ Pract. 2013;22(1):87–91.
26. Nugmanova D, Sokolova L, Feshchenko Y, Iashyna L, Gyrina O, Malynovska K, et al. The prevalence, burden and risk factors associated with bronchial asthma in commonwealth of independent states countries (Ukraine, Kazakhstan and Azerbaijan): results of the CORE study. BMC Pulm Med. 2018;18(1):110.
27. Dogruel D, Bingol G, Altintas DU, Seydaoglu G, Erkan A, Yilmaz M. The trend of change of allergic diseases over the years: three repeated surveys from 1994 to 2014. Int Arch Allergy Immunol. 2017;173(3):178–82.
28. Salarnia S, Momen T, Jari M. Prevalence and risk factors of allergic rhinitis in primary school students of Isfahan, Iran. Adv Biomed Res. 2018;7:157.
29. Shokouhi Shoormasti R, Pourpak Z, Fazlollahi MR, Kazemnejad A, Nadali F, Ebadi Z, et al. The prevalence of allergic rhinitis, allergic conjunctivitis, atopic dermatitis and asthma among adults of Tehran. Iran J Public Health. 2018;47(11):1749–55.

30. Fazlollahi MR, Najmi M, Fallahnezhad M, Sabetkish N, Kazemnejad A, Bidad K, et al. The prevalence of asthma in Iranian adults: the first national survey and the most recent updates. Clin Respir J. 2018;12(5):1872–81.

31. Janahi IA, Bener A, Bush A. Prevalence of asthma among Qatari schoolchildren: international study of asthma and allergies in childhood, Qatar. Pediatr Pulmonol. 2006;41(1):80–6.

32. Al-Ghobain MO, Al-Moamary MS, Al-Hajjaj MS, Al-Fayez AI, Basha SI. Prevalence of rhinitis symptoms among 16 to 18 years old adolescents in Saudi Arabia. Indian J Chest Dis Allied Sci. 2013;55(1):11–4.

33. Ziyab AH. Prevalence and risk factors of asthma, rhinitis, and eczema and their multimorbidity among young adults in Kuwait: a cross-sectional study. Biomed Res Int. 2017;2017:2184193.

34. Tamay Z, Akcay A, Ergin A, Guler N. Effects of dietary habits and risk factors on allergic rhinitis prevalence among Turkish adolescents. Int J Pediatr Otorhinolaryngol. 2013;77(9):1416–23.

35. El-Rab MO. Foods and food allergy: the prevalence of IgE antibodies specific for food allergens in Saudi patients. Saudi J Gastroenterol. 1998;4(1):25–9.

36. Dalal I, Binson I, Reifen R, Amitai Z, Shohat T, Rahmani S, et al. Food allergy is a matter of geography after all: sesame as a major cause of severe IgE-mediated food allergic reactions among infants and young children in Israel. Allergy. 2002;57(4):362–5.

37. Yangzong Y, Shi Z, Nafstad P, Haheim LL, Luobu O, Bjertness E. The prevalence of childhood asthma in China: a systematic review. BMC Public Health. 2012;12:860.

38. Bishwajit G, Tang S, Yaya S, Feng Z. Burden of asthma, dyspnea, and chronic cough in South Asia. Int J Chron Obstruct Pulmon Dis. 2017;12:1093–9.

39. Lam HT, Van TTN, Ekerljung L, Ronmark E, Lundback B. Allergic rhinitis in Northern Vietnam: increased risk of urban living according to a large population survey. Clin Transl Allergy. 2011;1(1):7.

40. Bunjean K, Sukkasem K, Noppacroh N, Yamkaew N, Janthayanont D, Theerapancharern W, et al. Prevalence of allergic rhinitis and types of sensitized allergen in adult at Wat Intaram community, Hua Raeu, Phra Nakhon Si Ayutthaya District, Phra Nakhon Si Ayutthaya Province, Thailand. J Med Assoc Thail. 2012;95(Suppl 5):S63–8.

41. Lee AJ, Thalayasingam M, Lee BW. Food allergy in Asia: how does it compare? Asia Pac Allergy. 2013;3(1):3–14.

42. Tang R, Wang ZX, Ji CM, Leung PSC, Woo E, Chang C, et al. Regional differences in food allergies. Clin Rev Allergy Immunol. 2019;57(1):98–110.

43. Arias SJ, Neffen H, Bossio JC, Calabrese CA, Videla AJ, Armando GA, et al. Prevalence and features of asthma in young adults in urban areas of Argentina. Arch Bronconeumol. 2018;54(3):134–9.

44. Roncada C, de Oliveira SG, Cidade SF, Sarria EE, Mattiello R, Ojeda BS, et al. Burden of asthma among inner-city children from Southern Brazil. J Asthma. 2016;53(5):498–504.

45. Menezes AM, Wehrmeister FC, Horta B, Szwarcwald CL, Vieira ML, Malta DC. Prevalence of asthma medical diagnosis among Brazilian adults: National Health Survey, 2013. Rev Bras Epidemiol. 2015;18(Suppl 2):204–13.

46. Ramirez-Soto M, Bedolla-Barajas M, Gonzalez-Mendoza T. Prevalence of asthma, allergic rhinitis and atopic dermatitis in school children of the Mexican Bajio region. Rev Alerg Mex. 2018;65(4):372–8.

47. Luna Mde F, Almeida PC, Silva MG. Asthma and rhinitis prevalence and co-morbidity in 13-14-year-old schoolchildren in the city of Fortaleza, Ceara State, Brazil. Cad Saude Publica. 2011;27(1):103–12.

48. Soto-Martinez ME, Yock-Corrales A, Camacho-Badilla K, Abdallah S, Duggan N, Avila-Benedictis L, et al. The current prevalence of asthma, allergic rhinitis, and eczema related symptoms in school-aged children in Costa Rica. J Asthma. 2019;56(4):360–8.

49. Penaranda A, Aristizabal G, Garcia E, Vasquez C, Rodriguez-Martinez CE, Satizabal CL. Allergic rhinitis and associated factors in schoolchildren from Bogota, Colombia. Rhinology. 2012;50(2):122–8.

50. Cabrera-Chavez F, Rodriguez-Bellegarrigue CI, Figueroa-Salcido OG, Lopez-Gallardo JA, Aramburo-Galvez JG, Vergara-Jimenez MJ, et al. Food allergy prevalence in Salvadoran school children estimated by parent-report. Int J Environ Res Public Health. 2018;15(11):2446.
51. Mehaudy R, Parisi C, Petriz N, Eymann A, Jauregui MB, Orsi M. Prevalence of cow's milk protein allergy among children in a university community hospital. Arch Argent Pediatr. 2018;116(3):219–23.
52. Bezzaoucha A. Epidemiology of asthma in children and young adults in Algiers. Rev Mal Respir. 1992;9(4):417–23.
53. Yemaneberhan H, Flohr C, Lewis SA, Bekele Z, Parry E, Williams HC, et al. Prevalence and associated factors of atopic dermatitis symptoms in rural and urban Ethiopia. Clin Exp Allergy. 2004;34(5):779–85.
54. Georgy V, Fahim HI, El-Gaafary M, Walters S. Prevalence and socioeconomic associations of asthma and allergic rhinitis in northern [corrected] Africa. Eur Respir J. 2006;28(4): 756–62.
55. Desalu OO, Salami AK, Iseh KR, Oluboyo PO. Prevalence of self reported allergic rhinitis and its relationship with asthma among adult Nigerians. J Investig Allergol Clin Immunol. 2009;19(6):474–80.
56. Belyhun Y, Amberbir A, Medhin G, Erko B, Hanlon C, Venn A, et al. Prevalence and risk factors of wheeze and eczema in 1-year-old children: the Butajira birth cohort, Ethiopia. Clin Exp Allergy. 2010;40(4):619–26.
57. Gray CL, Levin ME, Zar HJ, Potter PC, Khumalo NP, Volkwyn L, et al. Food allergy in south African children with atopic dermatitis. Pediatr Allergy Immunol. 2014;25(6):572–9.
58. Kumah DB, Lartey SY, Yemanyi F, Boateng EG, Awuah E. Prevalence of allergic conjunctivitis among basic school children in the Kumasi Metropolis (Ghana): a community-based cross-sectional study. BMC Ophthalmol. 2015;15:69.
59. Kiboneka A, Levin M, Mosalakatane T, Makone I, Wobudeya E, Makubate B, et al. Prevalence of asthma among school children in Gaborone, Botswana. Afr Health Sci. 2016;16(3):809–16.
60. Arrais M, Lulua O, Quifica F, Rosado-Pinto J, Gama JMR, Taborda-Barata L. Prevalence of asthma and allergies in 13-14-year-old adolescents from Luanda, Angola. Int J Tuberc Lung Dis. 2017;21(6):705–12.
61. Zeyrek CD, Zeyrek F, Sevinc E, Demir E. Prevalence of asthma and allergic diseases in Sanliurfa, Turkey, and the relation to environmental and socioeconomic factors: is the hygiene hypothesis enough? J Investig Allergol Clin Immunol. 2006;16(5):290–5.
62. Selcuk ZT, Demir AU, Tabakoglu E, Caglar T. Prevalence of asthma and allergic diseases in primary school children in Edirne, Turkey, two surveys 10 years apart. Pediatr Allergy Immunol. 2010;21(4 Pt 2):e711–7.
63. Khan AA, Tanzil S, Jamali T, Shahid A, Naeem S, Sahito A, et al. Burden of asthma among children in a developing megacity: childhood asthma study, Pakistan. J Asthma. 2014;51(9):891–9.
64. Cobanoglu HB, Isik AU, Topbas M, Ural A. Prevalence of allergic rhinitis in children in the Trabzon Province of the Black Sea Region of Turkey. Turk Arch Otorhinolaryngol. 2016;54(1):21–8.
65. Masoompour SM, Mahdaviazad H, Ghayumi SMA. Asthma and its related socioeconomic factors: the Shiraz adult respiratory disease study 2015. Clin Respir J. 2018;12(6):2110–6.
66. Tarraf H, Aydin O, Mungan D, Albader M, Mahboub B, Doble A, et al. Prevalence of asthma among the adult general population of five Middle Eastern countries: results of the SNAPSHOT program. BMC Pulm Med. 2018;18(1):68.
67. Chan-Yeung M, Zhan LX, Tu DH, Li B, He GX, Kauppinen R, et al. The prevalence of asthma and asthma-like symptoms among adults in rural Beijing, China. Eur Respir J. 2002;19(5):853–8.
68. Hassan MR, Kabir AR, Mahmud AM, Rahman F, Hossain MA, Bennoor KS, et al. Self-reported asthma symptoms in children and adults of Bangladesh: findings of the National Asthma Prevalence Study. Int J Epidemiol. 2002;31(2):483–8.

69. Vichyanond P, Sunthornchart S, Singhirannusorn V, Ruangrat S, Kaewsomboon S, Visitsunthorn N. Prevalence of asthma, allergic rhinitis and eczema among university students in Bangkok. Respir Med. 2002;96(1):34–8.
70. Lao-araya M, Trakultivakorn M. Prevalence of food allergy among preschool children in northern Thailand. Pediatr Int. 2012;54(2):238–43.
71. Agrawal S, Pearce N, Ebrahim S. Prevalence and risk factors for self-reported asthma in an adult Indian population: a cross-sectional survey. Int J Tuberc Lung Dis. 2013;17(2):275–82.
72. Zhao K, Song GH, Gu HQ, Liu S, Zhang Y, Guo YR. Epidemiological survey and risk factor analysis of asthma in children in urban districts of Zhengzhou, China. Zhongguo Dang Dai Er Ke Za Zhi. 2014;16(12):1220–5.
73. Huang J, Huang DM, Xiao XX, Fu SM, Luo CM, Zeng G, et al. Epidemiological survey of asthma among children aged 0-14 years in 2010 in urban Zhongshan, China. Zhongguo Dang Dai Er Ke Za Zhi. 2015;17(2):149–54.
74. Shi JB, Fu QL, Zhang H, Cheng L, Wang YJ, Zhu DD, et al. Epidemiology of chronic rhinosinusitis: results from a cross-sectional survey in seven Chinese cities. Allergy. 2015;70(5):533–9.
75. Zhang F, Hang J, Zheng B, Su L, Christiani DC. The changing epidemiology of asthma in Shanghai, China. J Asthma. 2015;52(5):465–70.
76. Fu QL, Du Y, Xu G, Zhang H, Cheng L, Wang YJ, et al. Prevalence and occupational and environmental risk factors of self-reported asthma: evidence from a cross-sectional survey in seven Chinese cities. Int J Environ Res Public Health. 2016;13(11):E1084.
77. Hu SJ, Wei P, Kou W, Wu XF, Liu MY, Chen C, et al. Prevalence and risk factors of allergic rhinitis: a Meta-analysis. Lin Chung Er Bi Yan Hou Tou Jing Wai Ke Za Zhi. 2017;31(19):1485–91.
78. Ma Q, Yang T. Prevalence and influential factors for asthma among adults in Chinese. Zhong Nan Da Xue Xue Bao Yi Xue Ban. 2017;42(9):1086–93.
79. Bunyavanich S, Soto-Quiros ME, Avila L, Laskey D, Senter JM, Celedon JC. Risk factors for allergic rhinitis in Costa Rican children with asthma. Allergy. 2010;65(2):256–63.
80. Borges WG, Burns DA, Felizola ML, Oliveira BA, Hamu CS, Freitas VC. Prevalence of allergic rhinitis among adolescents from Distrito Federal, Brazil: comparison between ISAAC phases I and III. J Pediatr. 2006;82(2):137–43.
81. Chhabra SK, Gupta CK, Chhabra P, Rajpal S. Risk factors for development of bronchial asthma in children in Delhi. Ann Allergy Asthma Immunol. 1999;83(5):385–90.
82. Tomac N, Demirel F, Acun C, Ayoglu F. Prevalence and risk factors for childhood asthma in Zonguldak, Turkey. Allergy Asthma Proc. 2005;26(5):397–402.
83. Breda D, Freitas PF, Pizzichini E, Agostinho FR, Pizzichini MM. Prevalence of asthma symptoms and risk factors among adolescents in Tubarao and Capivari de Baixo, Santa Catarina State, Brazil. Cad Saude Publica. 2009;25(11):2497–506.
84. Sun Y, Hou J, Sheng Y, Kong X, Weschler LB, Sundell J. Modern life makes children allergic. A cross-sectional study: associations of home environment and lifestyles with asthma and allergy among children in Tianjin region, China. Int Arch Occup Environ Health. 2019;92(4):587–98.
85. Xu D, Wang Y, Chen Z, Li S, Cheng Y, Zhang L, et al. Prevalence and risk factors for asthma among children aged 0-14 years in Hangzhou: a cross-sectional survey. Respir Res. 2016;17(1):122.
86. Liu SJ, Wang TT, Cao SY, Tan YQ, Chen LZ. A Meta analysis of risk factors for asthma in Chinese children. Zhongguo Dang Dai Er Ke Za Zhi. 2018;20(3):218–23.
87. Chatkin MN, Menezes AM, Victora CG, Barros FC. High prevalence of asthma in preschool children in Southern Brazil: a population-based study. Pediatr Pulmonol. 2003;35(4):296–301.
88. Chatkin MN, Menezes AM. Prevalence and risk factors for asthma in schoolchildren in southern Brazil. J Pediatr. 2005;81(5):411–6.
89. Gibbons L, Belizán JM, Lauer JA, Betrán AP, Merialdi M, Althabe F. The global numbers and costs of additionally needed and unnecessary caesarean sections performed per year: overuse as a barrier to universal coverage. World Health Report Background Paper, 30. Geneva; 2010.
90. El Kettani S, Lotfi AB, Aichane A. Prevalence of allergic rhinitis in a rural area of Settat, Morocco. East Mediterr Health J. 2009;15(1):167–77.

91. Droma Y, Kunii O, Yangzom Y, Shan M, Pingzo L, Song P. Prevalence and severity of asthma and allergies in schoolchildren in Lhasa, Tibet. Clin Exp Allergy. 2007;37(9):1326–33.
92. Song N, Shamssain M, Zhang J, Wu J, Fu C, Hao S, et al. Prevalence, severity and risk factors of asthma, rhinitis and eczema in a large group of Chinese schoolchildren. J Asthma. 2014;51(3):232–42.
93. Nakao M, Yamauchi K, Ishihara Y, Omori H, Solongo B, Ichinnorov D. Prevalence and risk factors of airflow limitation in a Mongolian population in Ulaanbaatar: cross-sectional studies. PLoS One. 2017;12(4):e0175557.
94. Cassol VE, Rizzato TM, Teche SP, Basso DF, Centenaro DF, Maldonado M, et al. Obesity and its relationship with asthma prevalence and severity in adolescents from southern Brazil. J Asthma. 2006;43(1):57–60.
95. Soto-Martinez M, Avila L, Soto N, Chaves A, Celedon JC, Soto-Quiros ME. Trends in hospitalizations and mortality from asthma in Costa Rica over a 12- to 15-year period. J Allergy Clin Immunol Pract. 2014;2(1):85–90.
96. Guddattu V, Swathi A, Nair NS. Household and environment factors associated with asthma among Indian women: a multilevel approach. J Asthma. 2010;47(4):407–11.
97. Sousa CA, Cesar CL, Barros MB, Carandina L, Goldbaum M, Pereira JC. Respiratory diseases and associated factors: population-based study in Sao Paulo, 2008–2009. Rev Saude Publica. 2012;46(1):16–25.
98. Baumann LM, Romero KM, Robinson CL, Hansel NN, Gilman RH, Hamilton RG, et al. Prevalence and risk factors for allergic rhinitis in two resource-limited settings in Peru with disparate degrees of urbanization. Clin Exp Allergy. 2015;45(1):192–9.
99. Gonzalez-Garcia M, Caballero A, Jaramillo C, Maldonado D, Torres-Duque CA. Prevalence, risk factors and underdiagnosis of asthma and wheezing in adults 40 years and older: a population-based study. J Asthma. 2015;52(8):823–30.
100. Hijazi N, Abalkhail B, Seaton A. Diet and childhood asthma in a society in transition: a study in urban and rural Saudi Arabia. Thorax. 2000;55(9):775–9.
101. Norback D, Zhao ZH, Wang ZH, Wieslander G, Mi YH, Zhang Z. Asthma, eczema, and reports on pollen and cat allergy among pupils in Shanxi province, China. Int Arch Occup Environ Health. 2007;80(3):207–16.
102. Gutierrez-Delgado RI, Barraza-Villarreal A, Escamilla-Nunez MC, Solano-Gonzalez M, Moreno-Macias H, Romieu I. Food consumption and asthma in school children in Cuernavaca, Morelos, Mexico. Salud Publica Mex. 2009;51(3):202–11.
103. Farrokhi S, Gheybi MK, Movahhed A, Dehdari R, Gooya M, Keshvari S, et al. Prevalence and risk factors of asthma and allergic diseases in primary schoolchildren living in Bushehr, Iran: phase I, III ISAAC protocol. Iran J Allergy Asthma Immunol. 2014;13(5): 348–55.
104. Alqahtani JM. Asthma and other allergic diseases among Saudi schoolchildren in Najran: the need for a comprehensive intervention program. Ann Saudi Med. 2016;36(6):379–85.
105. Poongadan MN, Gupta N, Kumar R. Dietary pattern and asthma in India. Pneumonol Alergol Pol. 2016;84(3):160–7.
106. Viinanen A, Munhbayarlah S, Zevgee T, Narantsetseg L, Naidansuren T, Koskenvuo M, et al. Prevalence of asthma, allergic rhinoconjunctivitis and allergic sensitization in Mongolia. Allergy. 2005;60(11):1370–7.
107. Nyembue TD, Jorissen M, Hellings PW, Muyunga C, Kayembe JM. Prevalence and determinants of allergic diseases in a Congolese population. Int Forum Allergy Rhinol. 2012;2(4):285–93.
108. Shimwela M, Mwita JC, Mwandri M, Rwegerera GM, Mashalla Y, Mugusi F. Asthma prevalence, knowledge, and perceptions among secondary school pupils in rural and urban coastal districts in Tanzania. BMC Public Health. 2014;14:387.
109. Morgan BW, Siddharthan T, Grigsby MR, Pollard SL, Kalyesubula R, Wise RA, et al. Asthma and allergic disorders in Uganda: a population-based study across urban and rural settings. J Allergy Clin Immunol Pract. 2018;6(5):1580–7.e2.

110. Ma Y, Zhao J, Han ZR, Chen Y, Leung TF, Wong GW. Very low prevalence of asthma and allergies in schoolchildren from rural Beijing, China. Pediatr Pulmonol. 2009;44(8):793–9.
111. Bartlett E, Parr J, Lindeboom W, Khanam MA, Koehlmoos TP. Sources and prevalence of self-reported asthma diagnoses in adults in urban and rural settings of Bangladesh. Glob Public Health. 2013;8(1):79–89.
112. Zheng M, Wang X, Bo M, Wang K, Zhao Y, He F, et al. Prevalence of allergic rhinitis among adults in urban and rural areas of China: a population-based cross-sectional survey. Allergy Asthma Immunol Res. 2015;7(2):148–57.
113. Wang XY, Zhuang Y, Ma TT, Zhang B, Wang XY. Prevalence of self-reported food allergy in six regions of inner Mongolia, northern China: a population-based survey. Med Sci Monit. 2018;24:1902–11.
114. Camargos PA, Castro RM, Feldman JS. Prevalence of symptoms related to asthma in school children of Campos Gerais, Brazil. Rev Panam Salud Publica. 1999;6(1):8–15.
115. Solis Soto MT, Patino A, Nowak D, Radon K. Prevalence of asthma, rhinitis and eczema symptoms in rural and urban school-aged children from Oropeza Province – Bolivia: a cross-sectional study. BMC Pulm Med. 2014;14:40.
116. Kalyoncu AF, Selcuk ZT, Enunlu T, Demir AU, Coplu L, Sahin AA, et al. Prevalence of asthma and allergic diseases in primary school children in Ankara, Turkey: two cross-sectional studies, five years apart. Pediatr Allergy Immunol. 1999;10(4):261–5.
117. Al Frayh AR, Shakoor Z, Gad El Rab MO, Hasnain SM. Increased prevalence of asthma in Saudi Arabia. Ann Allergy Asthma Immunol. 2001;86(3):292–6.
118. Ghozikali MG, Ansarin K, Naddafi K, Nodehi RN, Yaghmaeian K, Hassanvand MS, et al. Prevalence of asthma and associated factors among male late adolescents in Tabriz, Iran. Environ Sci Pollut Res Int. 2018;25(3):2184–93.
119. Razzaq S, Nafees AA, Rabbani U, Irfan M, Naeem S, Khan MA, et al. Epidemiology of asthma and associated factors in an urban Pakistani population: adult asthma study-Karachi. BMC Pulm Med. 2018;18(1):184.
120. Quah BS, Wan-Pauzi I, Ariffin N, Mazidah AR. Prevalence of asthma, eczema and allergic rhinitis: two surveys, 6 years apart, in Kota Bharu, Malaysia. Respirology. 2005;10(2):244–9.
121. Sharma SK, Banga A. Prevalence and risk factors for wheezing in children from rural areas of north India. Allergy Asthma Proc. 2007;28(6):647–53.
122. Pakhale S, Wooldrage K, Manfreda J, Anthonisen N. Prevalence of asthma symptoms in 7th- and 8th-grade school children in a rural region in India. J Asthma. 2008;45(2):117–22.
123. Agrawal S. Effect of indoor air pollution from biomass and solid fuel combustion on prevalence of self-reported asthma among adult men and women in India: findings from a nationwide large-scale cross-sectional survey. J Asthma. 2012;49(4):355–65.
124. Hong H, Yang Q, Zuo K, Chen X, Xia W, Lv M, et al. A hospital-based survey on the prevalence of bronchial asthma in patients with allergic rhinitis in southern China. Am J Rhinol Allergy. 2013;27(6):502–5.
125. Wang F, Wang M, Chen CB, Cai ZW, Wen DD, Chen FY, et al. Epidemiological analysis of childhood asthma in Yichang City, China. Zhongguo Dang Dai Er Ke Za Zhi. 2013;15(11):979–82.
126. Kumar P, Ram U. Patterns, factors associated and morbidity burden of asthma in India. PLoS One. 2017;12(10):e0185938.
127. Bhalla K, Nehra D, Nanda S, Verma R, Gupta A, Mehra S. Prevalence of bronchial asthma and its associated risk factors in school-going adolescents in Tier-III North Indian City. J Family Med Prim Care. 2018;7(6):1452–7.
128. Casagrande RR, Pastorino AC, Souza RG, Leone C, Sole D, Jacob CM. Asthma prevalence and risk factors in schoolchildren of the city of Sao Paulo, Brazil. Rev Saude Publica. 2008;42(3):517–23.
129. Soto-Quiros M, Bustamante M, Gutierrez I, Hanson LA, Strannegard IL, Karlberg J. The prevalence of childhood asthma in Costa Rica. Clin Exp Allergy. 1994;24(12):1130–6.

130. Dagoye D, Bekele Z, Woldemichael K, Nida H, Yimam M, Venn AJ, et al. Domestic risk factors for wheeze in urban and rural Ethiopian children. QJM. 2004;97(8):489–98.
131. Aggarwal AN, Chaudhry K, Chhabra SK, D'Souza GA, Gupta D, Jindal SK, et al. Prevalence and risk factors for bronchial asthma in Indian adults: a multicentre study. Indian J Chest Dis Allied Sci. 2006;48(1):13–22.
132. Dong GH, Ding HL, Ma YN, Jin J, Cao Y, Zhao YD, et al. Housing characteristics, home environmental factors and respiratory health in 14,729 Chinese children. Rev Epidemiol Sante Publique. 2008;56(2):97–107.
133. Gonzalez-Diaz SN, Del Rio-Navarro BE, Pietropaolo-Cienfuegos DR, Escalante-Dominguez AJ, Garcia-Almaraz RG, Merida-Palacio V, et al. Factors associated with allergic rhinitis in children and adolescents from northern Mexico: international study of asthma and allergies in childhood phase IIIB. Allergy Asthma Proc. 2010;31(4):e53–62.
134. Dhabadi BB, Athavale A, Meundi A, Rekha R, Suruliraman M, Shreeranga A, et al. Prevalence of asthma and associated factors among schoolchildren in rural South India. Int J Tuberc Lung Dis. 2012;16(1):120–5.
135. Coelho MA, de Pinho L, Marques PQ, Silveira MF, Sole D. Prevalence and factors associated with asthma in students from Montes Claros, Minas Gerais, Brazil. Cien Saude Colet. 2016;21(4):1207–16.
136. Bolat E, Arikoglu T, Sungur MA, Batmaz SB, Kuyucu S. Prevalence and risk factors for wheezing and allergic diseases in preschool children: a perspective from the Mediterranean coast of Turkey. Allergol Immunopathol (Madr). 2017;45(4):362–8.
137. Celedon JC, Soto-Quiros ME, Silverman EK, Hanson L, Weiss ST. Risk factors for childhood asthma in Costa Rica. Chest. 2001;120(3):785–90.
138. Al-Kubaisy W, Ali SH, Al-Thamiri D. Risk factors for asthma among primary school children in Baghdad, Iraq. Saudi Med J. 2005;26(3):460–6.
139. Uthaisangsook S. Risk factors for development of asthma in Thai adults in Phitsanulok: a university-based study. Asian Pac J Allergy Immunol. 2010;28(1):23–8.
140. Juca SC, Takano OA, Moraes LS, Guimaraes LV. Asthma prevalence and risk factors in adolescents 13 to 14 years of age in Cuiaba, Mato Grosso State, Brazil. Cad Saude Publica. 2012;28(4):689–97.
141. Bener A, al-Jawadi TQ, Ozkaragoz F, al-Frayh A, Gomes J. Bronchial asthma and wheeze in a desert country. Indian J Pediatr. 1993;60(6):791–7.
142. Civelek E, Sahiner UM, Yuksel H, Boz AB, Orhan F, Uner A, et al. Prevalence, burden, and risk factors of atopic eczema in schoolchildren aged 10–11 years: a national multicenter study. J Investig Allergol Clin Immunol. 2011;21(4):270–7.
143. Stephen GA, McRill C, Mack MD, O'Rourke MK, Flood TJ, Lebowitz MD. Assessment of respiratory symptoms and asthma prevalence in a U.S.-Mexico border region. Arch Environ Health. 2003;58(3):156–62.
144. Vedanthan PK, Mahesh PA, Vedanthan R, Holla AD, Liu AH. Effect of animal contact and microbial exposures on the prevalence of atopy and asthma in urban vs rural children in India. Ann Allergy Asthma Immunol. 2006;96(4):571–8.
145. Ngui R, Lim YA, Chow SC, de Bruyne JA, Liam CK. Prevalence of bronchial asthma among orang asli in peninsular Malaysia. Med J Malaysia. 2011;66(1):27–31.
146. Li J, Wang H, Chen Y, Zheng J, Wong GW, Zhong N. House dust mite sensitization is the main risk factor for the increase in prevalence of wheeze in 13- to 14-year-old schoolchildren in Guangzhou city, China. Clin Exp Allergy. 2013;43(10):1171–9.
147. Kurt E, Metintas S, Basyigit I, Bulut I, Coskun E, Dabak S, et al. Prevalence and risk factors of allergies in Turkey: results of a multicentric cross-sectional study in children. Pediatr Allergy Immunol. 2007;18(7):566–74.
148. Dong GH, Ma YN, Ding HL, Jin J, Cao Y, Zhao YD, et al. Effects of housing characteristics and home environmental factors on respiratory symptoms of 10,784 elementary school children from Northeast China. Respiration. 2008;76(1):82–91.

149. Zhang Y, Zhang L. Prevalence of allergic rhinitis in China. Allergy Asthma Immunol Res. 2014;6(2):105–13.
150. Yoshihara S, Munkhbayarlakh S, Makino S, Ito C, Logii N, Dashdemberel S, et al. Prevalence of childhood asthma in Ulaanbaatar, Mongolia in 2009. Allergol Int. 2016;65(1):62–7.
151. Rojas Molina N, Legorreta Soberanis J, Olvera GF. Prevalence and asthma risk factors in municipalities of the State of Guerrero, Mexico. Rev Alerg Mex. 2001;48(4):115–8.
152. Sriyaraj K, Priest N, Shutes B. Environmental factors influencing the prevalence of respiratory diseases and allergies among schoolchildren in Chiang Mai, Thailand. Int J Environ Health Res. 2008;18(2):129–48.
153. Kurt E, Metintas S, Basyigit I, Bulut I, Coskun E, Dabak S, et al. Prevalence and Risk Factors of Allergies in Turkey (PARFAIT): results of a multicentre cross-sectional study in adults. Eur Respir J. 2009;33(4):724–33.
154. Wang HY, Chen YZ, Ma Y, Wong GW, Lai CK, Zhong NS. Disparity of asthma prevalence in Chinese schoolchildren is due to differences in lifestyle factors. Zhonghua Er Ke Za Zhi. 2006;44(1):41–5.
155. Benicio MH, Ferreira MU, Cardoso MR, Konno SC, Monteiro CA. Wheezing conditions in early childhood: prevalence and risk factors in the city of Sao Paulo, Brazil. Bull World Health Organ. 2004;82(7):516–22.
156. Al-Mazam A, Mohamed AG. Risk factors of bronchial asthma in Bahrah, Saudi Arabia. J Family Community Med. 2001;8(1):33–9.
157. Dela Bianca A, Wandalsen G, Mallol J, Sole D. Risk factors for wheezing disorders in infants in the first year of life living in Sao Paulo, Brazil. J Trop Pediatr. 2012;58(6):501–4.
158. Baccioglu A, Sogut A, Kilic O, Beyhun E. The prevalence of allergic diseases and associated risk factors in school-age children and adults in Erzurum, Turkey. Turk Thorac J. 2015;16(2):68–72.
159. Wong GW, Ko FW, Hui DS, Fok TF, Carr D, von Mutius E, et al. Factors associated with difference in prevalence of asthma in children from three cities in China: multicentre epidemiological survey. BMJ. 2004;329(7464):486.
160. Hesse IF. Knowledge of asthma and its management in newly qualified doctors in Accra, Ghana. Respir Med. 1995;89(1):35–9.
161. Abudahish A, Bella H. Primary care physicians perceptions and practices on asthma care in Aseer region, Saudi Arabia. Saudi Med J. 2006;27(3):333–7.
162. Bhulani N, Lalani S, Ahmed A, Jan Y, Faheem U, Khan A, et al. Knowledge of asthma management by general practitioners in Karachi, Pakistan: comparison with international guidelines. Prim Care Respir J. 2011;20(4):448–51.
163. Jumbe Marsden E, Wa Somwe S, Chabala C, Soriano JB, Valles CP, Anchochea J. Knowledge and perceptions of asthma in Zambia: a cross-sectional survey. BMC Pulm Med. 2016; 16:33.
164. Kouotou EA, Nansseu JR, Ngangue Engome AD, Tatah SA, Zoung-Kanyi Bissek AC. Knowledge, attitudes and practices of the medical personnel regarding atopic dermatitis in Yaounde, Cameroon. BMC Dermatol. 2017;17(1):1.
165. Urrutia-Pereira M, Fernandez C, Valentin-Rostan M, Cruz A, Torres O, Simon L, et al. Primary care physicians' knowledge about allergic rhinitis and its impact on asthma (ARIA guidelines): a comparative Brazilian/Paraguayan/Uruguayan pilot study. Rev Alerg Mex. 2018;65(4):321–30.
166. Yilmaz O, Reisli I, Tahan F, Orhan F, Boz AB, Yuksel H. Influence of education on primary care physicians' knowledge on childhood allergy as a systemic disease and the atopic march. Allergol Immunopathol (Madr). 2011;39(2):73–8.
167. Hussein S, Partridge M. Perceptions of asthma in south Asians and their views on educational materials and self-management plans: a qualitative study. Patient Educ Couns. 2002;48(2):189–94.
168. Osaretin OW, Uchechukwu ND, Osawaru O. Asthma management by medical practitioners: the situation in a developing country. World J Pediatr. 2013;9(1):64–7.

169. Hussain SF, Zahid S, Khan JA, Haqqee R. Asthma management by general practitioners in Pakistan. Int J Tuberc Lung Dis. 2004;8(4):414–7.
170. Chan YC, Tay YK, Sugito TL, Boediardja SA, Chau DD, Nguyen KV, et al. A study on the knowledge, attitudes and practices of Southeast Asian dermatologists in the management of atopic dermatitis. Ann Acad Med Singap. 2006;35(11):794–803.
171. Neffen H, Baena-Cagnani CE, Malka S, Sole D, Sepulveda R, Caraballo L, et al. Asthma mortality in Latin America. J Investig Allergol Clin Immunol. 1997;7(4):249–53.
172. Hounkpati A, Hounkpati HY, Kpanla E, Balogou KA, Tidjani O. Evaluation of asthma care in Africa. Rev Mal Respir. 2009;26(1):11–20.
173. Opedun N, Ehlers VJ, Roos JH. Compliance amongst asthma patients registered for an asthma disease risk-management programme in South Africa. Curationis. 2011;34(1):E1–8.
174. Chima EI, Iroezindu MO, Uchenna NR, Mbata GO, Okwuonu CG. A survey of asthma management practices and implementation of global initiative for asthma guidelines among doctors in a resource-limited setting in Nigeria. Niger J Clin Pract. 2017;20(8):984–91.
175. Badoum G, Ouedraogo SM, Lankoande H, Ouedraogo G, Boncoungou K, Bambara M, et al. Knowledge, attitudes and practices of general practitioners about asthma in the city of Ouagadougou. Mali Med. 2012;27(1):10–3.
176. Kotwani A, Chhabra SK, Tayal V, Vijayan VK. Quality of asthma management in an urban community in Delhi, India. Indian J Med Res. 2012;135:184–92.
177. Justin-Temu M, Risha P, Abla O, Massawe A. Incidence, knowledge and health seeking behaviour for perceived allergies at household level: a case study in Ilala district Dar es Salaam Tanzania. East Afr J Public Health. 2008;5(2):90–3.
178. Zhao J. Asthma control status in children and related factors in 29 cities of China. Zhonghua Er Ke Za Zhi. 2013;51(2):90–5.
179. Al-Khateeb AJ, Al Khateeb JM. Research on psychosocial aspects of asthma in the Arab world: a literature review. Multidiscip Respir Med. 2015;10(1):15.
180. Alzaabi A, Idrees M, Behbehani N, Khaitov MR, Tunceli K, Urdaneta E, et al. Cross-sectional study on asthma insights and management in the Gulf and Russia. Allergy Asthma Proc. 2018;39(6):430–6.
181. Urrutia-Pereira M, Mocellin LP, de Oliveira RB, Simon L, Lessa L, Sole D. Knowledge on asthma, food allergies, and anaphylaxis: assessment of elementary school teachers, parents/caregivers of asthmatic children, and university students in Uruguaiana, in the state of Rio Grande do Sul, Brazil. Allergol Immunopathol (Madr). 2018;46(5):421–30.
182. Mavale-Manuel S, Duarte N, Alexandre F, Albuquerque O, Scheinmann P, Poisson-Salomon AS, et al. Knowledge, attitudes, and behavior of the parents of asthmatic children in Maputo. J Asthma. 2004;41(5):533–8.
183. Sy DQ, Thanh Binh MH, Quoc NT, Hung NV, Quynh Nhu DT, Bao NQ, et al. Prevalence of asthma and asthma-like symptoms in Dalat Highlands, Vietnam. Singapore Med J. 2007;48(4):294–303.
184. Rastogi D, Gupta S, Kapoor R. Comparison of asthma knowledge, management, and psychological burden among parents of asthmatic children from rural and urban neighborhoods in India. J Asthma. 2009;46(9):911–5.
185. Salama AA, Mohammed AA, El Okda el SE, Said RM. Quality of care of Egyptian asthmatic children: clinicians adherence to asthma guidelines. Ital J Pediatr. 2010;36:33.
186. Al-Busaidi N, Habibulla Z, Bhatnagar M, Al-Lawati N, Al-Mahrouqi Y. The burden of asthma in Oman. Sultan Qaboos Univ Med J. 2015;15(2):e184–90.
187. Rezvanfar MA, Kebriaeezadeh A, Moein M, Nikfar S, Gharibnaseri Z, Abdollahi-Asl A. Cost analysis of childhood asthma in Iran: a cost evaluation based on referral center data for asthma and allergies. J Res Pharm Pract. 2013;2(4):162–8.
188. Chuesakoolvanich K. Cost of hospitalizing asthma patients in a regional hospital in Thailand. Respirology. 2007;12(3):433–8.
189. Handa S, Jain N, Narang T. Cost of care of atopic dermatitis in India. Indian J Dermatol. 2015;60(2):213.

190. Ibrahim WH, Suleiman NN, El-Allus F, Suleiman J, Elbuzidi AA, Guerrero MD, et al. The burden of adult asthma in a high GDP per capita country: the QASMA study. Ann Allergy Asthma Immunol. 2015;114(1):12–7.

191. Ding B, DiBonaventura M, Karlsson N, Ling X. A cross-sectional assessment of the prevalence and burden of mild asthma in urban China using the 2010, 2012, and 2013 China National Health and Wellness Surveys. J Asthma. 2017;54(6):632–43.

192. Mungan D, Aydin O, Mahboub B, Albader M, Tarraf H, Doble A, et al. Burden of disease associated with asthma among the adult general population of five Middle Eastern countries: results of the SNAPSHOT program. Respir Med. 2018;139:55–64.

193. Bavbek S, Mungan D, Turktas H, Misirligil Z, Gemicioglu B. A cost-of-illness study estimating the direct cost per asthma exacerbation in Turkey. Respir Med. 2011;105(4):541–8.

194. Ding B, Small M. Disease burden of mild asthma in China. Respirology. 2018;23(4): 369–77.

195. Civelek E, Yavuz ST, Boz AB, Orhan F, Yuksel H, Uner A, et al. Epidemiology and burden of rhinitis and rhinoconjunctivitis in 9- to 11-year-old children. Am J Rhinol Allergy. 2010;24(5):364–70.

196. Nafti S, Taright S, El Ftouh M, Yassine N, Benkheder A, Bouacha H, et al. Prevalence of asthma in North Africa: the Asthma Insights and Reality in the Maghreb (AIRMAG) study. Respir Med. 2009;103(Suppl 2):S2–11.

197. Belhocine M, Ait-Khaled N. Prevalence of asthma in a region of Algeria. Bull Int Union Tuberc Lung Dis. 1991;66(2–3):91–3.

198. Arrais M, Lulua O, Quifica F, Rosado-Pinto J, Gama JMR, Taborda-Barata L. Prevalence of asthma, allergic rhinitis and eczema in 6–7-year-old schoolchildren from Luanda, Angola. Allergol Immunopathol (Madr). 2019;47(6):523–534.

199. Miningou SD, Zoubga AZ, Meda H, Meda N, Tiendrebeogo H. Prevalence of asthma in subjects aged 15-64 years in Bobo-Dioulasso (Burkina Faso) in 1998. Rev Pneumol Clin. 2002;58(6 Pt 1):341–5.

200. Pefura-Yone EW, Kengne AP, Balkissou AD, Boulleys-Nana JR, Efe-de-Melingui NR, Ndjeutcheu-Moualeu PI, et al. Prevalence of asthma and allergic rhinitis among adults in Yaounde, Cameroon. PLoS One. 2015;10(4):e0123099.

201. Mbatchou Ngahane BH, Afane Ze E, Nde F, Ngomo E, Mapoure Njankouo Y, Njock LR. Prevalence and risk factors for allergic rhinitis in bakers in Douala, Cameroon. BMJ Open. 2014;4(8):e005329.

202. Mugusi F, Edwards R, Hayes L, Unwin N, Mbanya JC, Whiting D, et al. Prevalence of wheeze and self-reported asthma and asthma care in an urban and rural area of Tanzania and Cameroon. Trop Dr. 2004;34(4):209–14.

203. Hailu S, Tessema T, Silverman M. Prevalence of symptoms of asthma and allergies in schoolchildren in Gondar town and its vicinity, northwest Ethiopia. Pediatr Pulmonol. 2003;35(6):427–32.

204. Melaku K, Berhane Y. Prevalence of wheeze and asthma related symptoms among school children in Addis Ababa, Ethiopia. Ethiop Med J. 1999;37(4):247–54.

205. Adeyemi AS, Akinboro AO, Adebayo PB, Tanimowo MO, Ayodele OE. The prevalence, risk factors and changes in symptoms of self reported asthma, rhinitis and eczema among pregnant women in Ogbomoso, Nigeria. J Clin Diagn Res. 2015;9(9):Oc01–7.

206. Hogewoning AA, Bouwes Bavinck JN, Amoah AS, Boakye DA, Yazdanbakhsh M, Kremsner PG, et al. Point and period prevalences of eczema in rural and urban schoolchildren in Ghana, Gabon and Rwanda. J Eur Acad Dermatol Venereol. 2012;26(4):488–94.

207. Roudaut M, Meda AH, Seka A, Fadiga D, Pigearias B, Akoto A. Prevalence of asthma and respiratory diseases in schools in Bouake (Ivory Coast): preliminary results. Med Trop (Mars). 1992;52(3):279–83.

208. Wolff PT, Arison L, Rahajamiakatra A, Raserijaona F, Niggemann B. High asthma prevalence and associated factors in urban malagasy schoolchildren. J Asthma. 2012;49(6):575–80.

209. Bouayad Z, Aichane A, Afif A, Benouhoud N, Trombati N, Chan-Yeung M, et al. Prevalence and trend of self-reported asthma and other allergic disease symptoms in Morocco: ISAAC phase I and III. Int J Tuberc Lung Dis. 2006;10(4):371–7.
210. Mavale-Manuel S, Joaquim O, Nunes E, Pedro A, Bandeira S, Eduardo E, et al. Prevalence of asthma-like symptoms by ISAAC video questionnaire in Mozambican schoolchildren. Monaldi Arch Chest Dis. 2006;65(4):189–95.
211. Falade AG, Ige OM, Yusuf BO, Onadeko MO, Onadeko BO. Trends in the prevalence and severity of symptoms of asthma, allergic rhinoconjunctivitis, and atopic eczema. J Natl Med Assoc. 2009;101(5):414–8.
212. Falade AG, Olawuyi JF, Osinusi K, Onadeko BO. Prevalence and severity of symptoms of asthma, allergic rhinoconjunctivitis, and atopic eczema in 6- to 7-year-old Nigerian primary school children: the international study of asthma and allergies in childhood. Med Princ Pract. 2004;13(1):20–5.
213. Falade AG, Olawuyi F, Osinusi K, Onadeko BO. Prevalence and severity of symptoms of asthma, allergic rhino-conjunctivitis and atopic eczema in secondary school children in Ibadan, Nigeria. East Afr Med J. 1998;75(12):695–8.
214. Hooper LG, Dieye Y, Ndiaye A, Diallo A, Fan VS, Neuzil KM, et al. Estimating pediatric asthma prevalence in rural senegal: a cross-sectional survey. Pediatr Pulmonol. 2017;52(3):303–9.
215. Herrant M, Loucoubar C, Boufkhed S, Bassene H, Sarr FD, Baril L, et al. Risk factors associated with asthma, atopic dermatitis and rhinoconjunctivitis in a rural Senegalese cohort. Allergy Asthma Clin Immunol. 2015;11(1):24.
216. Olaniyan T, Dalvie MA, Roosli M, Naidoo R, Kunzli N, de Hoogh K, et al. Asthma-related outcomes associated with indoor air pollutants among schoolchildren from four informal settlements in two municipalities in the Western Cape Province of South Africa. Indoor Air. 2019;29(1):89–100.
217. Teclessou JN, Mouhari-Toure A, Akakpo S, Bayaki S, Boukari OB, Elegbede YM, et al. Risk factors and allergic manifestations associated with atopic dermatitis in Lome (Togo): a multicenter study of 476 children aged 0–15 years. Med Sante Trop. 2016;26(1): 88–91.
218. Sonia T, Meriem M, Yacine O, Nozha BS, Nadia M, Bechir L, et al. Prevalence of asthma and rhinitis in a Tunisian population. Clin Respir J. 2018;12(2):608–15.
219. Khaldi F, Fakhfakh R, Mattoussi N, Ben Ali B, Zouari S, Khemiri M. Prevalence and severity of asthma, allergic rhinoconjunctivitis and atopic eczema in "Grand Tunis" schoolchildren: ISAAC. Tunis Med. 2005;83(5):269–73.
220. Nantanda R, Ostergaard MS, Ndeezi G, Tumwine JK. Factors associated with asthma among under-fives in Mulago hospital, Kampala Uganda: a cross sectional study. BMC Pediatr. 2013;13:141.
221. Bemanin MH, Fallahpour M, Arshi S, Nabavi M, Yousofi T, Shariatifar A. First report of asthma prevalence in Afghanistan using international standardized methods. East Mediterr Health J. 2015;21(3):194–8.
222. Fazlollahi MR, Najmi M, Fallahnezhad M, Sabetkish N, Kazemnejad A, Bidad K, et al. Paediatric asthma prevalence: the first national population-based survey in Iran. Clin Respir J. 2019;13(1):14–22.
223. Alavinezhad A, Boskabady MH. The prevalence of asthma and related symptoms in Middle East countries. Clin Respir J. 2018;12(3):865–77.
224. Fazlollahi MR, Souzanch G, Nourizadeh M, Sabetkish N, Tazesh B, Entezari A, et al. The prevalence of allergic rhinitis and it's relationship with second-hand tobacco smoke among adults in Iran. Acta Med Iran. 2017;55(11):712–7.
225. Varmaghani M, Farzadfar F, Sharifi F, Rashidian A, Moin M, Moradi-Lakeh M, et al. Prevalence of asthma, COPD, and chronic bronchitis in Iran: a systematic review and meta-analysis. Iran J Allergy Asthma Immunol. 2016;15(2):93–104.

226. Mehravar F, Rafiee S, Bazrafshan B, Khodadost M. Prevalence of asthma symptoms in Golestan schoolchildren aged 6–7 and 13–14 years in Northeast Iran. Front Med. 2016;10(3):345–50.

227. Mohammadbeigi A, Hassanzadeh J, Mousavizadeh A. Prevalence of asthma in elementary school age children in Iran--a systematic review and meta analysis study. Pak J Biol Sci. 2011;14(19):887–93.

228. Golshan M, Mohamad-Zadeh Z, Zahedi-Nejad N, Rostam-Poor B. Prevalence of asthma and related symptoms in primary school children of Isfahan, Iran, in 1998. Asian Pac J Allergy Immunol. 2001;19(3):163–70.

229. Khazaei HA, Hashemi SR, Aghamohammadi A, Farhoudi F, Rezaei N. The study of type 1 allergy prevalence among people of south-east of Iran by skin prick test using common allergens. Iran J Allergy Asthma Immunol. 2003;2(3):165–8.

230. Khatami A, Nassiri-Kashani M, Gorouhi F, Babakoohi S, Kazerouni-Timsar A, Davari P, et al. Allergic contact dermatitis to metal allergens in Iran. Int J Dermatol. 2013;52(12):1513–8.

231. Ahanchian H, Jafari S, Behmanesh F, Haghi NM, Nakhaei AA, Kiani MA, et al. Epidemiological survey of pediatric food allergy in Mashhad in Northeast Iran. Electron Physician. 2016;8(1):1727–32.

232. Moghtaderi M, Hosseini Teshnizi S, Farjadian S. Sensitization to common allergens among patients with allergies in major Iranian cities: a systematic review and meta-analysis. Epidemiol Health. 2017;39:e2017007.

233. Nabavi M, Lavavpour M, Arshi S, Bemanian MH, Esmaeilzadeh H, Molatefi R, et al. Characteristics, etiology and treatment of pediatric and adult anaphylaxis in Iran. Iran J Allergy Asthma Immunol. 2017;16(6):480–7.

234. Pereg D, Tirosh A, Lishner M, Goldberg A, Shochat T, Confino-Cohen R. Prevalence of asthma in a large group of Israeli adolescents: influence of country of birth and age at migration. Allergy. 2008;63(8):1040–5.

235. Magen E, Mishal J, Schlesinger M. Sensitizations to allergens of TRUE test in 864 consecutive eczema patients in Israel. Contact Dermatitis. 2006;55(6):370–1.

236. Abu-Ekteish F, Otoom S, Shehabi I. Prevalence of asthma in Jordan: comparison between Bedouins and urban schoolchildren using the international study of asthma and allergies in childhood phase III protocol. Allergy Asthma Proc. 2009;30(2):181–5.

237. Abdualrasool M, Al-Shanfari S, Booalayan H, Boujarwa A, Al-Mukaimi A, Alkandery O, et al. Exposure to environmental tobacco smoke and prevalence of atopic dermatitis among adolescents in Kuwait. Dermatology. 2018;234(5–6):186–91.

238. Ali F. A survey of self-reported food allergy and food-related anaphylaxis among young adult students at Kuwait University, Kuwait. Med Princ Pract. 2017;26(3):229–34.

239. Owayed A, Behbehani N, Al-Momen J. Changing prevalence of asthma and allergic diseases among Kuwaiti children. An ISAAC Study (Phase III). Med Princ Pract. 2008;17(4):284–9.

240. Behbehani NA, Abal A, Syabbalo NC, Abd Azeem A, Shareef E, Al-Momen J. Prevalence of asthma, allergic rhinitis, and eczema in 13- to 14-year-old children in Kuwait: an ISAAC study. International Study of Asthma and Allergies in Childhood. Ann Allergy Asthma Immunol. 2000;85(1):58–63.

241. Ramadan FM, Khoury MN, Hajjar TA, Mroueh SM. Prevalence of allergic diseases in children in Beirut: comparison to worldwide data. J Med Liban. 1999;47(4):216–21.

242. Qasem JA, Nasrallah H, Al-Khalaf BN, Al-Sharifi F, Al-Sherayfee A, Almathkouri SA, et al. Meteorological factors, aeroallergens and asthma-related visits in Kuwait: a 12-month retrospective study. Ann Saudi Med. 2008;28(6):435–41.

243. Almutairi N, Almutawa F. Allergic contact dermatitis pattern in Kuwait: nickel leads the pack. In-depth analysis of nickel allergy based on the results from a large prospective patch test series report. Postepy Dermatol Alergol. 2017;34(3):207–15.

244. Alkazemi D, Albeajan M, Kubow S. Early infant feeding practices as possible risk factors for immunoglobulin E-mediated food allergies in Kuwait. Int J Pediatr. 2018;2018:1701903.

245. Irani C, Maalouly G. Prevalence of self-reported food allergy in Lebanon: a Middle-Eastern taste. Int Sch Res Notices. 2015;2015:639796.
246. Musharrafieh U, Al-Sahab B, Zaitoun F, El-Hajj MA, Ramadan F, Tamim H. Prevalence of asthma, allergic rhinitis and eczema among Lebanese adolescents. J Asthma. 2009;46(4):382–7.
247. Waked M, Salameh P. Risk factors for asthma and allergic diseases in school children across Lebanon. J Asthma Allergy. 2008;2:1–7.
248. Al-Rawas OA, Al-Maniri AA, Al-Riyami BM. Home exposure to Arabian incense (bakhour) and asthma symptoms in children: a community survey in two regions in Oman. BMC Pulm Med. 2009;9:23.
249. Al-Rawas OA, Al-Riyami BM, Al-Kindy H, Al-Maniri AA, Al-Riyami AA. Regional variation in the prevalence of asthma symptoms among Omani school children: comparisons from two nationwide cross-sectional surveys six years apart. Sultan Qaboos Univ Med J. 2008;8(2):157–64.
250. Al-Riyami BM, Al-Rawas OA, Al-Riyami AA, Jasim LG, Mohammed AJ. A relatively high prevalence and severity of asthma, allergic rhinitis and atopic eczema in schoolchildren in the Sultanate of Oman. Respirology. 2003;8(1):69–76.
251. Shafique RH, Akhter S, Abbas S, Ismail M. Sensitivity to house dust mite allergens and prevalence of allergy-causing house dust mite species in Pothwar, Pakistan. Exp Appl Acarol. 2018;74(4):415–26.
252. Hasnain SM, Khan M, Saleem A, Waqar MA. Prevalence of asthma and allergic rhinitis among school children of Karachi, Pakistan, 2007. J Asthma. 2009;46(1):86–90.
253. Inam M, Shafique RH, Roohi N, Irfan M, Abbas S, Ismail M. Prevalence of sensitization to food allergens and challenge proven food allergy in patients visiting allergy centers in Rawalpindi and Islamabad, Pakistan. Springerplus. 2016;5(1):1330.
254. El-Sharif NA, Nemery B, Barghuthy F, Mortaja S, Qasrawi R, Abdeen Z. Geographical variations of asthma and asthma symptoms among schoolchildren aged 5 to 8 years and 12 to 15 years in Palestine: the International Study of Asthma and Allergies in Childhood (ISAAC). Ann Allergy Asthma Immunol. 2003;90(1):63–71.
255. El-Sharif N, Abdeen Z, Qasrawi R, Moens G, Nemery B. Asthma prevalence in children living in villages, cities and refugee camps in Palestine. Eur Respir J. 2002;19(6):1026–34.
256. Mohamed Hussain S, Ayesha Farhana S, Mohammed AS. Time trends and regional variation in prevalence of asthma and associated factors in Saudi Arabia: a systematic review and meta-analysis. Biomed Res Int. 2018;2018:8102527.
257. Alruwaili MF, Elwan A. Prevalence of asthma among male 16 to 18-year-old adolescents in the Northern Borders Region of Saudi Arabia. Electron Physician. 2018;10(6):6920–6.
258. Al Ghobain MO, Algazlan SS, Oreibi TM. Asthma prevalence among adults in Saudi Arabia. Saudi Med J. 2018;39(2):179–84.
259. Moradi-Lakeh M, El Bcheraoui C, Daoud F, Tuffaha M, Kravitz H, Al Saeedi M, et al. Prevalence of asthma in Saudi adults: findings from a national household survey, 2013. BMC Pulm Med. 2015;15:77.
260. Nahhas M, Bhopal R, Anandan C, Elton R, Sheikh A. Prevalence of allergic disorders among primary school-aged children in Madinah, Saudi Arabia: two-stage cross-sectional survey. PLoS One. 2012;7(5):e36848.
261. Al Ghobain MO, Al-Hajjaj MS, Al Moamary MS. Asthma prevalence among 16- to 18-year-old adolescents in Saudi Arabia using the ISAAC questionnaire. BMC Public Health. 2012;12:239.
262. Sobki SH, Zakzouk SM. Point prevalence of allergic rhinitis among Saudi children. Rhinology. 2004;42(3):137–40.
263. Bener A, al-Jawadi TQ, Ozkaragoz F, Anderson JA. Prevalence of asthma and wheeze in two different climatic areas of Saudi Arabia. Indian J Chest Dis Allied Sci. 1993;35(1):9–15.

264. Alqahtani JM, Asaad AM, Awadalla NJ, Mahfouz AA. Environmental determinants of bronchial asthma among Saudi school children in Southwestern Saudi Arabia. Int J Environ Res Public Health. 2016;14(1):22.
265. Dogruel D, Bingol G, Yilmaz M, Altintas DU. The ADAPAR birth cohort study: food allergy results at five years and new insights. Int Arch Allergy Immunol. 2016;169(1):57–61.
266. Dogruel D, Bingol G, Altintas DU, Yilmaz M, Kendirli SG. Prevalence of and risk factors for atopic dermatitis: a birth cohort study of infants in Southeast Turkey. Allergol Immunopathol (Madr). 2016;44(3):214–20.
267. Tamay Z, Akcay A, Ergin A, Guler N. Prevalence of allergic rhinitis and risk factors in 6- to 7-yearold children in Istanbul, Turkey. Turk J Pediatr. 2014;56(1):31–40.
268. Talay F, Kurt B, Tug T, Kurt OK, Goksugur N, Yasar Z. The prevalence of asthma and allergic diseases among adults 30–49 years of age in Bolu, Western Black Sea Region of Turkey. Clin Ter. 2014;165(1):e59–63.
269. Duksal F, Becerir T, Ergin A, Akcay A, Guler N. The prevalence of asthma diagnosis and symptoms is still increasing in early adolescents in Turkey. Allergol Int. 2014;63(2):189–97.
270. Duksal F, Akcay A, Becerir T, Ergin A, Becerir C, Guler N. Rising trend of allergic rhinitis prevalence among Turkish schoolchildren. Int J Pediatr Otorhinolaryngol. 2013;77(9):1434–9.
271. Civelek E, Cakir B, Boz AB, Yuksel H, Orhan F, Uner A, et al. Extent and burden of allergic diseases in elementary schoolchildren: a national multicenter study. J Investig Allergol Clin Immunol. 2010;20(4):280–8.
272. Gelincik A, Buyukozturk S, Gul H, Isik E, Issever H, Ozseker F, et al. Confirmed prevalence of food allergy and non-allergic food hypersensitivity in a Mediterranean population. Clin Exp Allergy. 2008;38(8):1333–41.
273. Selcuk ZT, Caglar T, Enunlu T, Topal T. The prevalence of allergic diseases in primary school children in Edirne, Turkey. Clin Exp Allergy. 1997;27(3):262–9.
274. Orhan F, Karakas T, Cakir M, Aksoy A, Baki A, Gedik Y. Prevalence of immunoglobulin E-mediated food allergy in 6-9-year-old urban schoolchildren in the eastern Black Sea region of Turkey. Clin Exp Allergy. 2009;39(7):1027–35.
275. Kurt E, Demir AU, Cadirci O, Yildirim H, Ak G, Eser TP. Occupational exposures as risk factors for asthma and allergic diseases in a Turkish population. Int Arch Occup Environ Health. 2011;84(1):45–52.
276. Akcay A, Tamay Z, Hocaoglu AB, Ergin A, Guler N. Risk factors affecting asthma prevalence in adolescents living in Istanbul, Turkey. Allergol Immunopathol (Madr). 2014;42(5):449–58.
277. Haktanir Abul M, Dereci S, Hacisalihoglu S, Orhan F. Is kiwifruit allergy a matter in kiwifruit-cultivating regions? A population-based study. Pediatr Allergy Immunol. 2017;28(1):38–43.
278. Ozdemir SK, Ozguvarsigmalu S. Pollen food allergy syndrome in Turkey: clinical characteristics and evaluation of its association with skin test reactivity to pollens. Asian Pac J Allergy Immunol. 2018;36(2):77–81.
279. Zhang Y, Chen Y, Zhao A, Li H, Mu Z, Zhang Y, et al. Prevalence of self-reported food allergy and food intolerance and their associated factors in 3–12 year-old children in 9 areas in China. Wei Sheng Yan Jiu. 2015;44(2):226–31.
280. Du EC, Li ZM, Sui C, Wang W, Zhang QX. Relationship between asthma and allergic antigens in rural houses. Biomed Environ Sci. 1993;6(1):27–30.
281. Norback D, Lu C, Wang J, Zhang Y, Li B, Zhao Z, et al. Asthma and rhinitis among Chinese children – indoor and outdoor air pollution and indicators of socioeconomic status (SES). Environ Int. 2018;115:1–8.
282. Guo X, Li Z, Ling W, Long J, Su C, Li J, et al. Epidemiology of childhood asthma in mainland China (1988–2014): a meta-analysis. Allergy Asthma Proc. 2018;39(3):15–29.
283. Guo Y, Li P, Tang J, Han X, Zou X, Xu G, et al. Prevalence of atopic dermatitis in Chinese children aged 1–7 ys. Sci Rep. 2016;6:29751.
284. Huang C, Liu W, Hu Y, Zou Z, Zhao Z, Shen L, et al. Updated prevalences of asthma, allergy, and airway symptoms, and a systematic review of trends over time for childhood asthma in Shanghai, China. PLoS One. 2015;10(4):e0121577.

285. Sha L, Shao M, Liu C, Li S, Li Z, Luo Y, et al. The prevalence of asthma in children: a comparison between the year of 2010 and 2000 in urban China. Zhonghua Jie He He Hu Xi Za Zhi. 2015;38(9):664–8.
286. Zeng GQ, Luo JY, Huang HM, Zheng PY, Luo WT, Wei NL, et al. Food allergy and related risk factors in 2540 preschool children: an epidemiological survey in Guangdong Province, southern China. World J Pediatr. 2015;11(3):219–25.
287. Yang Z, Zheng W, Yung E, Zhong N, Wong GW, Li J. Frequency of food group consumption and risk of allergic disease and sensitization in school children in urban and rural China. Clin Exp Allergy. 2015;45(12):1823–32.
288. Wang Y, Sai X, Sun Y, Zheng Y. A cross sectional survey on the prevalence of food intolerance and its determinants through physical checkup programs in the elderly. Zhonghua Liu Xing Bing Xue Za Zhi. 2014;35(11):1249–51.
289. Xiong M, Ni C, Pan JH, Wang Q, Zheng LL. Epidemiological survey of childhood asthma in Hefei City, China. Zhongguo Dang Dai Er Ke Za Zhi. 2013;15(2):109–11.
290. Chang ML, Shao B, Liu YH, Li LL, Pei LC, Wang BY. Analysis of allergens in 5 473 patients with allergic diseases in Harbin, China. Biomed Environ Sci. 2013;26(11):886–93.
291. Hao GD, Zheng YW, Gjesing B, Kong XA, Wang JY, Song ZJ, et al. Prevalence of sensitization to weed pollens of Humulus scandens, Artemisia vulgaris, and Ambrosia artemisiifolia in northern China. J Zhejiang Univ Sci B. 2013;14(3):240–6.
292. Chen J, Liao Y, Zhang HZ, Zhao H, Chen J, Li HQ. Prevalence of food allergy in children under 2 years of age in three cities in China. Zhonghua Er Ke Za Zhi. 2012;50(1):5–9.
293. Gu JL, Ma HL, Zheng YJ. Epidemiological survey of asthma in children aged 0–14 years in the Futian District of Shenzhen, China between 2010 and 2011. Zhongguo Dang Dai Er Ke Za Zhi. 2012;14(12):918–23.
294. Li F, Zhou Y, Li S, Jiang F, Jin X, Yan C, et al. Prevalence and risk factors of childhood allergic diseases in eight metropolitan cities in China: a multicenter study. BMC Public Health. 2011;11:437.
295. Sai XY, Zheng YS, Zhao JM, Hao W. A cross sectional survey on the prevalence of food intolerance and its determinants in Beijing, China. Zhonghua Liu Xing Bing Xue Za Zhi. 2011;32(3):302–5.
296. Zhao J, Bai J, Shen KL, Xiang L, Huang Y, Huang S, et al. Questionnaire-based survey of allergic diseases among children aged 0–14 years in the downtown of Beijing, Chongqing and Guangzhou. Zhonghua Er Ke Za Zhi. 2011;49(10):740–4.
297. Hu Y, Chen J, Li H. Comparison of food allergy prevalence among Chinese infants in Chongqing, 2009 versus 1999. Pediatr Int. 2010;52(5):820–4.
298. Zhao J, Bai J, Shen K, Xiang L, Huang S, Chen A, et al. Self-reported prevalence of childhood allergic diseases in three cities of China: a multicenter study. BMC Public Health. 2010;10:551.
299. Chen J, Hu Y, Allen KJ, Ho MH, Li H. The prevalence of food allergy in infants in Chongqing, China. Pediatr Allergy Immunol. 2011;22(4):356–60.
300. Han DM, Zhang L, Huang D, Wu YF, Dong Z, Xu G, et al. Self-reported prevalence of allergic rhinitis in eleven cities in China. Zhonghua Er Bi Yan Hou Tou Jing Wai Ke Za Zhi. 2007;42(5):378–84.
301. Wong GW, Leung TF, Ma Y, Liu EK, Yung E, Lai CK. Symptoms of asthma and atopic disorders in preschool children: prevalence and risk factors. Clin Exp Allergy. 2007;37(2):174–9.
302. Chen YZ. A nationwide survey in China on prevalence of asthma in urban children. Zhonghua Er Ke Za Zhi. 2003;41(2):123–7.
303. Wang W, Huang X, Chen Z, Zheng R, Chen Y, Zhang G, et al. Prevalence and trends of sensitisation to aeroallergens in patients with allergic rhinitis in Guangzhou, China: a 10-year retrospective study. BMJ Open. 2016;6(5):e011085.
304. Li J, Huang Y, Lin X, Zhao D, Tan G, Wu J, et al. Factors associated with allergen sensitizations in patients with asthma and/or rhinitis in China. Am J Rhinol Allergy. 2012;26(2):85–91.

305. Saha GK. House dust mite allergy in Calcutta, India: evaluation by RAST. Ann Allergy. 1993;70(4):305–9.
306. Chhabra SK, Gupta CK, Chhabra P, Rajpal S. Prevalence of bronchial asthma in schoolchildren in Delhi. J Asthma. 1998;35(3):291–6.
307. Awasthi S, Kalra E, Roy S, Awasthi S. Prevalence and risk factors of asthma and wheeze in school-going children in Lucknow, North India. Indian Pediatr. 2004;41(12):1205–10.
308. Kasera R, Singh BP, Lavasa S, Prasad KN, Sahoo RC, Singh AB. Kidney bean: a major sensitizer among legumes in asthma and rhinitis patients from India. PLoS One. 2011;6(11): e27193.
309. Dey D, Ghosh N, Pandey N, Gupta BS. A hospital-based survey on food allergy in the population of Kolkata, India. Int Arch Allergy Immunol. 2014;164(3):218–21.
310. Singh S, Sharma BB, Sharma SK, Sabir M, Singh V. Prevalence and severity of asthma among Indian school children aged between 6 and 14 years: associations with parental smoking and traffic pollution. J Asthma. 2016;53(3):238–44.
311. Shaikh WA, Shaikh SW. Allergies in India: an analysis of 3389 patients attending an allergy clinic in Mumbai, India. J Indian Med Assoc. 2008;106(4):220, 2, 4 passim.
312. Kumar GS, Roy G, Subitha L, Sahu SK. Prevalence of bronchial asthma and its associated factors among school children in urban Puducherry, India. J Nat Sci Biol Med. 2014;5(1): 59–62.
313. Nitin J, Palagani R, Shradha NH, Vaibhav J, Kowshik K, Manoharan R, et al. Prevalence, severity and risk factors of allergic disorders among people in south India. Afr Health Sci. 2016;16(1):201–9.
314. Phathammavong O, Ali M, Phengsavanh A, Xaysomphou D, Odajima H, Nishima S, et al. Prevalence and potential risk factors of rhinitis and atopic eczema among schoolchildren in Vientiane capital, Lao PDR: ISAAC questionnaire. Biosci Trends. 2008;2(5):193–9.
315. Quah BS, Razak AR, Hassan MH. Prevalence of asthma, rhinitis and eczema among schoolchildren in Kelantan, Malaysia. Acta Paediatr Jpn. 1997;39(3):329–35.
316. Sam CK, Kesavan P, Liam CK, Soon SC, Lim AL, Ong EK. A study of pollen prevalence in relation to pollen allergy in Malaysian asthmatics. Asian Pac J Allergy Immunol. 1998;16(1):1–4.
317. Quah BS, Mazidah AR, Hamzah AM, Simpson H. Prevalence of wheeze, night cough and doctor-diagnosed asthma in pre-school children in Kota Bharu. Asian Pac J Allergy Immunol. 2000;18(1):15–21.
318. Sonomjamts M, Dashdemberel S, Logii N, Nakae K, Chigusa Y, Ohhira S, et al. Prevalence of asthma and allergic rhinitis among adult population in Ulaanbaatar, Mongolia. Asia Pac Allergy. 2014;4(1):25–31.
319. Shek LP, Cabrera-Morales EA, Soh SE, Gerez I, Ng PZ, Yi FC, et al. A population-based questionnaire survey on the prevalence of peanut, tree nut, and shellfish allergy in 2 Asian populations. J Allergy Clin Immunol. 2010;126(2):324–31, 31.e1–7.
320. Connett GJ, Gerez I, Cabrera-Morales EA, Yuenyongviwat A, Ngamphaiboon J, Chatchatee P, et al. A population-based study of fish allergy in the Philippines, Singapore and Thailand. Int Arch Allergy Immunol. 2012;159(4):384–90.
321. Amarasekera ND, Gunawardena NK, de Silva NR, Weerasinghe A. Prevalence of childhood atopic diseases in the Western Province of Sri Lanka. Ceylon Med J. 2010;55(1):5–8.
322. de Silva NR, Dasanayake WM, Karunatilleke C, Malavige GN. Food dependant exercise induced anaphylaxis a retrospective study from 2 allergy clinics in Colombo, Sri Lanka. Allergy Asthma Clin Immunol. 2015;11(1):22.
323. Seneviratne R, Gunawardena NS. Prevalence and associated factors of wheezing illnesses of children aged three to five years living in under-served settlements of the Colombo Municipal Council in Sri Lanka: a cross-sectional study. BMC Public Health. 2018;18(1):127.
324. Vichyanond P, Jirapongsananuruk O, Visitsuntorn N, Tuchinda M. Prevalence of asthma, rhinitis and eczema in children from the Bangkok area using the ISAAC (International Study for Asthma and Allergy in Children) questionnaires. J Med Assoc Thail. 1998;81(3):175–84.

325. Teeratakulpisarn J, Wiangnon S, Kosalaraksa P, Heng S. Surveying the prevalence of asthma, allergic rhinitis and eczema in school-children in Khon Kaen, Northeastern Thailand using the ISAAC questionnaire: phase III. Asian Pac J Allergy Immunol. 2004;22(4): 175–81.
326. Uthaisangsook S. Prevalence of asthma, rhinitis, and eczema in the university population of Phitsanulok, Thailand. Asian Pac J Allergy Immunol. 2007;25(2–3):127–32.
327. Boonchai W, Iamtharachai P, Sunthonpalin P. Prevalence of allergic contact dermatitis in Thailand. Dermatitis. 2008;19(3):142–5.
328. Lam HT, Ronmark E, Tu'o'ng NV, Ekerljung L, Chuc NT, Lundback B. Increase in asthma and a high prevalence of bronchitis: results from a population study among adults in urban and rural Vietnam. Respir Med. 2011;105(2):177–85.
329. Lam HT, Ekerljung L, Bjerg A, Van TTN, Lundback B, Ronmark E. Sensitization to airborne allergens among adults and its impact on allergic symptoms: a population survey in northern Vietnam. Clin Transl Allergy. 2014;4(1):6.
330. Toizumi M, Hashizume M, Nguyen HAT, Yasunami M, Kitamura N, Iwasaki C, et al. Asthma, rhinoconjunctivitis, eczema, and the association with perinatal anthropometric factors in Vietnamese children. Sci Rep. 2019;9(1):2655.
331. Le TTK, Nguyen DH, Vu ATL, Ruethers T, Taki AC, Lopata AL. A cross-sectional, population-based study on the prevalence of food allergies among children in two different socio-economic regions of Vietnam. Pediatr Allergy Immunol. 2019;30(3):348–55.
332. Sole D, Yamada E, Vana AT, Costa-Carvalho BT, Naspitz CK. Prevalence of asthma and related symptoms in school-age children in Sao Paulo, Brazil–International Study of Asthma and Allergies in Children (ISAAC). J Asthma. 1999;36(2):205–12.
333. De Britto MC, Bezerra PG, Ferreira OS, Maranhao IC, Trigueiro GA. Asthma prevalence in schoolchildren in a city in north-east Brazil. Ann Trop Paediatr. 2000;20(2):95–100.
334. Vanna AT, Yamada E, Arruda LK, Naspitz CK, Sole D. International Study of Asthma and Allergies in Childhood: validation of the rhinitis symptom questionnaire and prevalence of rhinitis in schoolchildren in Sao Paulo, Brazil. Pediatr Allergy Immunol. 2001;12(2): 95–101.
335. Maia JG, Marcopito LF, Amaral AN, Tavares Bde F, Santos FA. Prevalence of asthma and asthma symptoms among 13 and 14-year-old schoolchildren, Brazil. Rev Saude Publica. 2004;38(2):292–9.
336. Rios JL, Boechat JL, Sant'Anna CC, Franca AT. Atmospheric pollution and the prevalence of asthma: study among schoolchildren of 2 areas in Rio de Janeiro, Brazil. Ann Allergy Asthma Immunol. 2004;92(6):629–34.
337. Sole D, Camelo-Nunes IC, Vana AT, Yamada E, Werneck F, de Freitas LS, et al. Prevalence of rhinitis and related-symptoms in schoolchildren from different cities in Brazil. Allergol Immunopathol (Madr). 2004;32(1):7–12.
338. Neto AC, Annes RD, Wolff NM, Klein AP, Dos Santos FC, Dullius JL, et al. Prevalence and severity of asthma, rhinitis, and atopic eczema in 13- to 14-year-old schoolchildren from southern Brazil. Allergy Asthma Clin Immunol. 2006;2(1):3–10.
339. Sole D, Wandalsen GF, Camelo-Nunes IC, Naspitz CK. Prevalence of symptoms of asthma, rhinitis, and atopic eczema among Brazilian children and adolescents identified by the International Study of Asthma and Allergies in Childhood (ISAAC) – Phase 3. J Pediatr. 2006;82(5):341–6.
340. Kuschnir FC, Cunha AJ, Braga Dde A, Silveira HH, Barroso MH, Aires ST. Asthma in 13-14-year-old schoolchildren in the city of Nova Iguacu, Rio de Janeiro State, Brazil: prevalence, severity, and gender differences. Cad Saude Publica. 2007;23(4):919–26.
341. Sole D, Camelo-Nunes IC, Wandalsen GF, Rosario Filho NA, Naspitz CK. Prevalence of rhinitis among Brazilian schoolchildren: ISAAC phase 3 results. Rhinology. 2007;45(2):122–8.
342. Sole D, Camelo-Nunes IC, Wandalsen GF, Mallozi MC, Naspitz CK. Is the prevalence of asthma and related symptoms among Brazilian children related to socioeconomic status? J Asthma. 2008;45(1):19–25.

343. Castro LK, Cerci Neto A, Ferreira Filho OF. Prevalence of symptoms of asthma, rhinitis and atopic eczema among students between 6 and 7 years of age in the city of Londrina, Brazil. J Bras Pneumol. 2010;36(3):286–92.

344. Wehrmeister FC, Peres KG. Regional inequalities in the prevalence of asthma diagnosis in children: an analysis of the Brazilian National Household Sample Survey, 2003. Cad Saude Publica. 2010;26(9):1839–52.

345. Toledo MF, Rozov T, Leone C. Prevalence of asthma and allergies in 13- to 14-year-old adolescents and the frequency of risk factors in carriers of current asthma in Taubate, Sao Paulo, Brazil. Allergol Immunopathol (Madr). 2011;39(5):284–90.

346. Sousa CA, Cesar CL, Barros MB, Carandina L, Goldbaum M, Pereira JC. Prevalence of asthma and risk factors associated: population based study in Sao Paulo, Southeastern Brazil, 2008–2009. Rev Saude Publica. 2012;46(5):825–33.

347. Oliveira-Santos S, Motta-Franco J, Barreto I, Sole D, Gurgel R. Asthma in adolescents--prevalence trends and associated factors in Northeast Brazil. Allergol Immunopathol (Madr). 2015;43(5):429–35.

348. Goncalves LC, Guimaraes TC, Silva RM, Cheik MF, de Ramos Napolis AC, Barbosa ESG, et al. Prevalence of food allergy in infants and pre-schoolers in Brazil. Allergol Immunopathol (Madr). 2016;44(6):497–503.

349. Toledo MF, Saraiva-Romanholo BM, Oliveira RC, Saldiva PH, Silva LF, Nascimento LF, et al. Changes over time in the prevalence of asthma, rhinitis and atopic eczema in adolescents from Taubate, Sao Paulo, Brazil (2005–2012): relationship with living near a heavily travelled highway. Allergol Immunopathol (Madr). 2016;44(5):439–44.

350. Kuschnir FC, Alves da Cunha AJ. Environmental and socio-demographic factors associated to asthma in adolescents in Rio de Janeiro, Brazil. Pediatr Allergy Immunol. 2007;18(2):142–8.

351. de Magalhaes Simoes S, da Cunha SS, Cruz AA, Dias KC, Alcantara-Neves NM, Amorim LD, et al. A community study of factors related to poorly controlled asthma among Brazilian urban children. PLoS One. 2012;7(5):e37050.

352. Barreto BA, Sole D. Prevalence of asthma and associated factors in adolescents living in Belem (Amazon region), Para, Brazil. Allergol Immunopathol (Madr). 2014;42(5):427–32.

353. Mallol J, Cortez E, Amarales L, Sanchez I, Calvo M, Soto S, et al. Prevalence of asthma in Chilean students. Descriptive study of 24,470 children. ISAAC-Chile. Rev Med Chil. 2000;128(3):279–85.

354. Hoyos-Bachiloglu R, Ivanovic-Zuvic D, Alvarez J, Linn K, Thone N, de los Angeles Paul M, et al. Prevalence of parent-reported immediate hypersensitivity food allergy in Chilean school-aged children. Allergol Immunopathol (Madr). 2014;42(6):527–32.

355. Caraballo L, Cadavid A, Mendoza J. Prevalence of asthma in a tropical city of Colombia. Ann Allergy. 1992;68(6):525–9.

356. Marrugo J, Hernandez L, Villalba V. Prevalence of self-reported food allergy in Cartagena (Colombia) population. Allergol Immunopathol (Madr). 2008;36(6):320–4.

357. Penaranda A, Aristizabal G, Garcia E, Vasquez C, Rodriguez-Martinez CE. Rhinoconjunctivitis prevalence and associated factors in school children aged 6-7 and 13-14 years old in Bogota, Colombia. Int J Pediatr Otorhinolaryngol. 2012;76(4):530–5.

358. Garcia E, Aristizabal G, Vasquez C, Rodriguez-Martinez CE, Sarmiento OL, Satizabal CL. Prevalence of and factors associated with current asthma symptoms in school children aged 6-7 and 13-14 yr old in Bogota, Colombia. Pediatr Allergy Immunol. 2008;19(4):307–14.

359. Soto-Quiros ME, Soto-Martinez M, Hanson LA. Epidemiological studies of the very high prevalence of asthma and related symptoms among school children in Costa Rica from 1989 to 1998. Pediatr Allergy Immunol. 2002;13(5):342–9.

360. Tatto-Cano MI, Sanin-Aguirre LH, Gonzalez V, Ruiz-Velasco S, Romieu I. Prevalence of asthma, rhinitis and eczema in school children in the city of Cuernavaca, Mexico. Salud Publica Mex. 1997;39(6):497–506.

361. Rodriguez A, Vaca M, Oviedo G, Erazo S, Chico ME, Teles C, et al. Urbanisation is associated with prevalence of childhood asthma in diverse, small rural communities in Ecuador. Thorax. 2011;66(12):1043–50.
362. Rodriguez A, Vaca MG, Chico ME, Rodrigues LC, Barreto ML, Cooper PJ. Lifestyle domains as determinants of wheeze prevalence in urban and rural schoolchildren in Ecuador: cross sectional analysis. Environ Health. 2015;14:15.
363. Thongkham D, Tran J, Clunes MT, Brahim F. Prevalence and severity of asthmatic symptoms in Grenadian school children: the Grenada National Asthma Survey. BMJ Open. 2015;5(10):e008557.
364. Draaisma E, Garcia-Marcos L, Mallol J, Sole D, Perez-Fernandez V, Brand PL. A multinational study to compare prevalence of atopic dermatitis in the first year of life. Pediatr Allergy Immunol. 2015;26(4):359–66.
365. Kahwa EK, Waldron NK, Younger NO, Edwards NC, Knight-Madden JM, Bailey KA, et al. Asthma and allergies in Jamaican children aged 2-17 years: a cross-sectional prevalence survey. BMJ Open. 2012;2(4):e001132.
366. Garcia CR. Air-borne allergens and respiratory allergy in the state of Oaxaca, Mexico. Rev Alerg. 1991;38(3):85–7.
367. Baeza Bacab MA, Grahma Zapata LF. Prevalence of asthma. Survey of a school population in Villahermosa, Tabasco, Mexico. Rev Alerg. 1992;39(2):32–6.
368. Avila Castanon L, Perez Lopez J, del Rio Navarro BE, Rosas Vargas MA, Lerma Ortiz L, Sienra Monge JJ. Hypersensitivity detected by skin tests to food in allergic patients in the Hospital Infantil de Mexico Federico Gomez. Rev Alerg Mex. 2002;49(3):74–9.
369. Cisneros Perez V, Alvarado EC. Prevalence of allergic rhinitis in Durango, Mexico. Rev Alerg Mex. 2004;51(2):49–53.
370. Baeza Bacab MA, Davila Velazquez JR, Loeza Medina SR. Prevalence of positive skin tests to indoor allergens in preschooler children with respiratory allergy in Merida, Yucatan, Mexico. Rev Alerg Mex. 2005;52(6):237–42.
371. Del-Rio-Navarro B, Del Rio-Chivardi JM, Berber A, Sienra-Monge JJ, Rosas-Vargas MA, Baeza-Bacab M. Asthma prevalence in children living in north Mexico City and a comparison with other Latin American cities and world regions. Allergy Asthma Proc. 2006;27(4):334–40.
372. Barraza-Villarreal A, Hernandez-Cadena L, Moreno-Macias H, Ramirez-Aguilar M, Romieu I. Trends in the prevalence of asthma and other allergic diseases in schoolchildren from Cuernavaca, Mexico. Allergy Asthma Proc. 2007;28(3):368–74.
373. Rodriguez Orozco AR, Nunez Tapia RM. Prevalence of atopic dermatitis in 6–14 year old children in Morelia, Michoacan, Mexico. Rev Alerg Mex. 2007;54(1):20–3.
374. Esquivel CA, Perez VC, Arredondo DM, Iturbide MS, Hernandez Ade L, Arellano AG. Prevalence of asthma in Tepehuano and Mestizo school children from Durango, Mexico. Rev Alerg Mex. 2008;55(5):189–95.
375. Lopez Campos C, Carrillo Lucero JM, Lopez Campos JE, Rincon Castaneda C, Velasco Gutierrez JM, Cairo Cueto SM, et al. Prevalence and severity of asthma in 6 and 7 year-old children from Torreon, Coahuila, Mexico. Rev Alerg Mex. 2008;55(4):148–52.
376. Bedolla Barajas M, Barrera Zepeda AT, Morales RJ. Atopic dermatitis in scholar children from Ciudad Guzman, Mexico. Prevalence and related factors. Rev Alerg Mex. 2010;57(3):71–8.
377. Bedolla-Barajas M, Cuevas-Rios G, Garcia-Barboza E, Barrera-Zepeda AT, Morales-Romero J. Prevalence and associated factors to allergic rhinitis in school children of ciudad Guzman, Mexico. Rev Investig Clin. 2010;62(3):244–51.
378. Bedolla-Barajas M, Morales-Romero J, Hernandez-Colin DD, Arevalo-Cruz D. Prevalence of sensitization to the most common allergens in elderly patients from the Western of Mexico. Rev Alerg Mex. 2012;59(3):131–8.
379. Bedolla-Barajas M, Morales-Romero J, Robles-Figueroa M, Fregoso-Fregoso M. Asthma in late adolescents of Western Mexico: prevalence and associated factors. Arch Bronconeumol. 2013;49(2):47–53.

380. Bedolla-Barajas M, Bedolla-Pulido TR, Macriz-Romero N, Morales-Romero J, Robles-Figueroa M. Prevalence of peanut, tree nut, sesame, and seafood allergy in Mexican adults. Rev Investig Clin. 2015;67(6):379–86.
381. Medina-Hernandez A, Huerta-Hernandez RE, Gongora-Melendez MA, Dominguez Silva MG, Mendoza-Hernandez DA, Romero-Tapia SJ, et al. Clinical-epidemiological profile of patients with suspicion of alimentary allergy in Mexico. Mexipreval study. Rev Alerg Mex. 2015;62(1):28–40.
382. Ontiveros N, Valdez-Meza EE, Vergara-Jimenez MJ, Canizalez-Roman A, Borzutzky A, Cabrera-Chavez F. Parent-reported prevalence of food allergy in Mexican schoolchildren: a population-based study. Allergol Immunopathol (Madr). 2016;44(6):563–70.
383. Mancilla-Hernandez E, Gonzalez-Solorzano EVM, Medina-Avalos MA, Barnica-Alvarado RH. Prevalence of allergic rhinitis and its symptoms in the school children population of Cuernavaca, Morelos, Mexico. Rev Alerg Mex. 2017;64(3):243–9.
384. Martin M, Sauer T, Alarcon JA, Vinoles J, Walter EC, Ton TG, et al. Prevalence and impact of asthma among school-aged students in Lima, Peru. Int J Tuberc Lung Dis. 2017;21(11):1201–5.
385. Bordel-Gomez MT, Miranda-Romero A, Castrodeza-Sanz J. Epidemiology of contact dermatitis: prevalence of sensitization to different allergens and associated factors. Actas Dermosifiliogr. 2010;101(1):59–75.
386. Monteil MA, Joseph G, Changkit C, Wheeler G, Antoine RM. Comparison of prevalence and severity of asthma among adolescents in the Caribbean islands of Trinidad and Tobago: results of a nationwide cross-sectional survey. BMC Public Health. 2005;5:96.

Chapter 3
Racial and Ethnic Disparity in Allergic Diseases in the United States: Example of a Large Country with a Diverse Population

Hendrik Sy and Anne Marie Ditto

Abbreviations

AR	Allergic rhinitis
GWAS	Genome-wide association studies
ICAS	Inner-City Asthma Study
NHANES	National Health and Nutrition Examination Survey
NHIS	National Health Interview Survey
SES	Socioeconomic status
SNP	single nucleotide polymorphism
ssIgE	serum-specific IgE

Introduction

Racial/ethnic minority groups are growing in the United States and comprise a significant part of the population. In 2016, the US Census Bureau estimated that the US race/ethnic proportions were 61.3% non-Hispanic Whites, 17.8% Hispanics, 13.3% Blacks or African Americans, 5.7% Asians, and 2.6% with two or more races. Minority groups will continue to grow with the US Census Bureau's population projection for 2060 comprising 44.3% non-Hispanic Whites, 27.5% Hispanics, 15% Blacks or African Americans, 9.1% Asians, and 6.2% with two or more races [1].

H. Sy
Department for Infectious Diseases and Pulmonary Medicine, Charité – University Medicine Berlin, Berlin, Germany

A. M. Ditto (✉)
Department of Medicine, Division of Allergy-Immunology, Northwestern University Feinberg School of Medicine, Chicago, IL, USA
e-mail: amditto@northwestern.edu

© Springer Nature Switzerland AG 2020
M. Mahdavinia (ed.), *Health Disparities in Allergic Diseases*,
https://doi.org/10.1007/978-3-030-31222-0_3

For the purpose of this book chapter, race and ethnicity follow the definitions of the 1997 Office of Management and Budget (OMB) standards. Thus, race follows a social rather than genetic or anthropologic definition. The concept of race differs from ethnicity, which refers to Hispanic origin. Hispanics can be of any race [2]. Race and ethnicity are associated with many sociodemographic factors such as poverty status, educational attainment, exposure and housing characteristics, psychological distress, insurance coverage, and cost barriers [3].

Over 50 million Americans suffer from allergies each year, which makes it the 6th leading cause of chronic illness in the United States. The annual cost is estimated to mount to $18 billion [4]. Racial/ethnic minorities are disproportionally affected by many allergic diseases compared to Whites with higher asthma morbidity [5–7], higher rates of anaphylaxis due to food or medication allergies [8, 9] as well as higher rates of atopic dermatitis [10]. Most data on racial/ethnic disparity in allergic diseases in the United States is derived from nationwide surveys, such as the National Health and Nutrition Examination Survey (NHANES) and the National Health Interview Survey (NHIS) or from smaller studies conducted throughout the country. There are relatively more studies addressing disparity in asthma compared to other allergic diseases.

This chapter will review the role of genetic predisposition as opposed to environmental, lifestyle, and socioeconomic factors that might contribute to the observed racial and ethnic disparities. Asthma will be used as an example to discuss genetic predisposition, as most data is available for this condition (Fig. 3.1). Disparities in other allergic diseases will be discussed for atopic dermatitis/eczema, food allergy, and anaphylaxis, as well as allergic rhinitis/hay fever. Lastly, examples for interventions and future directions to overcome racial and ethnic disparity in allergic diseases in the United States will be reviewed.

Racial and Ethnic Disparity by Allergic Disease

Asthma

According to the CDC, over 26 million people or 8.3% of US adults suffered from asthma in 2016 [11]. Racial/ethnic minorities are disproportionally affected by asthma. African American adults are two to three times more likely to die from asthma than any other racial or ethnic group, and Black children are two times more likely to have asthma than White children [5]. Blacks have a significantly higher emergency department (ED) visit rate and hospitalization rate for asthma compared to Whites (Figs. 3.1 and 3.2) [12].

Among Hispanics, Puerto Ricans show the highest prevalence of current asthma (14.3%), surpassing the rates for non-Hispanic Blacks (11.6%) and non-Hispanic Whites (8.3%), while Mexican Americans have a lower prevalence (5.7%) [11]. As of 2017, 5.5 million Puerto Ricans lived in the continental United States with 20.2%

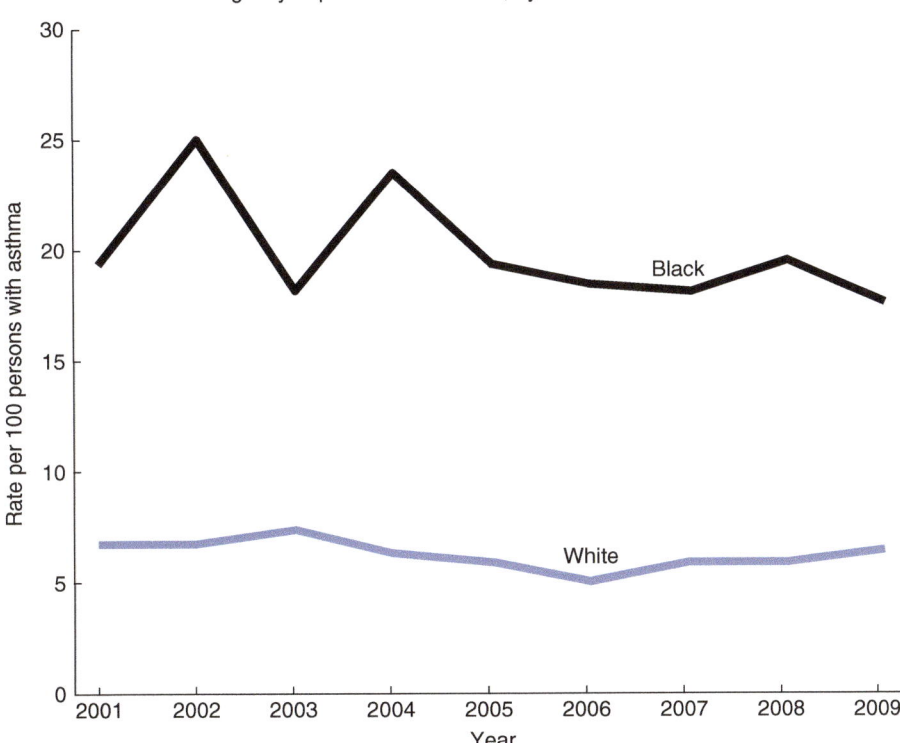

Asthma emergency department visit rates, by race: United States, 2001–2009

NOTES: Crude (unadjusted) risk-based rates are presented.
SOURCE: CDC/NCHS, National Hospital Ambulatory Medical Care Survey.

Fig. 3.1 Asthma emergency department visit rates, by race: United States, 2001–2009. (Adjusted from Moorman et al. [12])

living below the poverty line in 2016 [13, 14], while 3.2 million residents lived in the island of Puerto Rico, a US territory, 44% of those living in poverty as of 2018 [15]. A growing body of evidence supports a multifactorial etiology of asthma in Puerto Ricans with interactions between hereditary and environmental risk factors in this high-risk group, many of them still unidentified [16, 17].

Role of Genetic Predisposition

The high asthma morbidity among African Americans and Puerto Ricans compared to Mexican Americans raises the question of an association between genetic ancestry and asthma susceptibility. Puerto Ricans have been found to have a higher proportion of African and European ancestry compared to Mexican Americans who have a higher proportion of Native American ancestry. Native American ancestry is

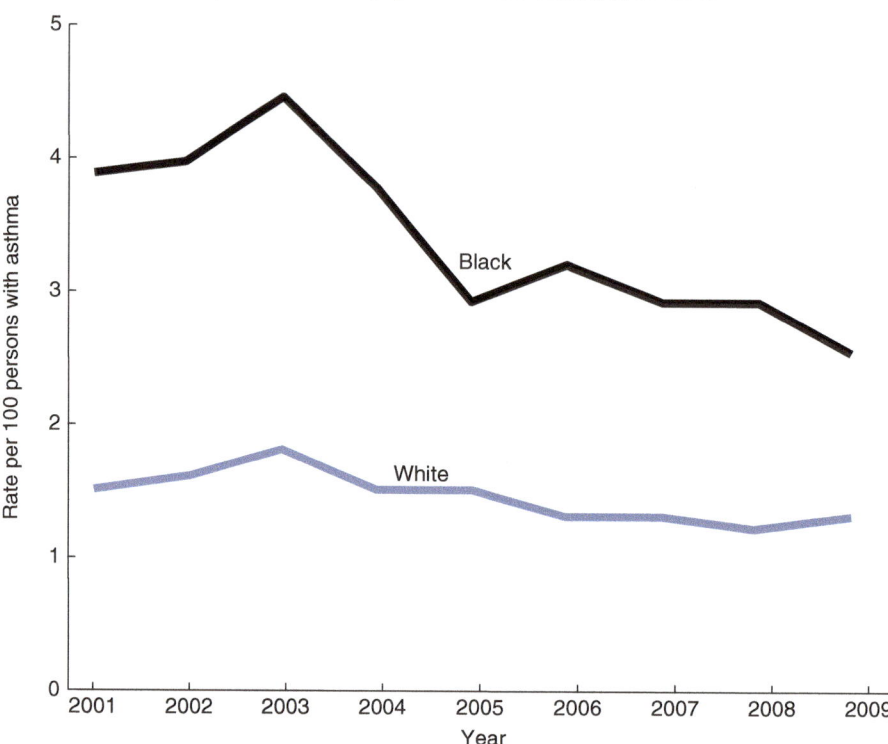

Asthma hospitalization rates, by race: United States, 2001–2009

NOTES: Crude (unadjusted) risk-based rates are presented.
SOURCE: CDC/NCHS, National Hospital Discharge Survey.

Fig. 3.2 Asthma hospitalization rates, by race: United States, 2001–2009. (Adjusted from Moorman et al. [12])

associated with lower odds of asthma, while African ancestry is associated with lower lung function and higher odds of asthma [18, 19]. Other studies have confirmed the association of African ancestry with increased asthma risk and lower lung function in Puerto Ricans and African Americans [20–22].

It is unknown whether ancestral effects are explained by allelic variants or environmental factors correlated with racial ancestry. Genome-wide association studies (GWAS) identified single nucleotide polymorphisms (SNPs) as asthma-susceptibility variants across ethnic groups that have been replicated in African Americans and individuals of Mexican and Puerto Rican descent. These SNPs were located in genes such as ORMDL3 and *GSDMB* on the 17q2 locus [23, 24] as well as *TSLP* and *IL33* [17, 25]. Other asthma-susceptibility variants have been identified for African Americans [25, 26] and Hispanics [27, 28]. Of note, variants detected in Hispanics, including Puerto Ricans and Mexican Americans, have previously been identified in subjects of European descent [24]. The lack of replication in some

GWAS studies that discovered ethnic-specific loci for asthma in Hispanics might be contributable to the high genetic variation in this population due to their complex ancestry. Furthermore, other technical variations such as the use of commercial genotyping assays developed specifically for European populations or small sample sizes leading to decreased statistical power can be the reason behind these controversial results. Admixture mapping that compares genetic ancestry at a given location in the genome may be a promising tool to overcome these challenges [17, 28].

Little is known about gene-environment interactions and epigenetic changes in racial/ethnic minorities with asthma, and studies lack replication or statistical power. DNA methylation marks in specific gene loci have been associated with childhood asthma [29]. In a Kansas City cohort, African American children with persistent asthma had higher levels of global DNA methylation than asthmatic children of other races/ethnicity. Low socioeconomic status, as measured by <50% mean family income, strongly correlated with higher global DNA methylation levels in African American children relative to children of other race/ethnicity with low socioeconomic status [30]. DNA methylation was also correlated with exposure to violence in Puerto Rican children [31]. The role of gene variants as risk factors for asthma and their interaction with environmental exposures are still poorly understood, and further studies are needed to identify susceptibility genes and the implications for racial/ethnic disparities in asthma.

Environmental and Lifestyle Factors

Socioeconomic Status

In the United States, ethnicity and race are strongly correlated to socioeconomic status (SES). African Americans and Hispanics are disproportionately affected by poverty, which has been shown to increase the rate of asthma [32, 33]. The effect of SES on asthma is likely mediated by multiple factors operating on individual and community levels such as environmental exposures, access to health care, psychosocial stress, and exposure to violence. However, different racial/ethnic groups have a widely divergent burden from asthma (Table 3.1) [33, 34]. Among children in California, African American children had 23% greater odds of asthma with each decrease in the SES index (derived from maternal educational attainment level, annual household income, and insurance status). Conversely, Mexican American children had 17% reduced odds of asthma with each decrease in the SES index [35]. In a study of Keet et al., household poverty increased the risk of asthma among non-Hispanic Blacks and Whites as well as Puerto Ricans but not among other Hispanics [7]. However, in a larger study with data on 1.5 million Medicaid-insured children, residence in poor neighborhoods among this low-income population was associated with more asthma-related ED visits and hospitalizations regardless of Hispanic status [36]. It is likely that racial/ethnic disparity in asthma arises from complex interactions between multiple risk factors related to SES and individual susceptibility.

Table 3.1 Asthma susceptibility factors in racial/ethnic minorities

Asthma susceptibility factors in racial/ethnic minorities	
Genetic predisposition	African ancestry Reduced bronchodilator response Epigenetic changes
Environmental and lifestyle factors	Inner-city residence Poor housing quality Indoor allergens Ambient air pollution Tobacco smoke Vitamin D deficiency Obesity Place of birth in the United States
Health-care access and management	Inadequate health insurance Lack of regular source of care Low health literacy Language barriers Undocumented immigration status Cultural influence on disease perception Lower use of controller medication
Psychosocial factors	Low socioeconomic status Exposure to psychological stress, discrimination, and violence

Inner-City Residence

Using data from the National Health Interview Survey (NHIS), 2009–2011, that included 23,065 children, Keet et al. found that the prevalence of current asthma was 12.9% in inner-city and 10.6% in non-inner-city areas. However, this difference was no longer significant after adjusting for confounders. Black race and Puerto Rican ethnicity were strong independent risk factors for asthma exacerbation and emergency room visits for asthma in this study [7]. Among children enrolled in Medicaid between 2009 and 2010, Keet et al. showed that living in inner-city areas does not increase asthma prevalence; however, it is significantly associated with asthma morbidity with higher asthma-related ED visits and hospitalizations. The increase in asthma morbidity in poor and urban areas is likely to be caused by multiple mechanisms including psychosocial stress and violence, ambient air pollution, housing conditions, and exposure to indoor allergens as well as possible barriers to health care in poor neighborhoods [36].

Psychosocial Stress and Violence

In the United States, racial/ethnic minorities are disproportionally affected by psychosocial stressors such as physical and sexual abuse, violence, and discrimination [31, 37–39]. These have been linked to asthma morbidity [40]. Among minority youths, experiencing discrimination was associated with greater odds of asthma and poor asthma control in African Americans [41]. Exposure to community violence is associated with a higher rate of asthma symptoms, hospitalizations, and ED visits [42, 43]. By following 28,456 African American women over the course of 16 years, Coogan et al. found a positive association between adult-onset asthma and childhood physical abuse among this group [44].

Parental stress and physical and sexual abuse were implicated in the development of asthma among Puerto Ricans [31, 45]. In school-aged Puerto Rican children, physical or sexual abuse was associated with almost twofold increase in odds of developing asthma as well as asthma morbidity [46]. The underlying mechanisms are unclear but might include a dysfunction of the hypothalamic-pituitary-adrenal axis, cortisol insensitivity, or production of inflammatory cytokines [47, 48]. Constituting a potential epigenetic factor, the exposure to violence was associated with DNA methylation of the *ADCYAP1R1* gene locus in Puerto Rican children, in whom such methylation changes were correlated with increased asthma. *ADCYAP1R1* was suggested to play a role in regulating expression of the glucocorticoid receptor gene [31, 49].

Ambient Air Pollution

Air pollution contributes to asthma mortality. In 2010, about 4% of the US population lived within 150 m of a major road and were exposed to traffic-related pollution. The proportion of non-Hispanic Blacks (4.4%) and Hispanics (5%) living near a major road is higher than that of non-Hispanic Whites (3.1%). Exposure to traffic-related pollution is also related to being born outside of the United States, speaking Spanish, and poverty [50]. In a study that included Hispanic and African American children from the US mainland and Puerto Rico, exposure to NO_2, a traffic-related air pollutant, in the first year of life was associated with greater odds for asthma [51]. A nationwide assessment of 100,000 schools found that those schools with predominantly Black students (>50%) were 18% (95% CI, 13–23%) more likely to be located within 250 m of a major roadway compared to schools with more heterogeneous student populations [52]. A possible detrimental synergistic effect exists between psychosocial stress and susceptibility to air pollution in asthma [53]. A retrospective cohort study among 413 children in Boston showed an elevated risk for asthma with increased NO_2 exposure for those subjects exposed to above-median violence as compared to those exposed to below-median violence [54]. Furthermore, traffic-related air pollution has been linked to allergic sensitization. Among 170 asthmatic children from Fresno, California, in utero exposure to 8-hour daily CO was associated with increased risk of sensitization to at least one outdoor allergen [55].

Housing Quality and Indoor Allergens

In 2011, a survey comprising 33,201 American households with children aged 6–17 years showed that non-Hispanic Black heads of household have higher odds of having a child diagnosed with asthma in comparison to non-Hispanic White heads of household (OR 1.72, 95% CI 1.50–1.96). Poor housing quality was associated with asthma diagnosis (adjusted OR 1.45, 95% CI 1.28–1.66) [6]. Certain housing types confer an elevated risk of asthma in urban areas. Among 5250 children living in New York City, the reported prevalence of current asthma was highest in public housing residents (21.8%) as compared to residents of private family dwellings (7.38%). Those living in public housing reported a much higher presence of cockroaches than residents of private family dwellings (68.7% vs. 21%). Minority children, especially African Americans and Puerto Ricans, and children from low-income households made up greater proportions of public housing residents compared to Whites and Asians [56]. In another study in Baltimore, mouse allergens as measured by mouse-specific IgE levels in children with asthma were associated with poor asthma outcomes, but cockroach sensitization was not [57]. Sun et al. found dampness (mold, floor moisture, water leakage) and living in small dwellings/mobile homes to be a risk factor for asthma among children in Northeastern **Texas,** with higher rates of asthma among African American children **as** compared to Mexican American and white children. This study also reported a higher rate of asthma among African American children compared to Mexican American and White children [58]. These studies underline the significance of poor housing quality and possibly indoor allergens such as cockroach and mice that disproportionally affect racial and ethnical minorities.

Environmental Tobacco Smoke

In 2016, 15.5% of US adults smoked cigarettes. Smoking rates vary widely among racial/ethnic groups with American Indians and Alaska Natives having the highest rates of 31.8%, followed by non-Hispanic Whites and African Americans with rates around 16%, Hispanics with rate of 10.7%, and Asians with rate of 9%. Among Hispanics, Puerto Ricans have higher rates of tobacco use than Mexican Americans. Smoking is also more prevalent for individuals living below the poverty line [59]. Among 3766 Northeast Texan children, exposure to tobacco smoke was strongly correlated with asthma and allergy. African American children were more often exposed to tobacco smoke (31.3%) than non-Hispanic White children (20.8%) [58]. Children exposed to tobacco smoke in utero have a higher risk of developing asthma and of having reduced lung function [60] In utero tobacco exposure has been shown to be associated with poor asthma control in Black and Hispanic children 8–17 years of age [61].

Vitamin D Deficiency

Vitamin D is an essential nutrient with immunomodulatory effects. Vitamin D deficiency shares common risk factors with asthma such as urban residence, obesity, and African American race. This has sparked interest in exploring the common link between these two conditions [62]. The prevalence of vitamin D deficiency shows large racial/ethnic differences. Using a cutoff of <30 ng/mL of 25(OH)D, the prevalence of vitamin D deficiency was higher in non-Hispanic Blacks (97%) and Mexican Americans (90%) compared to non-Hispanic Whites (71%) in a study published in 2004 [63]. A small case-control study in Washington DC among 106 African Americans 6–20 years of age found that vitamin D deficiency (<30 ng/mL) was associated with markedly higher odds of asthma (OR 42, 95% CI 4.4–399) [64]. Among 287 children with asthma in Puerto Rico, the odds of a severe asthma exacerbation was higher among children with a vitamin D level <30 ng/mL. The effect was greater in nonatopic children (OR 6.2, 95% CI 2–21.6) than in atopic children (OR 2.0, 95% CI 1–4.1) [65]. This suggests a possible role of nonatopic mechanisms. It was hypothesized that the protective effect of vitamin D is mediated by antiviral properties, better steroid responsiveness, or lung development in utero [62].

Obesity

In 2016, the prevalence of obesity in the United States among adults was 39.8%. The rate of obesity is significantly higher in Hispanics (47.0%) and non-Hispanic Blacks (46.8%) compared to non-Hispanic Whites (37.9%), and it is lowest in Asians (12.7%) [66]. Obesity is associated with asthma prevalence and asthma morbidity with higher rates of asthma-related ED visits, hospitalizations, worse symptom control, and higher need of controller medications [67–69].

In a study including African American and Hispanic children and adolescents, the effect of obesity on asthma control varied with race/ethnicity and gender. In boys, obesity was associated with poor asthma control, regardless of ethnicity. Among girls, however, obese African Americans were more likely to have better controlled asthma compared to nonobese (OR 0.65, 95% CI 0.41–1.05), while Mexican American girls had a 1.91 (95% CI 1.12–3.28) greater odds of worse asthma control [70]. In a study that included Puerto Rican children, increased body mass index (BMI), percent body fat, and waist circumference were associated with increased odds of asthma [71]. Akinbami et al. in contrast found most of the racial/ethnic disparity in asthma prevalence unexplained by weight status. Using NHANES data, from 1988–1994 to 2011–2014, he found that asthma prevalence increased more among non-Hispanic Black (8.4–18.0%) than in non-Hispanic White individuals (7.2–10.3%) aged 2–19 years. Obesity was a risk factor for asthma in all groups, and weight status did not modify the race/ethnicity association with asthma over time [72]. Although there is mounting evidence that obesity increases asthma risk in general, its effect in different racial/ethnic minorities is still controversial, and further studies are needed.

Nativity Effect

The risk of asthma might depend on the place of birth and time of residence in the United States. In Hispanics of Mexican origin, a nativity effect has been observed. Using data from NHANES III and NHIS, Holguin et al. found that US-born Mexican

Americans had higher rates of asthma compared to Mexican-born Mexican Americans. Interestingly, prolonged time of residence in the United States increased the prevalence of asthma in Mexican-born participants from 2% to 4% after 10 years [73]. This suggests that cumulative environmental exposures or lifestyle changes after immigration to the United States might constitute risk factors for developing asthma. The majority of immigration from Mexico is derived from rural areas to urban areas in the United States. In NHANES III and NHIS, those born in Mexico and those who lived in urban environments in the United States amounted to 68% and 55% of participants, respectively. The observed nativity effect and increase of asthma prevalence with prolonged residence in the United States might be due to risk factors encountered in urban areas such as ambient air pollution. The authors propose a protective role of higher rates of childhood infections in rural areas in Mexico that might confer an immunologic response, which fades over time [73].

A possible confounder may be a higher rate of asthma diagnoses due to better health-care access with longer residence in the United States. In NHANES III, 54% of Mexican-born participants with more than 10 years of residence in the United States had a regular source for health care compared with 46% of those residing fewer than 10 years in the United States. Additionally, for Mexican-born Mexican Americans, refraining from seeking health care due to their legal status might restrict health-care access [73]. However, Eldeirawi et al. found that the higher risk of asthma associated with being born in the United States persisted for Mexican American children after controlling for a regular place for health care [74]. Among Mexican Americans, higher rates of asthma and wheezing have also been associated with the degree of acculturation in the US and with an increase of obesity after immigration. In those with more than 10 years of residence in the United States, a BMI of 30 or greater was observed in 26% vs. 17% in those who resided fewer than 10 years in the United States. This increase in obesity might contribute to the higher asthma prevalence in this population [75]. Further prospective studies are needed to assess the temporal nature between asthma and place of birth.

Diagnosis and Management

Health-Care Access

Difficulties in health-care access contribute to disparities in allergic diseases, including asthma, in racial/ethnic minorities. Risk factors might include avoiding seeing a doctor regularly for asthma care for economic reasons [5], difficulties in disease management due to language barriers [76], and low health literacy [77]. Cultural influences on disease perception, lower trust in controller medication [78], and possibly, in health-care providers themselves [79, 80] might be contributory. Having less access to regular care may lead to different health-care utilization patterns with higher rates of ED visits and hospitalizations [5]. Among racial and ethnic minorities, undocumented immigrants in particular face challenges when accessing health care [81].

Language Barriers and Health Literacy

Language barriers contribute to a lower health-care access. In a survey among 1847 Hispanic children with asthma in New York City, those living in Spanish-speaking families were twice as likely to be hospitalized for asthma (9.4% vs. 4.4%, $P < 0.02$) than children in English-speaking families. Spanish-speaking households were more likely to be publicly insured, and parents were less likely to have communicated with their child's physician about recommended components of an asthma management plan, such as the use of rescue medication during an asthma attack and when to visit the ED [76]. In two inner-city clinics in East Harlem, limited English proficiency was associated with poorer asthma control, increased resource utilization, and lower quality of life scores. It resulted in lower self-efficacy, greater worries about asthma, and lower adherence to controller medication [82].

Inadequate health literacy and numeracy, and the mathematical knowledge required to understand instructions of health-care providers, have been shown to be risk factors for minority children. Among Puerto Rican children, low parental numeracy was associated with increased odds of ED visits for asthma (adjusted OR 1.7, 95% CI 1.03–2.7), and among those children not using inhaled corticosteroids, hospitalization rates were significantly higher with low parental numeracy [77]. It has been shown that some Mexican American parents of children with asthma face difficulties in understanding common Spanish words used in clinical settings to identify asthma, such as wheezing (sibilancia), and prefer using direct visualizations and sounds to describe symptoms [83]. A study of Shone et al. showed that among parents of children with asthma in Rochester, NY, low health literacy was associated with worry about their children's health and with a greater perceived asthma burden [84].

Perception of Asthma

Subjective perception of disease may vary by race/ethnicity [78]. In a study including 739 participants, parents of Black and Hispanic children had lower expectations for their child's asthma and worried more about their child's condition compared to Whites. Parents of Hispanic children had higher levels of concern about medications for asthma [78]. Furthermore, the subjective perception of lung function has been shown to differ between non-Hispanic White and Hispanic school-aged children. Perceptual accuracy of peak flow measurements was higher among non-Hispanic White children than in Hispanic children in Rhode Island, and for both groups, the accuracy was higher than for children living in Puerto Rico. Lower perceptual accuracy of lung function was associated with higher asthma morbidity and health-care use for asthma [85]. The culturally influenced perception that patients and their caretakers may have about asthma, including self-management and medication use, must be taken into account by health-care providers to communicate effectively.

Use of Controller Medication

The use of controller medication for asthma is lower among racial/ethnic minorities [86, 87]. Using data on 2499 children with asthma, a cross-sectional analysis for the periods 1988–2008 has shown lower use of preventive asthma medication among non-Hispanic Black (adjusted OR 0.5, 95% CI 0.4–0.7) and Mexican American children (adjusted OR 0.6, 95% CI 0.4–0.9) compared to non-Hispanic White children [86]. The reason for this disparity is not well understood. However, potential contributing factors are prescription patterns by health-care providers [88] as well as patient-driven factors such as cultural beliefs [78], patient preferences, and economic factors that influence the affordability of medication and routine doctor visits [5].

In a study that included Puerto Rican children with moderate to severe asthma, only 17% had used controller medications in the previous month [89]. Hispanic children from Rhode Island showed lower levels of adherence to controller medication than non-Hispanic White children. This was also the case for Hispanic children in Puerto Rico. Adherence was associated with parental belief regarding medication necessity and family routines around medications [90]. Furthermore, prescription patterns of controller medication by health-care providers may play a role. Disparities in dispensing asthma medication have been shown based on type of insurance coverage. Among 41,308 children with asthma, privately insured families were dispensed significantly more controller medication (48.3% vs. 12.0%) than publicly insured families. The differences were pronounced for inhaled corticosteroids (24.4% vs. 6.7%) as well as leukotriene modifiers and inhaled cromolyn (31.4% vs. 5.7%) [88].

Ethnic differences in response to controller medication have been proposed on the basis of pharmacogenetic differences between Mexican Americans and Puerto Ricans [91]. Susceptibility on the individual level interacts with environmental risk factors. One such factor is chronic stress, which has been associated with reduced expression of the β2-adrenergic receptor [47]. Among Puerto Rican children with asthma, high perceived stress has been shown to be associated with reduced bronchodilator response [92]. Further gene variations might contribute to differences in response to bronchodilators among Hispanics, but confirmatory studies are needed [91–93].

Health-Care Utilization

Racial and ethnic minorities have different health-care utilization patterns. Hispanics, especially undocumented immigrants and those not proficient in English, have been shown to be less likely to have a regular source of care [94, 95]. In a national survey, Spanish-speaking Hispanics were nearly three times as likely as Whites to report that their child did not have a usual source of care (OR 2.71, $P = 0.020$) [96].

Among minorities, alternative sources of health care are more utilized for asthma. Black and Hispanic children visit emergency departments for asthma care more often than White children [5]. Using data from Medicaid claims in 14 southern states, Malhotra et al. found a higher asthma prevalence and ED visit rate for Black compared to White children. However, when analyzing different counties, he found extensive geographic differences for both asthma prevalence and ED visit rates between Black and White children. The Black-White rate ratios of ED visits ranged from 0.25 in a county in Louisiana to 25.28 in a county in Kentucky. Of 556 counties included in the study, 68 showed ED visit rate ratios consistent with no racial disparities [97]. Keet et al. found higher odds of ED visits for asthma in Black as compared to White children (OR 3.02, 95% CI 2.29–3.99) [6]. In another study, Keet et al. analyzed data on 16,860,716 children aged 5–19 who were enrolled in Medicaid. Residence in inner-city areas and non-Hispanic Black race/ethnicity were associated with increased risk of ED visits and hospitalizations due to asthma. In contrast, Asian children had significantly fewer ED visits and hospitalizations than non-Hispanic White children [36].

Atopic Dermatitis/Eczema

Atopic dermatitis affects around 25% of children and 2–3% of adults [98]. Common comorbidities include food allergies, asthma, and allergic rhinitis. African Americans are disproportionally affected by atopic dermatitis [10]. Mahdavinia et al. found higher odds of having atopic dermatitis in African American and Hispanic children compared to White children. African American children had higher odds for eczema compared with both groups [9]. Risk factors for developing atopic dermatitis include a positive family history for atopy and a loss-of-function mutation in the filaggrin gene, and it has been associated with higher parental education [98]. No clear environmental exposure has been conclusively identified, although living in urban areas appears to increase the risk [99], while exposure to exotoxins, farm animals, and dogs may be protective [98]. Among children in Northeast Texas, a residential location in an urban area was a risk factor for eczema. In this study, African Americans had a significantly higher prevalence of eczema compared to Whites or Mexican Americans [58].

Wegienka et al. followed a cohort of African American and White children in the Detroit Metropolitan area in the first 2 years of life. In this cohort, atopic dermatitis was more common among African American than in White children (27.0% vs. 13.5%). African Americans also had higher total IgE levels and were more likely to have at least one positive skin prick test or positive serum-specific IgE (sIgE). These findings suggest that disparities in allergic diseases already exist at the age of 2 and are possibly related to exposures early in life [100]. Fischer et al. found different health-care utilization patterns for eczema care between non-Hispanic Black and White children in 2-year longitudinal cohorts. Non-Hispanic Blacks were less likely than Whites to report an ambulatory visit for eczema (adjusted OR 0.69, 95% CI 0.51–0.92). However, among those with ≥1 ambulatory visit for eczema, non-Hispanic Blacks reported more visits and prescriptions than Whites. Thus, despite reporting fewer ambulatory visits, the utilization pattern in Blacks suggested more severe disease. For Hispanic children, a similar trend was observed, but it was not statistically significant [101].

Janumpally et al. found that compared to Whites, Asians/Pacific Islanders were even more likely (OR 6.7, CI 4.8–9.5, $P < 0.001$) than African Americans (OR 3.4, CI 2.5–4.7, $P < 0.001$) to seek medical care for atopic dermatitis [102]. There is a paucity of literature on atopic dermatitis in Asian Americans despite the seemingly high prevalence of this condition. More research is needed to understand the observed disparity in eczema prevalence in this group.

Food Allergy and Anaphylaxis

The estimated prevalence of food allergy in the United States is 8.96% overall and 6.53% among children. In childhood, the most common allergies are to milk (1.94%), peanut (1.16%), and shellfish (0.87%), followed by egg (0.64%), tree nuts (0.52%), fish (0.43%), wheat (0.29%), corn (0.28%), and soy (0.25%) [103]. African Americans are at increased risk of likely/possible food allergy compared to Whites [103, 104].

When analyzing data from the CDC for the period 1988–2011, Keet et al. found an overall increase of food allergy prevalence of 1.2% per decade. However, the rate of increase varied by race/ethnicity. The estimated increase in food allergy prevalence per decade among Black children was 2.1% (95% CI 1.5–2.7%) compared to 1.2% (95% CI 0.7–1.7%) among Hispanics and 1.0% (95% CI 0.4–1.6%) among Whites. Until the late 2000s, Blacks reported food allergy with the same or lower frequency than Whites, with more frequent reporting in general and as compared to Whites thereafter [105]. Interestingly, in NHANES 2005–2006, sensitization to food allergens based on sIgE levels was 8.4% among Black children, compared to 2.5% among White and 4.2% among Hispanic children [104]. In NHIS, self-reported food allergy prevalence was 3.9–4.6% among Blacks, 4.3–4.8% among Whites, and 2.5–3.1% among Hispanics. Although there seems to be a predisposition based on sIgE levels, the lower self-reported prevalence might reflect lower recognition of food allergy in Blacks before the late 2000s or biologic differences in the correlation of sIgE with clinical symptoms in different racial/ethnic groups [105].

Within a cohort of 817 children in 2 urban tertiary care centers in the United States, Mahdavinia et al. showed that African American and Hispanic children had higher rates of food allergy-associated anaphylaxis and emergency department visits compared to White children. African American children had higher odds ratios of having allergy to wheat, soy, corn, fish, and shellfish. The rates of peanut, milk, and egg allergy were similar with lower rates of tree nut allergy as compared to White children. Hispanic children had higher odds of allergy to corn, fish, and shellfish [9]. In this study, minority children were more likely to have Medicaid insurance and were lost to follow-up at earlier ages, possibly a reflection of difficulties in access to health care. The authors hypothesized that the observed racial/ethnic variation in food allergen profiles may be due to differences in food introduction practices as well as differences in diets. Taveras et al. found that in African American and Hispanic infants, solid foods were more often introduced before 4 months of age (34% and 41%) as compared to White infants (13%). Additionally, exclusive breastfeeding at 6 months of age was significantly lower in African American and Hispanic infants [106]. Likewise, allergenic foods such as cow's milk, egg, fish, and peanut were introduced at an earlier age in a largely African American, urban, Medicaid-based population in Ohio than in a predominantly White suburban privately insured population [107]. In contrast to the assumption that early food introduction increases the rate of food allergy, the authors of the Learning Early About Peanut (LEAP) study, which included 640 children between the ages of 4 and 11 months, found a protective effect of peanut consumption during infancy. Of the children avoiding peanuts, 17.2% developed peanut allergy by the age of 5 years, while this was the case in only 3.2% of the children consuming peanuts [108].

Additionally, Mahdavinia et al. found higher rates of wheat allergy among African American children compared to White children. Eliminating wheat products completely can be a significant financial burden for low-income families, raising the risk for accidental exposures for allergic children. The higher rates of wheat allergy might thus contribute to higher rates of anaphylaxis and ED visits among African Americans. Rates of corn allergy are higher in children of Hispanic ethnicity than in White children. Thus, similar difficulties in eliminating corn-based products in families of Mexican origin might result in higher allergen exposure to corn-allergic children [9]. Further studies correlating food ingestion at the time of the food-related reaction are needed to confirm these hypotheses. Interestingly, the observed elevated rates of shellfish allergy among African Americans and Hispanics seen by Mahdavinia et al. might be contributed to tropomyosins from cockroach and HDM allergens. African American and Hispanic children in inner-city areas are exposed to higher levels of HDM and cockroach allergens [109, 110], which have both been proposed to function as a sensitizer to shellfish due to a high degree of homology [9, 111, 112].

In the period from 1999 to 2010, Jerchow et al. found 6.7% of all anaphylaxis-related deaths in the United States to be caused by food allergies. African Americans were most commonly affected with rates of 0.09 (95% CI 0.07–0.12) per million cases compared to 0.04 (95% CI 0.03–0.05) per million in Whites and 0.02 (95% CI 0.01–0.03) per million in Hispanics. African Americans showed the largest increase in anaphylaxis-related deaths due to food allergy over time. Except for venom-induced anaphylaxis, African Americans were more likely to die from all causes of anaphylaxis, including medication-related anaphylaxis, which accounts for the majority (58.8%) of anaphylaxis-related deaths [8].

In summary, racial/ethnic disparities in food allergy are increasing over time with higher rates of anaphylaxis among African Americans. Risk factors may include individual genetic predisposition, early food introduction practices with diet-specific sensitization patterns, exposure to indoor allergens, and differences in health-care access and utilization patterns.

Allergic Rhinitis/Hay Fever

According to data from the NHIS, allergic rhinitis (AR) was diagnosed in 19.9 million adults and 5.6 million children as of 2017. In adults, the prevalence of AR was highest among Whites (8.2%), followed by Asians (7.1%), and lowest in Blacks (4.8%). For children, the prevalence was found to be similar in Whites, lower in Asians (6.2%), and slightly higher in Blacks (5.3%) [113]. A study including 173,659 individuals in northern California found a higher risk in Asians compared to Whites. Chen et al. found strongly elevated odds for hay fever for Asians compared to Whites, with 1.5-fold excess odds for women and twofold excess odds for men. Also, Asian men had a 30% increased odds of asthma with AR as compared to White men. The prevalence of AR in Blacks did not differ significantly from that in Whites. In this study, birthplace outside of the United States was associated with a decreased risk of asthma and AR [114].

Allergic rhinitis is an independent risk factor for the development of asthma. Approximately 38% of patients with AR have asthma and up to 78% of asthma patients have AR [115]. Additionally, AR may function as a mediator for other risk factors related to asthma. A study among Puerto Rican children found that AR together with other markers of atopy such as skin test reactivity to cockroach significantly mediated the association between obesity and risk of asthma [71]. Further studies are needed to investigate the observed disparities in AR, especially among Asian Americans, and to quantify comorbidities such as asthma in different racial/ethnic groups.

Interventions to Address Racial and Ethnic Disparities in Allergic Diseases in the United States

Addressing disparities in allergic diseases between racial and ethnic groups will require a multifactorial approach at the levels of public health policy, health-care providers, and individuals. Interventions should be aimed at decreasing risk factors that disproportionally affect racial/ethnic minorities. These include campaigns to reduce air pollution in inner-city areas, control indoor allergen exposure, promote smoking cessation, and prevent violence in neighborhoods. Comorbidities should be treated such as obesity, PTSD, and depression. Health-care providers should aim to remove barriers to care by taking the patient's language fluency and health literacy into account. To foster adherence, health-care providers should inquire about cultural beliefs and fears related to management, such as concerns about use of controller medication for asthma [90]. Intervention programs that are culturally adapted to racial/ethnic minorities have shown to be beneficial.

To address health literacy among minority children, a longitudinal intervention program in Los Angeles taught asthma self-management skills to 110 minority children in a weekly Saturday school format. The intervention resulted in a significant decrease in ED visits through higher self-efficacy and improvement in reading ability, while a reduction in hospitalizations was associated with higher self-efficacy but not with improved reading ability [116]. Another asthma management intervention addressed low-income Puerto Rican families with culturally specific educational home visits. Children in families receiving the intervention were less likely to visit the ED or to be hospitalized for asthma compared to a control group. Also, caregivers reported feeling less helpless and frustrated with their children's asthma [117].

In an observational study, a culturally adapted 12-month intervention was conducted among children with asthma in two housing projects in Puerto Rico. Through home visits, community workers educated patients and caretakers about the reduction of allergen exposure including cockroach allergens and fostered the adherence to controller medication. After a 1-year follow-up period, asthma-related hospitalizations and ED visits were significantly reduced, and parents reported improved symptom control [89]. The study design was adapted from earlier home-based environmental interventions [118, 119] such as the Inner-City Asthma Study (ICAS), a randomized-controlled trial that included predominantly Black and Hispanic children with atopic asthma in seven US cities. Compared to the control group, those who received regular home visits with education about exposure to indoor allergens such as cockroach and house dust mites showed better symptom control of their asthma during the intervention year (3.39 vs. 4.20 days, $P < 0.001$) and the year after (2.62 vs. 3.21 days, $P < 0.001$). Further randomized-controlled trials are needed to identify the effectiveness of culturally adapted interventions in racial and ethnic minority groups [119].

While ancestral genetic factors may contribute to an increase in risk for allergic diseases for racial and ethnic minorities, the current disease burden is likely caused by interactions between individual predisposition and environmental exposures, psychosocial stressors, and comorbidities. Barriers to health care intensify the impact on health outcomes. The distribution of these factors is linked to historical and current structural discrimination. To understand health disparities in allergic diseases, the impact of structural discrimination on health should be further investigated. The complex interaction between environmental exposures and individual susceptibility on a genetic and epigenetic level will be of interest in future studies. Lastly, a focus on culturally competent interventions to decrease detrimental environmental exposures and improve health-care access and health management in racial and ethnic minorities will be crucial.

References

1. Vespa J, Armstrong DM [Internet]. Washington, DC: Demographic turning points for the United States: population projections for 2020 to 2060: United States Census Bureau. 2018 [cited 2019 Jan 10]. Available from: https://www.census.gov/content/dam/Census/library/publications/2018/demo/P25_1144.pdf.
2. Office of Management and Budget [Internet]. Washington, DC: Revisions to the standards for the classification of federal data on race and ethnicity. Federal Register Notice. 1997 [cited

2019 Dec 30]. Available from: https://www.whitehouse.gov/wp-content/uploads/2017/11/Revisions-to-the-Standards-for-the-Classification-of-Federal-Data-on-Race-and-Ethnicity-October30-1997.pdf.

3. CDC [Internet]. Washington, DC: Measures to identify and track racial disparities in childhood asthma: Asthma Disparities Workgroup Subcommittee Recommendations. 2016 [cited 2018 Dec 20]. Available from: https://www.cdc.gov/asthma/pdfs/Racial_Disparities_in_Childhood_Asthma.pdf.

4. CDC [Internet]. Washington, DC: Gateway to health communication and social marketing practice. Allergies. 2017 [cited 2019 Jan 10] Aviailable from: https://www.cdc.gov/health-communication/toolstemplates/entertainmented/tips/Allergies.html.

5. CDC [Internet]. Washington, DC: Asthma's impact on the nation. 2016 [cited 2019 Jan 3]. Available from: https://www.cdc.gov/asthma/impacts_nation/asthmafactsheet.pdf.

6. Hughes HK, Matsui EC, Tschudy MM, Pollack CE, Keet CA. Pediatric asthma health disparities: race, hardship, housing, and asthma in a national survey. Acad Pediatr. 2017;17(2):127–34.

7. Keet CA, McCormack MC, Pollack CE, Peng RD, McGowan E, Matsui EC. Neighborhood poverty, urban residence, race/ethnicity, and asthma: rethinking the inner-city asthma epidemic. J Allergy Clin Immunol. 2015;135(3):655–62.

8. Jerschow E, Lin RY, Scaperotti MM, McGinn AP. Fatal anaphylaxis in the United States, 1999–2010: temporal patterns and demographic associations. J Allergy Clin Immunol. 2014;134(6):1318–28. e7

9. Mahdavinia M, Fox SR, Smith BM, James C, Palmisano EL, Mohammed A, et al. Racial differences in food allergy phenotype and health care utilization among US children. J Allergy Clin Immunol Pract. 2017;5(2):352–7 e1.

10. Shaw TE, Currie GP, Koudelka CW, Simpson EL. Eczema prevalence in the United States: data from the 2003 National Survey of Children's Health. J Invest Dermatol. 2011;131(1):67–73.

11. CDC [Internet]. Washington, DC: Most recent asthma data. 2016 [cited 2019 Jan 17]. Available from: https://www.cdc.gov/asthma/most_recent_data.htm [Internet].

12. Moorman JE, Akinbami LJ, Bailey CM, Zahran HS, King ME, Johnson CA, et al. National surveillance of asthma: United States, 2001–2010. National Center for Health Statistics. Vital Health Stat 3 Anal Epidemiol Stud. 2012;(35):1–58.

13. Center for Puerto Rican Studies [Internet]. New York City: Datasheet. Puerto Ricans keep on growing! 2018 [cited 2019 Jan 19]. Available from: https://centropr.hunter.cuny.edu/sites/default/files/data_sheets/DS2018-08_DATASHEET_2017ACS_1YR.pdf.

14. Center for Puerto Rican Studies [Internet]. New York City: Puerto Ricans in the United States: 2010–2016. 2018 [cited 2019 Jan 19]. Available from: https://centropr.hunter.cuny.edu/sites/default/files/PDF/National_Report_2018_march.pdf.

15. United States Census Bureau [Internet]. Washington, DC: QuickFacts Puerto Rico. 2018 [cited 2019 Jan 19]. Available from: https://www.census.gov/quickfacts/fact/table/pr/PST045218#PST045218 [Internet].

16. Szentpetery SE, Forno E, Canino G, Celedon JC. Asthma in Puerto Ricans: lessons from a high-risk population. J Allergy Clin Immunol. 2016;138(6):1556–8.

17. Rosser FJ, Forno E, Cooper PJ, Celedon JC. Asthma in Hispanics. An 8-year update. Am J Respir Crit Care Med. 2014;189(11):1316–27.

18. Pino-Yanes M, Thakur N, Gignoux CR, Galanter JM, Roth LA, Eng C, et al. Genetic ancestry influences asthma susceptibility and lung function among Latinos. J Allergy Clin Immunol. 2015;135(1):228–35.

19. Salari K, Choudhry S, Tang H, Naqvi M, Lind D, Avila PC, et al. Genetic admixture and asthma-related phenotypes in Mexican American and Puerto Rican asthmatics. Genet Epidemiol. 2005;29(1):76–86.

20. Flores C, Ma SF, Pino-Yanes M, Wade MS, Perez-Mendez L, Kittles RA, et al. African ancestry is associated with asthma risk in African Americans. PLoS One. 2012;7(1):e26807.

21. Brehm JM, Acosta-Perez E, Klei L, Roeder K, Barmada MM, Boutaoui N, et al. African ancestry and lung function in Puerto Rican children. J Allergy Clin Immunol. 2012;129(6):1484–90 e6.
22. Rumpel JA, Ahmedani BK, Peterson EL, Wells KE, Yang M, Levin AM, et al. Genetic ancestry and its association with asthma exacerbations among African American subjects with asthma. J Allergy Clin Immunol. 2012;130(6):1302–6.
23. Galanter JM, Torgerson D, Gignoux CR, Sen S, Roth LA, Via M, et al. Cosmopolitan and ethnic-specific replication of genetic risk factors for asthma in 2 Latino populations. J Allergy Clin Immunol. 2011;128(1):37–43 e12.
24. Galanter J, Choudhry S, Eng C, Nazario S, Rodriguez-Santana JR, Casal J, et al. ORMDL3 gene is associated with asthma in three ethnically diverse populations. Am J Respir Crit Care Med. 2008;177(11):1194–200.
25. Torgerson DG, Ampleford EJ, Chiu GY, Gauderman WJ, Gignoux CR, Graves PE, et al. Meta-analysis of genome-wide association studies of asthma in ethnically diverse North American populations. Nat Genet. 2011;43(9):887–92.
26. Mathias RA, Grant AV, Rafaels N, Hand T, Gao L, Vergara C, et al. A genome-wide association study on African-ancestry populations for asthma. J Allergy Clin Immunol. 2010;125(2):336–46 e4.
27. Galanter JM, Gignoux CR, Torgerson DG, Roth LA, Eng C, Oh SS, et al. Genome-wide association study and admixture mapping identify different asthma-associated loci in Latinos: the Genes-environments & admixture in Latino Americans study. J Allergy Clin Immunol. 2014;134(2):295–305.
28. Torgerson DG, Gignoux CR, Galanter JM, Drake KA, Roth LA, Eng C, et al. Case-control admixture mapping in Latino populations enriches for known asthma-associated genes. J Allergy Clin Immunol. 2012;130(1):76–82 e12.
29. Yang IV, Pedersen BS, Liu A, O'Connor GT, Teach SJ, Kattan M, et al. DNA methylation and childhood asthma in the inner city. J Allergy Clin Immunol. 2015;136(1):69–80.
30. Chan MA, Ciaccio CE, Gigliotti NM, Rezaiekhaligh M, Siedlik JA, Kennedy K, et al. DNA methylation levels associated with race and childhood asthma severity. J Asthma. 2017;54(8):825–32.
31. Rosenberg SL, Miller GE, Brehm JM, Celedon JC. Stress and asthma: novel insights on genetic, epigenetic, and immunologic mechanisms. J Allergy Clin Immunol. 2014;134(5):1009–15.
32. Ramsey CD, Celedon JC, Sredl DL, Weiss ST, Cloutier MM. Predictors of disease severity in children with asthma in Hartford, Connecticut. Pediatr Pulmonol. 2005;39(3):268–75.
33. Forno E, Celedon JC. Asthma and ethnic minorities: socioeconomic status and beyond. Curr Opin Allergy Clin Immunol. 2009;9(2):154–60.
34. Forno E, Celedon JC. Health disparities in asthma. Am J Respir Crit Care Med. 2012;185(10):1033–5.
35. Thakur N, Oh SS, Nguyen EA, Martin M, Roth LA, Galanter J, et al. Socioeconomic status and childhood asthma in urban minority youths. The GALA II and SAGE II studies. Am J Respir Crit Care Med. 2013;188(10):1202–9.
36. Keet CA, Matsui EC, McCormack MC, Peng RD. Urban residence, neighborhood poverty, race/ethnicity, and asthma morbidity among children on Medicaid. J Allergy Clin Immunol. 2017;140(3):822–7.
37. Matthews KA, Gallo LC. Psychological perspectives on pathways linking socioeconomic status and physical health. Annu Rev Psychol. 2011;62:501–30.
38. Torres JM, Wallace SP. Migration circumstances, psychological distress, and self-rated physical health for Latino immigrants in the United States. Am J Public Health. 2013;103(9):1619–27.
39. Byrd DR. Race/ethnicity and self-reported levels of discrimination and psychological distress, California, 2005. Prev Chronic Dis. 2012;9:E156.
40. Yonas MA, Lange NE, Celedon JC. Psychosocial stress and asthma morbidity. Curr Opin Allergy Clin Immunol. 2012;12(2):202–10.

41. Thakur N, Barcelo NE, Borrell LN, Singh S, Eng C, Davis A, et al. Perceived discrimination associated with asthma and related outcomes in minority youth: the GALA II and SAGE II studies. Chest. 2017;151(4):804–12.
42. Apter AJ, Garcia LA, Boyd RC, Wang X, Bogen DK, Ten Have T. Exposure to community violence is associated with asthma hospitalizations and emergency department visits. J Allergy Clin Immunol. 2010;126(3):552–7.
43. Wright RJ, Mitchell H, Visness CM, Cohen S, Stout J, Evans R, et al. Community violence and asthma morbidity: the Inner-City Asthma Study. Am J Public Health. 2004;94(4):625–32.
44. Coogan PF, Wise LA, O'Connor GT, Brown TA, Palmer JR, Rosenberg L. Abuse during childhood and adolescence and risk of adult-onset asthma in African American women. J Allergy Clin Immunol. 2013;131(4):1058–63.
45. Lange NE, Bunyavanich S, Silberg JL, Canino G, Rosner BA, Celedon JC. Parental psychosocial stress and asthma morbidity in Puerto Rican twins. J Allergy Clin Immunol. 2011;127(3):734–40 e1–7.
46. Cohen RT, Canino GJ, Bird HR, Celedon JC. Violence, abuse, and asthma in Puerto Rican children. Am J Respir Crit Care Med. 2008;178(5):453–9.
47. Miller GE, Chen E. Life stress and diminished expression of genes encoding glucocorticoid receptor and beta2-adrenergic receptor in children with asthma. Proc Natl Acad Sci U S A. 2006;103(14):5496–501.
48. Marin TJ, Chen E, Munch JA, Miller GE. Double-exposure to acute stress and chronic family stress is associated with immune changes in children with asthma. Psychosom Med. 2009;71(4):378–84.
49. Chen W, Boutaoui N, Brehm JM, Han YY, Schmitz C, Cressley A, et al. ADCYAP1R1 and asthma in Puerto Rican children. Am J Respir Crit Care Med. 2013;187(6):584–8.
50. CDC [Internet]. Washington, DC: CDC health disparities and inequalities report – United States, 2013. 2013 [cited 2019 Jan 2]. Available from: https://www.cdc.gov/mmwr/pdf/other/su6203.pdf.
51. Nishimura KK, Galanter JM, Roth LA, Oh SS, Thakur N, Nguyen EA, et al. Early-life air pollution and asthma risk in minority children. The GALA II and SAGE II studies. Am J Respir Crit Care Med. 2013;188(3):309–18.
52. Kingsley SL, Eliot MN, Carlson L, Finn J, MacIntosh DL, Suh HH, et al. Proximity of US schools to major roadways: a nationwide assessment. J Expo Sci Environ Epidemiol. 2014;24(3):253–9.
53. Nardone A, Neophytou AM, Balmes J, Thakur N. Ambient air pollution and asthma-related outcomes in children of color of the USA: a scoping review of literature published between 2013 and 2017. Curr Allergy Asthma Rep. 2018;18(5):29.
54. Clougherty JE, Levy JI, Kubzansky LD, Ryan PB, Suglia SF, Canner MJ, et al. Synergistic effects of traffic-related air pollution and exposure to violence on urban asthma etiology. Environ Health Perspect. 2007;115(8):1140–6.
55. Mortimer K, Neugebauer R, Lurmann F, Alcorn S, Balmes J, Tager I. Early-lifetime exposure to air pollution and allergic sensitization in children with asthma. J Asthma. 2008;45(10):874–81.
56. Northridge J, Ramirez OF, Stingone JA, Claudio L. The role of housing type and housing quality in urban children with asthma. J Urban Health. 2010;87(2):211–24.
57. Ahluwalia SK, Peng RD, Breysse PN, Diette GB, Curtin-Brosnan J, Aloe C, et al. Mouse allergen is the major allergen of public health relevance in Baltimore City. J Allergy Clin Immunol. 2013;132(4):830–5 e1–2.
58. Sun Y, Sundell J. Life style and home environment are associated with racial disparities of asthma and allergy in Northeast Texas children. Sci Total Environ. 2011;409(20):4229–34.
59. CDC [Internet]. Washington, DC: Burden of tobacco use in the U.S. 2016 [cited 2019 Jan 15]. Available from: https://www.cdc.gov/tobacco/campaign/tips/resources/data/cigarette-smoking-in-united-states.html.

60. National Asthma Education and Prevention Program. Expert Panel Report 3 (EPR-3): guidelines for the diagnosis and management of asthma-summary report 2007. J Allergy Clin Immunol. 2007;120(5 Suppl):S94–138.
61. Oh SS, Tcheurekdjian H, Roth LA, Nguyen EA, Sen S, Galanter JM, et al. Effect of secondhand smoke on asthma control among black and Latino children. J Allergy Clin Immunol. 2012;129(6):1478–83 e7.
62. Paul G, Brehm JM, Alcorn JF, Holguin F, Aujla SJ, Celedon JC. Vitamin D and asthma. Am J Respir Crit Care Med. 2012;185(2):124–32.
63. Schleicher RL, Sternberg MR, Lacher DA, Sempos CT, Looker AC, Durazo-Arvizu RA, et al. The vitamin D status of the US population from 1988 to 2010 using standardized serum concentrations of 25-hydroxyvitamin D shows recent modest increases. Am J Clin Nutr. 2016;104(2):454–61.
64. Freishtat RJ, Iqbal SF, Pillai DK, Klein CJ, Ryan LM, Benton AS, et al. High prevalence of vitamin D deficiency among inner-city African American youth with asthma in Washington, DC. J Pediatr. 2010;156(6):948–52.
65. Brehm JM, Acosta-Perez E, Klei L, Roeder K, Barmada M, Boutaoui N, et al. Vitamin D insufficiency and severe asthma exacerbations in Puerto Rican children. Am J Respir Crit Care Med. 2012;186(2):140–6.
66. CDC [Internent]. Washington, DC: Prevalence of obesity among adults and youth: United States, 2015–2016. 2016 [cited 2019 Jan 15]. Available from: https://www.cdc.gov/obesity/data/adult.html.
67. Beuther DA, Sutherland ER. Overweight, obesity, and incident asthma: a meta-analysis of prospective epidemiologic studies. Am J Respir Crit Care Med. 2007;175(7):661–6.
68. Carroll CL, Bhandari A, Zucker AR, Schramm CM. Childhood obesity increases duration of therapy during severe asthma exacerbations. Pediatr Crit Care Med. 2006;7(6):527–31.
69. Vangeepuram N, Teitelbaum SL, Galvez MP, Brenner B, Doucette J, Wolff MS. Measures of obesity associated with asthma diagnosis in ethnic minority children. J Obes. 2011;2011:517417.
70. Borrell LN, Nguyen EA, Roth LA, Oh SS, Tcheurekdjian H, Sen S, et al. Childhood obesity and asthma control in the GALA II and SAGE II studies. Am J Respir Crit Care Med. 2013;187(7):697–702.
71. Forno E, Acosta-Perez E, Brehm JM, Han YY, Alvarez M, Colon-Semidey A, et al. Obesity and adiposity indicators, asthma, and atopy in Puerto Rican children. J Allergy Clin Immunol. 2014;133(5):1308–14, 14 e1–5.
72. Akinbami LJ, Rossen LM, Fakhouri THI, Simon AE, Kit BK. Contribution of weight status to asthma prevalence racial disparities, 2–19 year olds, 1988–2014. Ann Epidemiol. 2017;27(8):472–8 e3.
73. Holguin F, Mannino DM, Anto J, Mott J, Ford ES, Teague WG, et al. Country of birth as a risk factor for asthma among Mexican Americans. Am J Respir Crit Care Med. 2005;171(2):103–8.
74. Eldeirawi K, McConnell R, Freels S, Persky VW. Associations of place of birth with asthma and wheezing in Mexican American children. J Allergy Clin Immunol. 2005;116(1):42–8.
75. Eldeirawi KM, Persky VW. Associations of acculturation and country of birth with asthma and wheezing in Mexican American youths. J Asthma. 2006;43(4):279–86.
76. Claudio L, Stingone JA. Primary household language and asthma care among Latino children. J Health Care Poor Underserved. 2009;20(3):766–79.
77. Rosas-Salazar C, Ramratnam SK, Brehm JM, Han YY, Acosta-Perez E, Alvarez M, et al. Parental numeracy and asthma exacerbations in Puerto Rican children. Chest. 2013;144(1):92–8.
78. Wu AC, Smith L, Bokhour B, Hohman KH, Lieu TA. Racial/ethnic variation in parent perceptions of asthma. Ambul Pediatr. 2008;8(2):89–97.

79. Musa D, Schulz R, Harris R, Silverman M, Thomas SB. Trust in the health care system and the use of preventive health services by older black and white adults. Am J Public Health. 2009;99(7):1293–9.
80. Armstrong K, Ravenell KL, McMurphy S, Putt M. Racial/ethnic differences in physician distrust in the United States. Am J Public Health. 2007;97(7):1283–9.
81. Hacker K, Anies M, Folb BL, Zallman L. Barriers to health care for undocumented immigrants: a literature review. Risk Manag Healthc Policy. 2015;8:175–83.
82. Wisnivesky JP, Kattan M, Evans D, Leventhal H, Musumeci-Szabo TJ, McGinn T, et al. Assessing the relationship between language proficiency and asthma morbidity among inner-city asthmatics. Med Care. 2009;47(2):243–9.
83. Bialostozky A, Barkin SL. Understanding sibilancias (wheezing) among Mexican American parents. J Asthma. 2012;49(4):366–71.
84. Shone LP, Conn KM, Sanders L, Halterman JS. The role of parent health literacy among urban children with persistent asthma. Patient Educ Couns. 2009;75(3):368–75.
85. Fritz GK, McQuaid EL, Kopel SJ, Seifer R, Klein RB, Mitchell DK, et al. Ethnic differences in perception of lung function: a factor in pediatric asthma disparities? Am J Respir Crit Care Med. 2010;182(1):12–8.
86. Kit BK, Simon AE, Ogden CL, Akinbami LJ. Trends in preventive asthma medication use among children and adolescents, 1988–2008. Pediatrics. 2012;129(1):62–9.
87. Lieu TA, Lozano P, Finkelstein JA, Chi FW, Jensvold NG, Capra AM, et al. Racial/ethnic variation in asthma status and management practices among children in managed medicaid. Pediatrics. 2002;109(5):857–65.
88. Vila D, Rand CS, Cabana MD, Quinones A, Otero M, Gamache C, et al. Disparities in asthma medication dispensing patterns: the case of pediatric asthma in Puerto Rico. J Asthma. 2010;47(10):1136–41.
89. Lara M, Ramos-Valencia G, Gonzalez-Gavillan JA, Lopez-Malpica F, Morales-Reyes B, Marin H, et al. Reducing quality-of-care disparities in childhood asthma: La Red de Asma Infantil intervention in San Juan, Puerto Rico. Pediatrics. 2013;131(Suppl 1):S26–37.
90. McQuaid EL, Everhart RS, Seifer R, Kopel SJ, Mitchell DK, Klein RB, et al. Medication adherence among Latino and non-Latino white children with asthma. Pediatrics. 2012;129(6):e1404–10.
91. Choudhry S, Ung N, Avila PC, Ziv E, Nazario S, Casal J, et al. Pharmacogenetic differences in response to albuterol between Puerto Ricans and Mexicans with asthma. Am J Respir Crit Care Med. 2005;171(6):563–70.
92. Brehm JM, Ramratnam SK, Tse SM, Croteau-Chonka DC, Pino-Yanes M, Rosas-Salazar C, et al. Stress and bronchodilator response in children with asthma. Am J Respir Crit Care Med. 2015;192(1):47–56.
93. Drake KA, Torgerson DG, Gignoux CR, Galanter JM, Roth LA, Huntsman S, et al. A genome-wide association study of bronchodilator response in Latinos implicates rare variants. J Allergy Clin Immunol. 2014;133(2):370–8.
94. Scott G, Ni H. Access to health care among Hispanic/Latino children: United States, 1998–2001. Adv Data. 2004;(344):1–20.
95. Ortega AN, Fang H, Perez VH, Rizzo JA, Carter-Pokras O, Wallace SP, et al. Health care access, use of services, and experiences among undocumented Mexicans and other Latinos. Arch Intern Med. 2007;167(21):2354–60.
96. Greek AA, Kieckhefer GM, Kim H, Joesch JM, Baydar N. Family perceptions of the usual source of care among children with asthma by race/ethnicity, language, and family income. J Asthma. 2006;43(1):61–9.
97. Malhotra K, Baltrus P, Zhang S, McRoy L, Immergluck LC, Rust G. Geographic and racial variation in asthma prevalence and emergency department use among Medicaid-enrolled children in 14 southern states. J Asthma. 2014;51(9):913–21.

98. Eichenfield LF, Tom WL, Chamlin SL, Feldman SR, Hanifin JM, Simpson EL, et al. Guidelines of care for the management of atopic dermatitis: section 1. Diagnosis and assessment of atopic dermatitis. J Am Acad Dermatol. 2014;70(2):338–51.
99. Schram ME, Tedja AM, Spijker R, Bos JD, Williams HC, Spuls PI. Is there a rural/urban gradient in the prevalence of eczema? A systematic review. Br J Dermatol. 2010;162(5):964–73.
100. Wegienka G, Havstad S, Joseph CL, Zoratti E, Ownby D, Woodcroft K, et al. Racial disparities in allergic outcomes in African Americans emerge as early as age 2 years. Clin Exp Allergy. 2012;42(6):909–17.
101. Fischer AH, Shin DB, Margolis DJ, Takeshita J. Racial and ethnic differences in health care utilization for childhood eczema: an analysis of the 2001–2013 Medical Expenditure Panel Surveys. J Am Acad Dermatol. 2017;77(6):1060–7.
102. Janumpally SR, Feldman SR, Gupta AK, Fleischer AB Jr. In the United States, blacks and Asian/Pacific Islanders are more likely than whites to seek medical care for atopic dermatitis. Arch Dermatol. 2002;138(5):634–7.
103. McGowan EC, Keet CA. Prevalence of self-reported food allergy in the National Health and Nutrition Examination Survey (NHANES) 2007–2010. J Allergy Clin Immunol. 2013;132(5):1216–9. e5
104. Liu AH, Jaramillo R, Sicherer SH, Wood RA, Bock SA, Burks AW, et al. National prevalence and risk factors for food allergy and relationship to asthma: results from the National Health and Nutrition Examination Survey 2005–2006. J Allergy Clin Immunol. 2010;126(4):798–806 e13.
105. Keet CA, Savage JH, Seopaul S, Peng RD, Wood RA, Matsui EC. Temporal trends and racial/ethnic disparity in self-reported pediatric food allergy in the United States. Ann Allergy Asthma Immunol. 2014;112(3):222–9. e3
106. Taveras EM, Gillman MW, Kleinman KP, Rich-Edwards JW, Rifas-Shiman SL. Reducing racial/ethnic disparities in childhood obesity: the role of early life risk factors. JAMA Pediatr. 2013;167(8):731–8.
107. Hartman H, Dodd C, Rao M, DeBlasio D, Labowsky C, D'Souza S, et al. Parental timing of allergenic food introduction in urban and suburban populations. Ann Allergy Asthma Immunol. 2016;117(1):56–60 e2.
108. Du Toit G, Roberts G, Sayre PH, Bahnson HT, Radulovic S, Santos AF, et al. Randomized trial of peanut consumption in infants at risk for peanut allergy. N Engl J Med. 2015;372(9):803–13.
109. Call RS, Smith TF, Morris E, Chapman MD, Platts-Mills TA. Risk factors for asthma in inner city children. J Pediatr. 1992;121(6):862–6.
110. Findley S, Lawler K, Bindra M, Maggio L, Penachio MM, Maylahn C. Elevated asthma and indoor environmental exposures among Puerto Rican children of East Harlem. J Asthma. 2003;40(5):557–69.
111. Wong L, Huang CH, Lee BW. Shellfish and house dust mite allergies: is the link tropomyosin? Allergy, Asthma Immunol Res. 2016;8(2):101–6.
112. Santos AB, Chapman MD, Aalberse RC, Vailes LD, Ferriani VP, Oliver C, et al. Cockroach allergens and asthma in Brazil: identification of tropomyosin as a major allergen with potential cross-reactivity with mite and shrimp allergens. J Allergy Clin Immunol. 1999;104(2 Pt 1):329–37.
113. CDC [Internet]. Washington, DC: Summary health statistics tables for U.S. adults: National Health Interview Survey, 2017, Tables A-2b, A-2c. 2017 [cited 2019 Jan 17]. Available from: https://ftp.cdc.gov/pub/Health_Statistics/NCHS/NHIS/SHS/2017_SHS_Table_A-2.pdf.
114. Chen JT, Krieger N, Van Den Eeden SK, Quesenberry CP. Different slopes for different folks: socioeconomic and racial/ethnic disparities in asthma and hay fever among 173,859 U.S. men and women. Environ Health Perspect. 2002;110(Suppl 2):211–6.
115. Dykewicz MS, Wallace DV, Baroody F, Bernstein J, Craig T, Finegold I, et al. Treatment of seasonal allergic rhinitis: an evidence-based focused 2017 guideline update. Ann Allergy Asthma Immunol. 2017;119(6):489–511 e41.

116. Robinson LD Jr, Calmes DP, Bazargan M. The impact of literacy enhancement on asthma-related outcomes among underserved children. J Natl Med Assoc. 2008;100(8):892–6.
117. Canino G, Vila D, Normand SL, Acosta-Perez E, Ramirez R, Garcia P, et al. Reducing asthma health disparities in poor Puerto Rican children: the effectiveness of a culturally tailored family intervention. J Allergy Clin Immunol. 2008;121(3):665–70.
118. Thyne SM, Rising JP, Legion V, Love MB. The Yes We Can Urban Asthma Partnership: a medical/social model for childhood asthma management. J Asthma. 2006;43(9):667–73.
119. Morgan WJ, Crain EF, Gruchalla RS, O'Connor GT, Kattan M, Evans R 3rd, et al. Results of a home-based environmental intervention among urban children with asthma. N Engl J Med. 2004;351(11):1068–80.

Chapter 4
Disparity in Access to Care and Its Impact on Diagnosis and Outcomes of Allergic Diseases

Nima Parvaneh

Introduction

Allergic diseases comprise a significant cause of morbidity worldwide and a considerable burden on the health and medical systems [1]. Allergies affect a third of the population and their prevalence is increasing globally [2–4]. However, there are millions of people worldwide who do not have access to care by allergy specialists [2]. Moreover, epinephrine auto-injectors (EAIs), allergen-specific immunotherapy, and new biologic drugs are not available in many parts of the world. Even in affluent populations, there are enormous inequalities in access to allergic care. Health disparities are breaches in the quality of health and health care across racial, ethnic, and socioeconomic groups. Access to health care is strongly associated with socioeconomic features, including income, education, and employment [5–7]. There are even more restrictions for access to health care among racial and ethnic minorities. Ethnic and socioeconomic disparities in access to care in allergy practice are the result of multiple factors working at the individual and community levels. Disparities in access to appropriate medical care could result in different outcomes among specific groups [8, 9]. Much research has been conducted to understand allergic disease disparities considering access to care and its consequences. In this chapter, we will discuss these differential outcomes linked to access to care in multiple allergic diseases including asthma, food allergy, atopic dermatitis, and hymenoptera (stinging insects) allergy.

N. Parvaneh (✉)
Division of Allergy and Clinical Immunology, Department of Pediatrics, Tehran University of Medical Sciences, Tehran, Iran

Research Center for Immunodeficiencies, Children's Medical Center, Tehran University of Medical Sciences, Tehran, Iran
e-mail: nparvaneh@tums.ac.ir

© Springer Nature Switzerland AG 2020
M. Mahdavinia (ed.), *Health Disparities in Allergic Diseases*,
https://doi.org/10.1007/978-3-030-31222-0_4

Asthma Outcomes

Asthma is a common chronic lung disease affecting more than 8% of the adult and nearly 10% of the pediatric population of the United States [10]. Extensive evidence documents the significant differences in asthma prevalence by age, sex, race/ethnicity, and socioeconomic status (SES) [11–16]. The emergence of disparities in access to care and its health outcomes has been the topic of several studies during the last two decades (Table 4.1).

Table 4.1 Studies evaluating disparities in access to care and its outcomes among asthmatics during the last two decades

Study	Population	No	Outcome measures	Reported findings
Grant et al. [69]	5–34 years NCHS data for mortality 1991–1996	–	Asthma annual mortality rates	Higher standardized mortality ratios were seen for blacks vs whites (3.34 vs 0.65), low vs high educational level (1.51 vs 0.69), and low vs high income (1.46 vs 0.71)
Lieu et al. [37]	Children, the American Academy of Pediatrics (AAP) Children's Health Survey for Asthma	1658	Several asthma outcomes	After adjusting for sociodemographic variables and asthma status, black and Latino children were less likely to be using inhaled anti-inflammatory medication than white children
Cabana et al. [27]	<18 year children with asthma enrolled in a university-based managed care organization 1998–2000	3163	Receiving care from specialist	Compared with Medicaid patients, both non-Medicaid patients with copayment (OR, 2.52; 95% CI, 1.85–4.43) and non-Medicaid patients without any copayment (OR, 3.40; 95% CI, 2.35–4.93) were more likely to receive care from an asthma subspecialist
Boudreaux et al. [47]	Adult asthmatics from Multicenter Airway Research Collaboration (MARC) 1996–1998	1847	ED rates ED management Hospitalization rates	Black and Hispanic asthma patients had a history of more hospitalizations than did whites (ever-hospitalized patients: Black, 66%; Hispanic, 63%; white, 54%; $P < 0.001$; patients hospitalized in the past year: Black, 31%; Hispanic, 33%; white, 25%; $P < 0.05$) and more frequent ED use (median use in past year: Black, three visits; Hispanic, three visits; white, one visit; $P < 0.001$)

Table 4.1 (continued)

Study	Population	No	Outcome measures	Reported findings
Gupta et al. [67]	5–34 years National Hospital Discharge Survey and the US vital statistics system 1980–2002	–	Hospitalizations Mortality	For children, there have been notable increases in asthma B/W differences in hospitalizations and mortality since 1980, whereas for adults, the increase has been smaller
Ferris et al. [32]	National Ambulatory Medical Care Surveys (NAMCS)	3671	ICS usage	Minority patients with asthma were less than half as likely as nonminority patients to have had a steroid MDI prescribed during 1989–1990. By 1995–1996, minority and nonminority patients with asthma were equally likely to have had a steroid MDI prescribed. Although differences between black and white patients resolved, differences between white and Hispanic patients persisted even after adjusting for insurance
Kruse et al. [44]	Children 1–19 years Asthma ED and hospitalization rates in New Jersey 2004 and 2005	37,216	ED rates, ED admissions and hospitalization rates	ED rates among black NH children were 3.4 times higher and almost twice as high among Hispanic children compared to white NH children. Hospitalization rates were 3.3 times higher among black NH children and 1.9 times higher among Hispanic children compared to white NH children. The ED and hospitalization rates were highest among the youngest children (ages 1–4)
Peters et al. [51]	Adults, TENOR 2001–2003	1315	HCU, defined as ED visits and/or hospitalization	Medicaid insurance is not associated with increased HCU in patients with severe asthma once demographic factors have been taken into account but remains modestly associated with poorer asthma control

(continued)

Table 4.1 (continued)

Study	Population	No	Outcome measures	Reported findings
Stingone and Claudio [20]	5–12 years 2002–2003	5250	Allergy testing	The frequency of a reported allergy diagnosis varied with race/ethnicity, ranging from 14.4% in Mexican American children to 67.9% in white children. Only 54.9% of asthmatic children with an allergy diagnosis reported allergy testing. Children from lower-/middle-income households and children with public forms of health insurance were the least likely to report testing (adjusted ORs, 0.18 and 0.46)
Ginde et al. [43]	Data from the National Hospital Ambulatory Medical Care Survey 1993–2005	6850	ED visits	The overall asthma-related ED visit rate per 1000 US population was highest among the following groups: age <10 years (13), women (7.2), black subjects (19), Hispanic subjects (7.1), and subjects in the Northeast (9.2)
Haselkorn et al. [72]	≥18 years TENOR study 2001–2004	2128	Multiple asthma outcomes in severe-to-treat asthma	Blacks were more likely to have severe asthma and to be treated with 3 or more long-term controllers. Poorer quality of life, more asthma control problems, and higher risk of emergency department visits were observed in blacks compared with whites
Chandra et al. [60]	Children and adults hospitalized with a physician diagnosis of acute asthma at 30 hospitals in 22 US states	1232	Inpatient care and discharge plan	There were no significant racial/ethnic differences in the choice of inpatient medications or length of stay among either children or adults. At hospital discharge, Hispanic children were less likely to receive an asthma action plan (37%) compared to white children (60%) or black children (63%; $P < 0.001$)
Stingone and Claudio [38]	Children A parent-report survey conducted in 26 randomly selected New York City public elementary schools	912	Usage of long-term controller medication	Children of Spanish-speaking parents, African American children, and children with no health insurance were the least likely to use long-term control medication (ORs: 0.51, 0.49, 0.20, respectively)

Table 4.1 (continued)

Study	Population	No	Outcome measures	Reported findings
Gorman and Chu [9]	Adults Behavioral Risk Factor Surveillance System [BRFSS] 2004	133,509	Four measures of asthma-related medical care	Considerable racial/ethnic differences in asthma-related problems and medical care are also present, with Asians doing as well or better than whites, while blacks, Hispanics, and especially Native Americans report more asthma-related problems and medical care use
Roy et al. [49]	Data from the Mississippi Asthma Surveillance System 2003–2005	4242	Asthma hospitalization risk factors	Asthma hospitalization rates were significantly higher among all demographic groups in the rural Delta region compared with the urban Jackson Metropolitan Statistical Area ($P < 0.001$). In both regions, hospitalization rates were higher among blacks and females ($P < 0.001$) Asthma hospitalization rates were highest among children (0–17 years) and older adults (>65 years). In both regions, blacks were more likely to have three or more asthma hospitalizations ($P < 0.001$). Residents of the Delta had higher odds for multiple hospitalizations controlling for race, sex, age, and household income ($P < 0.05$)
Galbraith et al. [35]	Children with persistent asthma	563	ICS prescription	No racial differences in ICS prescription Children with persistent asthma are less likely to receive inhaled steroids if they receive care in community health centers or hospital clinics
Piper et al. [29]	0–17 years National Health Interview Survey (NHIS) 2000	1630	Utilization of health-care services	It was found that black children were highly associated with not visiting a general doctor in the past 12 months (OR 0.47; 95% CI 0.30, 0.75). Uninsured asthmatic children were associated with the risk of not seeing a general doctor in the past 12 months (OR 0.40; 95% CI 0.23, 0.69)

(continued)

Table 4.1 (continued)

Study	Population	No	Outcome measures	Reported findings
Piper et al. [23]	<18 years National Health Interview Survey 2002–2003	3102	Having an asthma management plan	Whites were significantly more likely than non-Hispanic blacks and Hispanics to have an asthma management plan (OR, 1.66; $P = 0.0031$). In this study, children who reported Children's Health Insurance Program (CHIP) coverage were twice as likely to have an asthma management plan (OR, 2.67; $P = 0.0004$)
Largent et al. [16]	Children 0–14 years living in Orange County 2000–2007	–	ED visits Hospital admissions	Rates of asthma hospital admissions and ED visits were highest among children aged 0–14 years, males, and African Americans and lowest among Asian/Pacific islanders Rates of hospital admissions and ED visits were significantly higher in low-SES groups
Gold et al. [73]	12-year-old asthmatics Asthma Insights and Management (AIM) survey 2009	2493	Asthma control	Having lower annual income was associated with asthma that was classified as partly or uncontrolled. Additionally, subjects/parents who owned their own homes and who were employed had higher rates of well-controlled asthma compared to subjects/parents who did not own their own homes or who were unemployed at the time of the survey. Having a high-school education or less was associated with asthma that was classified as uncontrolled. Finally, not having health insurance was associated with uncontrolled asthma compared to patients who did not have health insurance; similarly, having little or no trouble paying for health-related expenses was associated with well-controlled asthma

Table 4.1 (continued)

Study	Population	No	Outcome measures	Reported findings
Akinbami et al. [66]	0–17 years NCHS data 2001–2010	–	Trends in asthma outcomes: Asthma attack prevalence ED rates Hospitalizations deaths	Analysis with at-risk rates, which account for differences in asthma prevalence, showed that disparities in asthma outcomes remained stable (deaths), decreased (ED visits, hospitalizations), or did not exist (asthma attack prevalence)
Venkat et al. [61]	18–54 years old adults from Multicenter Airway Research Collaboration (MARC) study, 2011–2012	1785	ED care utilization	Non-Hispanic blacks with increased chronic asthma severity were only as likely ($P > 0.05$) as non-Hispanic whites or Hispanics to utilize controller medications or see asthma specialists before ED presentation and to be prescribed recommended inhaled corticosteroids at ED discharge.
Kharat et al. [34]	>4 years asthmatics from Medical Expenditure Panel Survey (MEPS) data 2009	1469	ICS prescription	Hispanic patients aged 18 years or older had 43% lower odds (OR, 0.6; 95% CI, 0.3–0.9) of having a receipt of an ICS prescription compared with non-Hispanic white patients, independent of other factors. There was no significant difference in receipt of an ICS prescription between Hispanic and non-Hispanic white children with asthma (aged 4–17 years)
Mitchell et al. [31]	Children Patient registry data from Baltimore, Maryland 2007–2010	273	Five morbidity outcomes: Hospitalization ICU admission FEV1, FEV1/FVC Asthma control	African American patients had worse asthma morbidity than their white counterparts, including higher rates of ICU admission, worse asthma control, and poorer lung function as indicated by lower FEV_1

(continued)

Table 4.1 (continued)

Study	Population	No	Outcome measures	Reported findings
Glick et al [55]	2–18 years US Nationwide Inpatient Sample 2007–2011	97,379	Mortality LOS Total costs	Native American race, older age (13–18 years), and West region were significant independent predictors of mortality. Intubation rate was lower in Hispanic compared with white children ($P = 0.028$). LOS was shorter in Asian compared with white children ($P = 0.022$) but longer in children with public insurance and from low-income areas ($P < 0.001$). Average costs were higher in black, Hispanic, and Asian compared with white children ($P < 0.05$)
Beck et al. [63]	1–16 years Greater Cincinnati Asthma Risk Study cohort	695	Time to asthma-related readmission	African American children were 2.26 times more likely to be readmitted than white children (95% CI, 1.56–3.26). The addition of biologic, environmental, disease management, and access variables resulted in 80% of the readmission disparity being explained
Silber et al. [52]	3–18 years Medicaid Analytic eXtract (MAX) database 2009–2010	11,079 pairs	Revisits, readmissions, LOS, and ICU use	Ten-day revisit rates were 3.8% in black patients versus 4.2% in white patients ($P = 0.12$); 30-day revisit and readmission rates were also not significantly different by race (10.5% in black patients versus 10.8% in white patients; $P = 0.49$). LOS was also similar However, ICU use was higher in black patients than white patients (22.2% versus 17.5%; $P < 0.001$)
Zhang et al. [45]	2–17 years Asthma Call-Back Survey (ACBS) in 2006–2010	5535	ED visits	Minority children with current asthma had higher risks of ED visits compared with white children in 2009 and 2010, e.g., the prevalence ratio (PR) (95% CI) for black children in 2009 was 3.64 (1.79, 7.41)

Table 4.1 (continued)

Study	Population	No	Outcome measures	Reported findings
Franklin et al. [48]	6–17-year-old children with persistent asthma lived in metropolitan Atlanta, Georgia 2016	276	Predictors of ED visit	ED use was disproportionately higher in black (38.7%) vs white (26.1%) children ($P = 0.04$) and children with public (40.4%) vs private (23.4%) insurance ($P = 0.005$), irrespective of race. In white children, an ED visit in the previous year and sensitization to dust mites and pets were associated with ED use during the study period. White children were also more likely than black children to report having a cat (27.5% vs 9.5%, $P = 0.001$) or dog (58.2% vs 34.3%, $P < 0.001$) inside the home. However, in black children, the variables associated with ED use during the study period included an ED visit in the previous year, the number of asthma controller medications, FEV1 less than 80% predicted, blood eosinophil count greater than 4%, and mold sensitization
Trent et al. [62]	Random sample of 2–54 years old asthmatics from Multicenter Airway Research Collaboration (MARC) 2011–2012	913	Provision of guideline-concordant asthma care in the hospital and after discharge	NHB children were significantly less likely to receive a written asthma action plan (OR 0.48; 95% CI 0.31–0.76) than NHW children. In contrast, among adults, we found no statistically significant difference in the provision of asthma action plan. Additionally, we found no difference in the provision of a new inhaled corticosteroid prescription or referral to asthma specialist among children or adults

(continued)

Table 4.1 (continued)

Study	Population	No	Outcome measures	Reported findings
Hughes et al. [50]	6–17 years American Housing Survey 2011	33,201	ED visits	Non-Hispanic black heads of household had a higher odds of having a child diagnosed with asthma in the home in comparison to non-Hispanic white heads of household (OR 1.72, 95%CI 1.50–1.96), and a higher odds of ED visits for asthma (OR 3.02, 95%CI 2.29–3.99)
Trivedi et al. [30]	Study of parent surveys of asthmatic children within the Population-Based Effectiveness in Asthma and Lung Diseases Network 2011	647	Family-provider interactions	Black children had fewer visits in the previous 12 months for asthma than white children: OR 0.63 (95% CI 0.40, 0.99). Additionally, black children were less likely to have a written asthma treatment plan given/ reviewed by a provider than their white peers, OR 0.44 (95% CI 0.26, 0.75)
Washington et al. [8]	8–15 years Chicago Initiative to Raise ASTHMA Health Equity (CHIRAH) cohort	544	Several asthma outcomes	African American race and Hispanic/Latino ethnicity were significantly associated with all outcomes when compared to whites. Adjusting for sociodemographic factors resulted in the most significant mediation of racial/ethnic disparities in all outcomes
Guilbert et al. [71]	6–11 years The Epidemiology and Natural History of Asthma: Outcomes and Treatment Regimens (TENOR) 2001–2004	348	Asthma control ED visits Long-term steroid use	Black children had higher geometric mean IgE levels (434.8 vs 136.8 IU/mL; $P < 0.001$), were more likely to have very poorly controlled asthma (72.1% vs 53.4%), use long-term systemic corticosteroids (30.2% vs 9.2%; $P < 0.001$), have poorer quality of life (5.5 vs 6.1; $P < 0.001$), and have an emergency department visit (27.4% vs 7.7%, $P < 0.001$) in the 3 months before month 12. Differences in asthma control and the severity of exacerbations persisted even after accounting for all confounding factors

Table 4.1 (continued)

Study	Population	No	Outcome measures	Reported findings
Zook et al. [46]	2–18-year-old children presented to EDs in the upper Midwest 2011–2012	1755	30-day ED revisits Steroid administration Ordering radiology tests	African American (adjusted OR, 1.78; 95% CI, 1.40–2.26) and Hispanic (aOR, 1.64; 95% CI, 1.22–2.22) patients had higher odds of receiving steroids compared with whites. African Americans (aOR, 0.58; 95% CI, 0.46–0.74) also had lower odds of radiological testing compared with whites. Asians had the lowest odds of 30-day ED revisits (aOR, 0.26; 95% CI, 0.08–0.84)

B/W, Black/white; *CI*, Confidence interval; *ED*, Emergency department; *HCU*, Health care utilization, *ICS*, Inhaled corticosteroid; *ICU*, Intensive care unit; *LOS*, Length of stay; *MDI*, Metered dose inhaler; *NHB*, non-Hispanic black; *NHW*, non-Hispanic white; *OR*, Odds ratio

Successful asthma management includes proper diagnosis of allergic sensitizations using allergy testing. Allergy testing can be used to tailor allergen avoidance directions and guide some patients to receive immunotherapy [17–19]. These could have beneficial effects on the health outcomes of asthma. However, there is a gap to receive proper allergy diagnosis among different racial and income groups. A study described that Mexican American children, children from lower-/middle-income households, and those with public forms of health insurance were the least likely to report allergy testing [20].

Asthma management plans are an essential component for the long-term treatment of pediatric asthma and beneficial for self-management [21–23]. Having an asthma management plan is also associated with fewer asthmatic episodes [24]. Receipt of specialty care by asthmatic children can affect cost and quality of care and is associated with substantial reductions in asthma emergency department (ED) visits and hospitalizations [25, 26]. Poor and Medicaid-covered children have significantly lower odds of receiving asthma subspecialty care [27, 28].

Racial disparities exist in access to health-care services among asthmatic children. Black children with asthma are seen less frequently by asthma providers and are less likely to have a written asthma treatment plan reviewed than white children with asthma. This can impact the morbidity gap between black and white asthmatic children [29–31]. Moreover, uninsured asthmatic children are less likely to visit a doctor and receive preventive care [23, 29]. Another important factor is whether there are racial disparities related to asthma decision-making during outpatient visits [30]. Inhaled corticosteroids (ICS) are the most efficient controller medications for patients who have persistent asthma [32]. Studies assessing ICS usage among racial minorities have reported conflicting results. Some studies described that black and Hispanic patients are less likely to receive a prescription for ICS [33, 34]. However, other studies did not find a significant racial difference in receiving an ICS prescription [35].The disparity in receipt of ICS prescriptions might also be attributed to racial differences in health beliefs and fears about steroids [36]. Moreover, younger asthmatics are less likely to receive a prescription for ICS medications [33, 34]. Insured patients have higher odds of having a receipt of an ICS prescription compared with uninsured patients [34, 37, 38].

Poor asthma control is associated with increased ED visits, hospital admissions, and significant medical costs [39]. Asthma-related ED visits present a measure of the asthma burden and morbidity [40]. ED visits add significantly to the financial burden of asthma, costing as much as five times more per visit than outpatient office visits for asthma [41, 42].

There is growing evidence of the presence of racial disparities in ED visits and hospitalization rates among patients with asthma in all age groups with more ED rates and inpatient admissions documented for minority groups [43–46]. ED rates and hospitalizations are higher among black non-Hispanic and Hispanic children compared to white non-Hispanic children [44, 45, 47–50]. Extremes of age are also risk factors for more frequent asthma-related ED rates [43, 44, 49]. Gender disparities reported being different in various studies. ED visits and hospitalizations are more common for females in Mississippi but less common for females living in Orange County [16, 49]. Living in rural and some geographical areas produces a gap in ED rates as well [43, 49]. ED rates and hospital admissions are higher among asthmatics who are not insured or use public insurances than those who have private insurances [16, 48].

Analysis of data from large observational TENOR (The Epidemiology and Natural History of Asthma: Outcomes and Treatment Regimens) study showed that Medicaid insurance is not associated with increased health-care utilization in patients with severe asthma once demographic factors have been taken into account but remains modestly associated with poorer asthma control [51]. Interestingly, in patients with Medicaid, race does not influence revisits, readmissions, or deaths, and blacks are found to have only a small, but significant, difference in ICU use [52].

Some factors may explain the disparities in asthma-related ED visits [45]. Patients with different sociodemographic factors may have variable exposure to environmental risks, such as living in households with poor air quality [53, 54]. The other possible explanation is a disparity in access to health care across race/ethnicity [55, 56].

Even with equal access to health care, the underlying health beliefs, attitudes, and educational level may trigger different health-care usage behaviors among patients and/or caregivers [57, 58].

Background socioeconomic factors also contribute to ED rate disparities. For example, there is an inverse relationship between income levels and ED visits among adults with asthma [12, 59]. Despite declining trends of pediatric asthma ED visits and hospitalizations, these rates are significantly higher in children living in low-SES areas [16].

Despite inequities in ED rates, the quality of care for a patient seen in the ED for asthma and the decision to admit the patient are the same regardless of race/ethnicity [44].

ED admission rates are similar across race/ethnicity groups. However, there are differences in the diagnostic and therapeutic interventions [44, 47, 60, 61]. In the ED setting, children from minority racial/ethnic groups were more likely to receive steroids and less likely to receive radiology tests than white children [46].

Another significant disparity in asthma care is the provision of the discharge plan, provision of a new prescription of an ICS, and referral to an asthma specialist. Non-Hispanic black and Hispanic children are significantly less likely to receive a written asthma action plan than non-Hispanic white children [60, 62]. After asthma-related ED admission, African American children are more likely to be readmitted than white children. However, up to 80% of this disparity is explained by biologic, environmental, disease management, and access to care variables [63, 64].

Adverse asthma outcomes, such as hospitalization and death, are mostly preventable, but rates are higher among some minority children than among white children [65–68].

Racial/ethnic disparities in asthma mortality rates are well described [69, 70]. Black and Native American races are independent risk factors of asthma mortality in different studies [55, 66, 67, 69]. Low SES is also contributing to asthma mortality independent of race [69].

A recent study analyzing US Nationwide Inpatient Samples for 2007–2011 studied factors associated with mortality and morbidity in children hospitalized for asthma [55]. Native American race, older age (13–18 years), and the West region were significant independent predictors of mortality. Hospital length of stay was shorter in Asian compared with white children but longer in children with public insurance and from low-income areas. The average costs were lower in white children compared with other ethnicities.

A large study on national datasets from the National Center for Health Statistics (NCHS) disclosed that population-based rates show stable or increasing racial disparities in asthma outcome. However at-risk rates which account for differences in asthma prevalence show stable mortalities and decreasing ED rates and hospitalizations gaps during recent years [66]. The TENOR study documented worse outcome measures in black patients compared with whites in both children and adults. Black asthmatics were more likely to have very poorly controlled asthma, use long-term systemic corticosteroids/several controllers, and have a more inferior quality of life [71, 72]. Using a large population of US asthma patients, Asthma Insights and Management (AIM) study demonstrated that poorly controlled asthma was strongly associated with indicators of low SES [73].

Differences in asthma-related health outcomes in different racial groups despite accounting for the demographic features and SES substantiate the role of other factors such as physiologic differences and pharmacogenetics [66, 71]. Ancestry seems significantly associated with lung function; African Americans have smaller lung function compared with whites [74]. Moreover, black subjects with asthma have been shown to require higher concentrations of glucocorticoid to suppress the activation of T-lymphocytes, suggesting that black subjects have a racial predisposition to reduced glucocorticoid response [75].

Food Allergy Outcomes

Childhood food allergy (FA) is a significant public health issue resulting in relatively high rates of severe allergic reactions and ED visits [76].

Recent large-scale epidemiologic studies suggest that there may be higher rates of FA in some ethnic/racial groups independent of household income or other atopic comorbidities [77–79].

Several studies examined FA-associated hospital admissions or ED events to assess potential ethnic/racial disparities. These studies demonstrated variable results from no ethnic differences to higher rates of food-induced anaphylaxis in black children [80–84].

Potential racial disparities exist in access to care which may create underdiagnosis/misdiagnosis of a potential FA and may daunt the ability to receive proper care [85]. This could significantly underestimate the rate of FA within certain population segments (Table 4.2).

A large study assessing knowledge about FA among caregivers noted a significant difference in correctly identifying the signs of a reaction, identifying

Table 4.2 Studies evaluating disparities in access to care and its outcomes among patients with food allergy

Study	Population	No	Outcome measures	Reported findings
Hannaway et al. [88]	Students from 3 Massachusetts school districts	21,875	Amount of dispensed EAI among schoolchildren	Males were more likely to be dispensed injectable epinephrine than females (odds ratio [OR], 1.44; $P < 0.02$). Whites were more likely to have been dispensed injectable epinephrine than nonwhites (OR, 4.76; $P < 0.001$)
Soller et al. [90]	Canadian study on the prevalence of FA 2008–2009	105,96	Position of EAI	Individuals with allergy residing in a household where the respondent was married/living with a partner were more likely to have an EAI: Probable group (OR, 3.8; 95% CI, 1.4–9.1) Diagnosed group (OR, 3.6; 95% CI, 1.1–9.4)
Johns and Savage [87]	Data from the 2011–2012 NHIS	26,021	Access to health care and food among subjects with FA	Black respondents with food allergy were significantly more likely to have low food security (OR, 2.15; 95% CI, 1.30–3.53), to have problems paying family medical bills (OR, 1.68; 95% CI, 1.09–2.59), and to have trouble affording prescriptions for the child (OR, 2.40; 95% CI, 1.14–5.05), and Hispanic respondents with food allergy were significantly more likely to have trouble affording follow-up care (OR, 3.02; 95% CI, 1.34–6.81 compared with white respondents with food allergy

Table 4.2 (continued)

Study	Population	No	Outcome measures	Reported findings
Shah et al. [89]	Students from 89 HISD schools 2010–2011 school year	69,310	Presence of EAI in school	When considered simultaneously, both SES ($P < 0.001$) and proficiency of the English language ($P < 0.01$) were found to be independently associated with the number of epinephrine injectors
Szychlinski et al. [91]	Illinois state schools 2012–2013	460 school nurses	School nurses' responses to FA emergencies	Rural schools were least likely to have a written plan or protocol to outline staff procedure in the event of a severe allergic reaction (59.4% of respondents working at rural schools were aware of a written plan or protocol vs 81.7% for suburban vs 71.9% for urban, $P < 0.0019$). Additionally, rural schools were least likely to report undesignated epinephrine policies (35.6% of rural, 47.5% of suburban, and 64.0% of urban schools, $P < 0.005$)
Bilaver et al. [92]	US caregivers with a food allergic child 2011–2012	1643	Economic impacts of FA	Children in the lowest-income stratum incurred 2.5 times the amount of emergency department and hospitalization costs as a result of their food allergy than higher-income children ($1021, SE ± $209, vs $416, SE ± $94; $P < 0.05$). Costs incurred for specialist visits were lower in the lowest-income group ($228, SE ± $21) compared with the highest income group ($311, SE ± $18; $P < 0.01$) as was spending on out-of-pocket medication costs ($117, SE ± $26, lowest income; $366, SE ± $44, highest income; $P < 0.001$)
Mahdavinia et al. [79]	2 FA patient cohorts followed at RUMC and CCHMC	717	Disease phenotype and disparities in health-care utilization	55%, 18%, and 11% of African American, Hispanic, and white children were covered by Medicaid, respectively ($P < 0.00001$). Compared with whites, African American and Hispanic children had a shorter duration of follow-up for FA with an allergy specialist and higher rates of FA-related anaphylaxis and ED visits ($P < 0.01$)

CCHMC, Cincinnati Children's Hospital Medical Center; *CI*, confidence interval; *EAI*, Epinephrine auto-injector; *FA*, Food allergy; *HISD*, Houston Independent School District; *OR*, Odds ratio; *RUMC*, Rush University Medical Center; *SE*, Standard error; *SES*, Socioeconomic status

FA triggers, and recognizing the need for food avoidance in parents of different races [86]. Another national study showed that parents of black children had significantly lower odds of receiving a formal diagnosis of FA by a physician [76].

Recent studies suggest there might be a barrier to accessing health care and food in children with FA, particularly among nonwhite children. Poor access to health care and food might increase morbidity, especially among minority children, by imposing poor nutrition and delayed treatment for allergic reactions.

A US large national survey examined access to health care and food among subjects with FA [87]. Even after adjusting for income and education, black respondents with FA were significantly more likely to report low food security and trouble affording prescriptions, and Hispanic respondents with FA were significantly more likely to report trouble affording follow-up care compared with white respondents.

There is a need to apply strategies to provide better access to outpatient specialist care for all children with FA, especially those from lower income families with lower access to care [85]. Some studies evaluate the possession and usage of EAI as an indicator of access to care for severe FA reactions. It seems that there are socioeconomic, gender, racial, and geographical inequities in access to EAI.

A study of Massachusetts school students showed that white schoolchildren were six times more likely to be dispensed EAIs than all other races [88]. Moreover, males were more likely to be dispensed injectable epinephrine than females.

Another study conducted in the Houston independent school district (HISD) showed both socioeconomic status and proficiency of the English language to be independently associated with the availability of EAIs in schools [89].

A Canadian national study demonstrated that individuals with allergy residing in a household where the respondent was living with a partner were more likely to have EAIs. Furthermore, children and females were more likely to have an EAI [90].

A study conducted in Illinois schools uncovered geographical disparity in the implementation of FA guidelines and access to undesignated epinephrine [91]. Nurses from rural schools reported the least experience with FA reactions and were least likely to recall a written policy for handling of FA emergencies.

Finally, the disparity in health-care utilization depicted as access to insurances and the availability of specialty care endanger children with FA from some minority groups.

Low-income children experience higher costs for ED visits and hospitalization and spend less on specialty care [92]. Compared with whites, African Americans and Hispanic children with a higher rate of Medicaid coverage have a shorter duration of follow-up for FA with a specialist and higher rates of FA-related anaphylaxis and ED visits [79].

Atopic Dermatitis

Atopic dermatitis (AD) is a chronic inflammatory skin condition that classically develops during infancy and early childhood. AD occurs worldwide with different prevalence, showing higher rates in Africa and Oceania, as opposed to India and Northern and Eastern Europe [93].

In the United States, AD prevalence is higher in African American (AA) children compared to European American (EA) children. AA children are three times more likely to be diagnosed with AD during a dermatologist visit; however, they are less likely to seek dermatological care [94, 95]. The association between race/ethnicity and AD persistence is limited and shows conflicting results [96, 97]. Results of a recent American cohort demonstrate that compared with non-Hispanic whites, Hispanics and non-Hispanic blacks with early childhood AD are more likely to have persistent disease into mid-childhood [98].

Considering access to medical care, non-Hispanic black children show low rates of overall health-care use for AD, but more outpatient visits and prescriptions for AD, suggesting a greater disease severity [99].

In the American population, ED visits for dermatological care are more often seen in black and Hispanic patients compared with white patients [100]. Moreover, hospitalization for AD and increased costs are more likely to occur in patients with nonwhite race/ethnicity, a lower income, and public or no insurance [101]. These differences may be due to the higher prevalence of and more severe AD and/or less access to appropriate outpatient care. Unfortunately, there are little data on the efficacy of conventional therapies for AD in nonwhite ethnic groups [102–104].

Less than 60% of AD clinical trials published between 2000 and 2009 included race and ethnicity as baseline information. Only about 10% of studies considered race or ethnicity in the final interpretation [104].

Emerging ethnic groups with different epidemiologic, clinical, and molecular differences have important, but limited therapeutic cues [94]. Topical anti-inflammatory drugs are the mainstay treatment for AD. There is some concern that the use of topical corticosteroids in darker skin types may worsen hypopigmentation; however, hypopigmentation is more likely related to postinflammatory changes than a medication effect [105]. However, topical calcineurin inhibitors showed no difference in treatment outcome among ethnic groups [106, 107].

Pharmacogenetic and pharmacokinetic differences among various populations may affect the optimal dose and side effects of systemic immunomodulators used in AD [105].

Narrowband (NB)-UVB, which is used in severe AD, requires higher doses in more pigmented skin types [108–110], but UVA1,which is an alternative for treating acute AD, does not require dose adjustments between different skin types [111, 112]. Recent Phase III trials of dupilumab (a fully human monoclonal antibody targeting the shared α-subunit of the IL-4 and IL-13 receptors) in moderate-to-severe AD showed comparable results among white, black, and Asian individuals [113–115]. These new medications are associated with very high cost and need close access to specialty care. Therefore, differential use of them will inevitably impact the outcome and persistence of AD and could be the underlying cause of the observed disparities in outcome of AD. Furthermore, due to its chronicity and fluctuating symptoms, treatment and outcome of AD are closely linked to support and rapport provided by physicians and health-care providers which is another potential factor impacting the outcome of disease that can be impacted by inequity in health care.

Stinging Insect Allergy

Many adults and children experience systemic reactions to Hymenoptera stings each year.

It is recommended that patients with systemic reactions to venom receive an epinephrine auto-injector and be referred to an allergist [116]. A study showed that males were more likely to have been given epinephrine auto-injector for stinging insect allergy than females [88]. Whites were nearly nine times more likely to have been dispensed EAI than nonwhites. Venom immunotherapy (VIT) by an allergist is indicated for confirmed cases of IgE-mediated systemic reactions to Hymenoptera venom [117]. Recent venom shortage due to a manufacturing delay of a leading supplier had an international impact on VIT practice [118, 119]. There is a potential for the emergence of disparities in access to VIT among different groups under this situation; however, no study has addressed it yet.

Conclusion

Access to equal health care is a prominent and unfair contributor to allergic disease disparities. Racial disparities persist in health-care access and quality of care in multiple settings. Low-income and impoverished populations utilize emergency department facilities more frequently for allergy-related needs as they have lower access to outpatient specialty care; however, this is not optimal care, and the problem goes beyond that. Racial inequalities in the use of urgent care were reported to exist even after controlling for accessibility and socioeconomic factors. This differential health-care utilization has resulted in poor outcome across all allergic conditions.

Effectively addressing disparities in allergy care requires a collective effort that includes the full range of public health and health-care systems. Moreover, it calls for the development and implementation of individualized programs intended to educate affected families considering their cultural and socioeconomic setting.

References

1. Sanchez-Borges M, Martin BL, Muraro AM, Wood RA, Agache IO, Ansotegui IJ, et al. The importance of allergic disease in public health: an iCAALL statement. World Allergy Organ J. 2018;11(1):8. https://doi.org/10.1186/s40413-018-0187-2.
2. Asher MI, Montefort S, Bjorksten B, Lai CK, Strachan DP, Weiland SK, et al. Worldwide time trends in the prevalence of symptoms of asthma, allergic rhinoconjunctivitis, and eczema in childhood: ISAAC Phases One and Three repeat multicountry cross-sectional surveys. Lancet Lond Engl. 2006;368(9537):733–43. https://doi.org/10.1016/s0140-6736(06)69283-0.
3. Bjorksten B, Clayton T, Ellwood P, Stewart A, Strachan D. Worldwide time trends for symptoms of rhinitis and conjunctivitis: Phase III of the International Study of Asthma and Allergies in Childhood. Pediatr Allergy Immunol. 2008;19(2):110–24. https://doi.org/10.1111/j.1399-3038.2007.00601.x.
4. Prescott SL, Pawankar R, Allen KJ, Campbell DE, Sinn J, Fiocchi A, et al. A global survey of changing patterns of food allergy burden in children. World Allergy Organ J. 2013;6(1):21. https://doi.org/10.1186/1939-4551-6-21.
5. Baicker K, Taubman SL, Allen HL, Bernstein M, Gruber JH, Newhouse JP, et al. The Oregon experiment--effects of Medicaid on clinical outcomes. N Engl J Med. 2013;368(18):1713–22. https://doi.org/10.1056/NEJMsa1212321.
6. Griffith K, Evans L, Bor J. The affordable care act reduced socioeconomic disparities in health care access. Health Aff (Project Hope). 2017;36(8):1503–10. https://doi.org/10.1377/hlthaff.2017.0083.
7. Pappas G, Queen S, Hadden W, Fisher G. The increasing disparity in mortality between socioeconomic groups in the United States, 1960 and 1986. N Engl J Med. 1993;329(2):103–9. https://doi.org/10.1056/nejm199307083290207.
8. Washington DM, Curtis LM, Waite K, Wolf MS, Paasche-Orlow MK. Sociodemographic factors mediate race and ethnicity-associated childhood asthma health disparities: a longitudinal analysis. J Racial Ethn Health Disparities. 2018;5(5):928–38. https://doi.org/10.1007/s40615-017-0441-2.
9. Gorman BK, Chu M. Racial and ethnic differences in adult asthma prevalence, problems, and medical care. Ethn Health. 2009;14(5):527–52. https://doi.org/10.1080/13557850902954195.
10. Akinbami LJ, Moorman JE, Bailey C, Zahran HS, King M, Johnson CA, et al. Trends in asthma prevalence, health care use, and mortality in the United States, 2001–2010. NCHS Data Brief. 2012;(94):1–8.
11. Beck AF, Moncrief T, Huang B, Simmons JM, Sauers H, Chen C, et al. Inequalities in neighborhood child asthma admission rates and underlying community characteristics in one US county. J Pediatr. 2013;163(2):574–80. https://doi.org/10.1016/j.jpeds.2013.01.064.
12. Bhan N, Kawachi I, Glymour MM, Subramanian SV. Time trends in racial and ethnic disparities in asthma prevalence in the United States from the Behavioral Risk Factor Surveillance System (BRFSS) Study (1999–2011). Am J Public Health. 2015;105(6):1269–75. https://doi.org/10.2105/ajph.2014.302172.
13. Brim SN, Rudd RA, Funk RH, Callahan DB. Asthma prevalence among US children in underrepresented minority populations: American Indian/Alaska Native, Chinese, Filipino, and Asian Indian. Pediatrics. 2008;122(1):e217–22. https://doi.org/10.1542/peds.2007-3825.
14. Jensen ME, Gibson PG, Collins CE, Wood LG. Airway and systemic inflammation in obese children with asthma. Eur Respir J. 2013;42(4):1012–9. https://doi.org/10.1183/09031936.00124912.
15. Keet CA, McCormack MC, Pollack CE, Peng RD, McGowan E, Matsui EC. Neighborhood poverty, urban residence, race/ethnicity, and asthma: rethinking the inner-city asthma epidemic. J Allergy Clin Immunol. 2015;135(3):655–62. https://doi.org/10.1016/j.jaci.2014.11.022.

16. Largent J, Nickerson B, Cooper D, Delfino RJ. Paediatric asthma hospital utilization varies by demographic factors and area socio-economic status. Public Health. 2012;126(11):928–36. https://doi.org/10.1016/j.puhe.2012.04.011.
17. Abramson MJ, Puy RM, Weiner JM. Allergen immunotherapy for asthma. Cochrane Database Syst Rev. 2003;(4):CD001186. https://doi.org/10.1002/14651858.CD001186.
18. Roberts G, Hurley C, Turcanu V, Lack G. Grass pollen immunotherapy as an effective therapy for childhood seasonal allergic asthma. J Allergy Clin Immunol. 2006;117(2):263–8. https://doi.org/10.1016/j.jaci.2005.09.054.
19. Weinmayr G, Weiland SK, Bjorksten B, Brunekreef B, Buchele G, Cookson WO, et al. Atopic sensitization and the international variation of asthma symptom prevalence in children. Am J Respir Crit Care Med. 2007;176(6):565–74. https://doi.org/10.1164/rccm.200607-994OC.
20. Stingone JA, Claudio L. Disparities in allergy testing and health outcomes among urban children with asthma. J Allergy Clin Immunol. 2008;122(4):748–53. https://doi.org/10.1016/j.jaci.2008.08.001.
21. Bryant-Stephens T, Li Y. Community asthma education program for parents of urban asthmatic children. J Natl Med Assoc. 2004;96(7):954–60.
22. Krishna S, Francisco BD, Balas EA, Konig P, Graff GR, Madsen RW. Internet-enabled interactive multimedia asthma education program: a randomized trial. Pediatrics. 2003;111(3):503–10.
23. Piper CN, Elder K, Glover S, Baek JD, Murph K. Disparities between asthma management and insurance type among children. J Natl Med Assoc. 2010;102(7):556–61.
24. Piper CN, Elder K, Glover S, Baek JD. Racial influences associated with asthma management among children in the United States. Ethn Dis. 2008;18(2):225–7.
25. Diette GB, Skinner EA, Nguyen TT, Markson L, Clark BD, Wu AW. Comparison of quality of care by specialist and generalist physicians as usual source of asthma care for children. Pediatrics. 2001;108(2):432–7.
26. Vollmer WM, O'Hollaren M, Ettinger KM, Stibolt T, Wilkins J, Buist AS, et al. Specialty differences in the management of asthma. A cross-sectional assessment of allergists' patients and generalists' patients in a large HMO. Arch Intern Med. 1997;157(11):1201–8.
27. Cabana M, Bruckman D, Rushton JL, Bratton SL, Green L. Receipt of asthma subspecialty care by children in a managed care organization. Ambul Pediatr. 2002;2(6):456–61.
28. Flores G, Snowden-Bridon C, Torres S, Perez R, Walter T, Brotanek J, et al. Urban minority children with asthma: substantial morbidity, compromised quality and access to specialists, and the importance of poverty and specialty care. J Asthma. 2009;46(4):392–8. https://doi.org/10.1080/02770900802712971.
29. Piper CN, Glover S, Elder K, Baek JD, Wilkinson L. Disparities in access to care among asthmatic children in relation to race and socioeconomic status. J Child Health Care. 2010;14(3):271–9. https://doi.org/10.1177/1367493510371629.
30. Trivedi M, Fung V, Kharbanda EO, Larkin EK, Butler MG, Horan K, et al. Racial disparities in family-provider interactions for pediatric asthma care. J Asthma. 2018;55(4):424–9. https://doi.org/10.1080/02770903.2017.1337790.
31. Mitchell SJ, Bilderback AL, Okelo SO. Racial disparities in asthma morbidity among pediatric patients seeking asthma specialist care. Acad Pediatr. 2016;16(1):64–7. https://doi.org/10.1016/j.acap.2015.06.010.
32. Becker AB, Abrams EM. Asthma guidelines: the global initiative for asthma in relation to national guidelines. Curr Opin Allergy Clin Immunol. 2017;17(2):99–103. https://doi.org/10.1097/aci.0000000000000346.
33. Ferris TG, Kuhlthau K, Ausiello J, Perrin J, Kahn R. Are minority children the last to benefit from a new technology? Technology diffusion and inhaled corticosteroids for asthma. Med Care. 2006;44(1):81–6.
34. Kharat AA, Borrego ME, Raisch DW, Roberts MH, Blanchette CM, Petersen H. Assessing disparities in the receipt of inhaled corticosteroid prescriptions for asthma by Hispanic and non-Hispanic white patients. Ann Am Thorac Soc. 2015;12(2):174–83. https://doi.org/10.1513/AnnalsATS.201405-186OC.

35. Galbraith AA, Smith LA, Bokhour B, Miroshnik IL, Sawicki GS, Glauber JH, et al. Asthma care quality for children with minority-serving providers. Arch Pediatr Adolesc Med. 2010;164(1):38–45. https://doi.org/10.1001/archpediatrics.2009.243.
36. Shanawani H. Health disparities and differences in asthma: concepts and controversies. Clin Chest Med. 2006;27(1):17–28, v. https://doi.org/10.1016/j.ccm.2005.11.002.
37. Lieu TA, Lozano P, Finkelstein JA, Chi FW, Jensvold NG, Capra AM, et al. Racial/ethnic variation in asthma status and management practices among children in managed Medicaid. Pediatrics. 2002;109(5):857–65.
38. Stingone JA, Claudio L. Components of recommended asthma care and the use of long-term control medication among urban children with asthma. Med Care. 2009;47(9):940–7. https://doi.org/10.1097/MLR.0b013e318199300c.
39. Bender B, Zhang L. Negative affect, medication adherence, and asthma control in children. J Allergy Clin Immunol. 2008;122(3):490–5. https://doi.org/10.1016/j.jaci.2008.05.041.
40. Grant EN, Wagner R, Weiss KB. Observations on emerging patterns of asthma in our society. J Allergy Clin Immunol. 1999;104(2 Pt 2):S1–9.
41. Coventry JA, Weston MS, Collins PM. Emergency room encounters of pediatric patients with asthma: cost comparisons with other treatment settings. J Ambul Care Manage. 1996;19(2):9–21.
42. Weiss KB, Sullivan SD, Lyttle CS. Trends in the cost of illness for asthma in the United States, 1985-1994. J Allergy Clin Immunol. 2000;106(3):493–9. https://doi.org/10.1067/mai.2000.109426.
43. Ginde AA, Espinola JA, Camargo CA Jr. Improved overall trends but persistent racial disparities in emergency department visits for acute asthma, 1993–2005. J Allergy Clin Immunol. 2008;122(2):313–8. https://doi.org/10.1016/j.jaci.2008.04.024.
44. Kruse LK, Deshpande S, Vezina M. Disparities in asthma hospitalizations among children seen in the emergency department. J Asthma. 2007;44(10):833–7. https://doi.org/10.1080/02770900701750163.
45. Zhang Q, Lamichhane R, Diggs LA. Disparities in emergency department visits in American children with asthma: 2006–2010. J Asthma. 2017;54(7):679–86. https://doi.org/10.1080/02770903.2016.1263315.
46. Zook HG, Payne NR, Puumala SE, Ziegler KM, Kharbanda AB. Racial/ethnic variation in emergency department care for children with asthma. Pediatr Emerg Care. 2019;35(3):209–15. https://doi.org/10.1097/pec.0000000000001282.
47. Boudreaux ED, Emond SD, Clark S, Camargo CA Jr. Acute asthma among adults presenting to the emergency department: the role of race/ethnicity and socioeconomic status. Chest. 2003;124(3):803–12.
48. Franklin JM, Grunwell JR, Bruce AC, Smith RC, Fitzpatrick AM. Predictors of emergency department use in children with persistent asthma in metropolitan Atlanta, Georgia. Ann Allergy Asthma Immunol. 2017;119(2):129–36. https://doi.org/10.1016/j.anai.2017.04.008.
49. Roy SR, McGinty EE, Hayes SC, Zhang L. Regional and racial disparities in asthma hospitalizations in Mississippi. J Allergy Clin Immunol. 2010;125(3):636–42. https://doi.org/10.1016/j.jaci.2009.11.046.
50. Hughes HK, Matsui EC, Tschudy MM, Pollack CE, Keet CA. Pediatric asthma health disparities: race, hardship, housing, and asthma in a national survey. Acad Pediatr. 2017;17(2):127–34. https://doi.org/10.1016/j.acap.2016.11.011.
51. Peters AT, Klemens JC, Haselkorn T, Weiss ST, Grammer LC, Lee JH, et al. Insurance status and asthma-related health care utilization in patients with severe asthma. Ann Allergy Asthma Immunol. 2008;100(4):301–7. https://doi.org/10.1016/s1081-1206(10)60590-x.
52. Silber JH, Rosenbaum PR, Calhoun SR, Reiter JG, Hill AS, Guevara JP, et al. Racial disparities in medicaid asthma hospitalizations. Pediatrics. 2017;139(1). https://doi.org/10.1542/peds.2016-1221.
53. Milligan KL, Matsui E, Sharma H. Asthma in urban children: epidemiology, environmental risk factors, and the public health domain. Curr Allergy Asthma Rep. 2016;16(4):33. https://doi.org/10.1007/s11882-016-0609-6.

54. Williams DR, Sternthal M, Wright RJ. Social determinants: taking the social context of asthma seriously. Pediatrics. 2009;123(Suppl 3):S174–84. https://doi.org/10.1542/peds.2008-2233H.

55. Glick AF, Tomopoulos S, Fierman AH, Trasande L. Disparities in mortality and morbidity in pediatric asthma hospitalizations, 2007 to 2011. Acad Pediatr. 2016;16(5):430–7. https://doi.org/10.1016/j.acap.2015.12.014.

56. Winer RA, Qin X, Harrington T, Moorman J, Zahran H. Asthma incidence among children and adults: findings from the Behavioral Risk Factor Surveillance system asthma call-back survey--United States, 2006–2008. J Asthma. 2012;49(1):16–22. https://doi.org/10.3109/02770903.2011.637594.

57. Sidora-Arcoleo K, Yoos HL, McMullen A, Kitzman H. Complementary and alternative medicine use in children with asthma: prevalence and sociodemographic profile of users. J Asthma. 2007;44(3):169–75. https://doi.org/10.1080/02770900701209640.

58. Griffiths C, Kaur G, Gantley M, Feder G, Hillier S, Goddard J, et al. Influences on hospital admission for asthma in south Asian and white adults: qualitative interview study. BMJ. 2001;323(7319):962–6.

59. Law HZ, Oraka E, Mannino DM. The role of income in reducing racial and ethnic disparities in emergency room and urgent care center visits for asthma-United States, 2001-2009. J Asthma. 2011;48(4):405–13. https://doi.org/10.3109/02770903.2011.565849.

60. Chandra D, Clark S, Camargo CA Jr. Race/ethnicity differences in the inpatient management of acute asthma in the United States. Chest. 2009;135(6):1527–34. https://doi.org/10.1378/chest.08-1812.

61. Venkat A, Hasegawa K, Basior JM, Crandall C, Healy M, Inboriboon PC, et al. Race/ethnicity and asthma management among adults presenting to the emergency department. Respirology (Carlton). 2015;20(6):994–7. https://doi.org/10.1111/resp.12572.

62. Trent SA, Hasegawa K, Ramratnam SK, Bittner JC, Camargo CA Jr. Variation in asthma care at hospital discharge by race/ethnicity groups. J Asthma. 2017:1–10. https://doi.org/10.1080/02770903.2017.1378356.

63. Beck AF, Huang B, Auger KA, Ryan PH, Chen C, Kahn RS. Explaining racial disparities in child asthma readmission using a causal inference approach. JAMA Pediatr. 2016;170(7):695–703. https://doi.org/10.1001/jamapediatrics.2016.0269.

64. Beck AF, Huang B, Simmons JM, Moncrief T, Sauers HS, Chen C, et al. Role of financial and social hardships in asthma racial disparities. Pediatrics. 2014;133(3):431–9. https://doi.org/10.1542/peds.2013-2437.

65. Akinbami LJ, Moorman JE, Garbe PL, Sondik EJ. Status of childhood asthma in the United States, 1980–2007. Pediatrics. 2009;123(Suppl 3):S131–45. https://doi.org/10.1542/peds.2008-2233C.

66. Akinbami LJ, Moorman JE, Simon AE, Schoendorf KC. Trends in racial disparities for asthma outcomes among children 0 to 17 years, 2001–2010. J Allergy Clin Immunol. 2014;134(3):547–53.e5. https://doi.org/10.1016/j.jaci.2014.05.037.

67. Gupta RS, Carrion-Carire V, Weiss KB. The widening black/white gap in asthma hospitalizations and mortality. J Allergy Clin Immunol. 2006;117(2):351–8. https://doi.org/10.1016/j.jaci.2005.11.047.

68. Newacheck PW, Halfon N. Prevalence, impact, and trends in childhood disability due to asthma. Arch Pediatr Adolesc Med. 2000;154(3):287–93.

69. Grant EN, Lyttle CS, Weiss KB. The relation of socioeconomic factors and racial/ethnic differences in US asthma mortality. Am J Public Health. 2000;90(12):1923–5.

70. Mannino DM, Homa DM, Akinbami LJ, Moorman JE, Gwynn C, Redd SC. Surveillance for asthma--United States, 1980–1999. MMWR Surveill Summ. 2002;51(1):1–13.

71. Guilbert T, Zeiger RS, Haselkorn T, Iqbal A, Alvarez C, Mink DR, et al. Racial disparities in asthma-related health outcomes in children with severe/difficult-to-treat asthma. J Allergy Clin Immunol Pract. 2019;7(2):568–77. https://doi.org/10.1016/j.jaip.2018.07.050.

72. Haselkorn T, Lee JH, Mink DR, Weiss ST. Racial disparities in asthma-related health outcomes in severe or difficult-to-treat asthma. Ann Allergy Asthma Immunol. 2008;101(3):256–63. https://doi.org/10.1016/s1081-1206(10)60490-5.

73. Gold LS, Yeung K, Smith N, Allen-Ramey FC, Nathan RA, Sullivan SD. Asthma control, cost and race: results from a national survey. J Asthma. 2013;50(7):783–90. https://doi.org/10.3109/02770903.2013.795589.

74. Menezes AM, Wehrmeister FC, Hartwig FP, Perez-Padilla R, Gigante DP, Barros FC, et al. African ancestry, lung function and the effect of genetics. Eur Respir J. 2015;45(6):1582–9. https://doi.org/10.1183/09031936.00112114.

75. Federico MJ, Covar RA, Brown EE, Leung DY, Spahn JD. Racial differences in T-lymphocyte response to glucocorticoids. Chest. 2005;127(2):571–8. https://doi.org/10.1378/chest.127.2.571.

76. Gupta RS, Springston EE, Warrier MR, Smith B, Kumar R, Pongracic J, et al. The prevalence, severity, and distribution of childhood food allergy in the United States. Pediatrics. 2011;128(1):e9–17. https://doi.org/10.1542/peds.2011-0204.

77. Gupta RS, Warren CM, Smith BM, Blumenstock JA, Jiang J, Davis MM, et al. The public health impact of parent-reported childhood food allergies in the United States. Pediatrics. 2018;142(6). https://doi.org/10.1542/peds.2018-1235.

78. Liu AH, Jaramillo R, Sicherer SH, Wood RA, Bock SA, Burks AW, et al. National prevalence and risk factors for food allergy and relationship to asthma: results from the National Health and Nutrition Examination Survey 2005–2006. J Allergy Clin Immunol. 2010;126(4):798–806.e13. https://doi.org/10.1016/j.jaci.2010.07.026.

79. Mahdavinia M, Fox SR, Smith BM, James C, Palmisano EL, Mohammed C, et al. Racial differences in food allergy phenotype and health care utilization among US children. J Allergy Clin Immunol Pract. 2017;5(2):352–7.e1. https://doi.org/10.1016/j.jaip.2016.10.006.

80. Banerji A, Rudders SA, Corel B, Garth AP, Clark S, Camargo CA Jr. Predictors of hospital admission for food-related allergic reactions that present to the emergency department. Ann Allergy Asthma Immunol. 2011;106(1):42–8. https://doi.org/10.1016/j.anai.2010.10.011.

81. Harduar-Morano L, Simon MR, Watkins S, Blackmore C. A population-based epidemiologic study of emergency department visits for anaphylaxis in Florida. J Allergy Clin Immunol. 2011;128(3):594–600 e1. https://doi.org/10.1016/j.jaci.2011.04.049.

82. Lin RY, Anderson AS, Shah SN, Nurruzzaman F. Increasing anaphylaxis hospitalizations in the first 2 decades of life: New York State, 1990–2006. Ann Allergy Asthma Immunol. 2008;101(4):387–93. https://doi.org/10.1016/S1081-1206(10)60315-8.

83. Ross MP, Ferguson M, Street D, Klontz K, Schroeder T, Luccioli S. Analysis of food-allergic and anaphylactic events in the National Electronic Injury Surveillance System. J Allergy Clin Immunol. 2008;121(1):166–71. https://doi.org/10.1016/j.jaci.2007.10.012.

84. Rudders SA, Espinola JA, Camargo CA Jr. North-south differences in US emergency department visits for acute allergic reactions. Ann Allergy Asthma Immunol. 2010;104(5):413–6. https://doi.org/10.1016/j.anai.2010.01.022.

85. Greenhawt M, Weiss C, Conte ML, Doucet M, Engler A, Camargo CA Jr. Racial and ethnic disparity in food allergy in the United States: a systematic review. J Allergy Clin Immunol Pract. 2013;1(4):378–86. https://doi.org/10.1016/j.jaip.2013.04.009.

86. Gupta RS, Kim JS, Springston EE, Smith B, Pongracic JA, Wang X, et al. Food allergy knowledge, attitudes, and beliefs in the United States. Ann Allergy Asthma Immunol. 2009;103(1):43–50. https://doi.org/10.1016/S1081-1206(10)60142-1.

87. Johns CB, Savage JH. Access to health care and food in children with food allergy. J Allergy Clin Immunol. 2014;133(2):582–5. https://doi.org/10.1016/j.jaci.2013.12.006.

88. Hannaway PJ, Connelly ME, Cobbett RM, Dobrow PJ. Differences in race, ethnicity, and socioeconomic status in schoolchildren dispensed injectable epinephrine in 3 Massachusetts school districts. Ann Allergy Asthma Immunol. 2005;95(2):143–8. https://doi.org/10.1016/S1081-1206(10)61203-3.

89. Shah SS, Parker CL, O'Brian Smith E, Davis CM. Disparity in the availability of inject-able epinephrine in a large, diverse US school district. J Allergy Clin Immunol Pract. 2014;2(3):288–93.e1. https://doi.org/10.1016/j.jaip.2013.09.016.

90. Soller L, Fragapane J, Ben-Shoshan M, Harrington DW, Alizadehfar R, Joseph L, et al. Possession of epinephrine auto-injectors by Canadians with food allergies. J Allergy Clin Immunol. 2011;128(2):426–8. https://doi.org/10.1016/j.jaci.2011.05.015.

91. Szychlinski C, Schmeissing KA, Fuleihan Z, Qamar N, Syed M, Pongracic JA, et al. Food allergy emergency preparedness in Illinois schools: rural disparity in guideline imple-mentation. J Allergy Clin Immunol Pract. 2015;3(5):805–7.e8. https://doi.org/10.1016/j.jaip.2015.04.017.

92. Bilaver LA, Kester KM, Smith BM, Gupta RS. Socioeconomic disparities in the eco-nomic impact of childhood food allergy. Pediatrics. 2016;137(5). https://doi.org/10.1542/peds.2015-3678.

93. Odhiambo JA, Williams HC, Clayton TO, Robertson CF, Asher MI. Global variations in prev-alence of eczema symptoms in children from ISAAC Phase Three. J Allergy Clin Immunol. 2009;124(6):1251–8.e23. https://doi.org/10.1016/j.jaci.2009.10.009.

94. Kaufman BP, Guttman-Yassky E, Alexis AF. Atopic dermatitis in diverse racial and eth-nic groups-variations in epidemiology, genetics, clinical presentation and treatment. Exp Dermatol. 2018;27(4):340–57. https://doi.org/10.1111/exd.13514.

95. Shaw TE, Currie GP, Koudelka CW, Simpson EL. Eczema prevalence in the United States: data from the 2003 National Survey of Children's Health. J Invest Dermatol. 2011;131(1):67–73. https://doi.org/10.1038/jid.2010.251.

96. Abuabara K, Hoffstad O, Troxel AB, Gelfand JM, McCulloch CE, Margolis DJ. Patterns and predictors of atopic dermatitis disease control past childhood: an observational cohort study. J Allergy Clin Immunol. 2018;141(2):778–80.e6. https://doi.org/10.1016/j.jaci.2017.05.031.

97. Margolis JS, Abuabara K, Bilker W, Hoffstad O, Margolis DJ. Persistence of mild to mod-erate atopic dermatitis. JAMA Dermatol. 2014;150(6):593–600. https://doi.org/10.1001/jamadermatol.2013.10271.

98. Kim Y, Blomberg M, Rifas-Shiman SL, Camargo CA Jr, Gold DR, Thyssen JP, et al. Racial/ethnic differences in incidence and persistence of childhood atopic dermatitis. J Invest Dermatol. 2018. https://doi.org/10.1016/j.jid.2018.10.029.

99. Fischer AH, Shin DB, Margolis DJ, Takeshita J. Racial and ethnic differences in health care utilization for childhood eczema: an analysis of the 2001–2013 Medical Expenditure Panel Surveys. J Am Acad Dermatol. 2017;77(6):1060–7. https://doi.org/10.1016/j.jaad.2017.08.035.

100. Abokwidir M, Davis SA, Fleischer AB, Pichardo-Geisinger RO. Use of the emergency department for dermatologic care in the United States by ethnic group. J Dermatolog Treat. 2015;26(4):392–4. https://doi.org/10.3109/09546634.2014.991674.

101. Narla S, Hsu DY, Thyssen JP, Silverberg JI. Predictors of hospitalization, length of stay, and costs of care among adult and pediatric inpatients with atopic dermatitis in the United States. Dermatitis. 2018;29(1):22–31. https://doi.org/10.1097/der.0000000000000323.

102. Bhattacharya T, Silverberg JI. Efficacy of systemic treatments for atopic dermatitis in racial and ethnic minorities in the United States. JAMA Dermatol. 2014;150(11):1232–4. https://doi.org/10.1001/jamadermatol.2014.1674.

103. Charrow A, Xia FD, Joyce C, Mostaghimi A. Diversity in dermatology clinical trials: a sys-tematic review. JAMA Dermatol. 2017. https://doi.org/10.1001/jamadermatol.2016.4129.

104. Hirano SA, Murray SB, Harvey VM. Reporting, representation, and subgroup analy-sis of race and ethnicity in published clinical trials of atopic dermatitis in the United States between 2000 and 2009. Pediatr Dermatol. 2012;29(6):749–55. https://doi.org/10.1111/j.1525-1470.2012.01797.x.

105. Vachiramon V, Tey HL, Thompson AE, Yosipovitch G. Atopic dermatitis in African American children: addressing unmet needs of a common disease. Pediatr Dermatol. 2012;29(4):395–402. https://doi.org/10.1111/j.1525-1470.2012.01740.x.

106. Eichenfield LF, Lucky AW, Langley RG, Lynde C, Kaufmann R, Todd G, et al. Use of pimecrolimus cream 1% (Elidel) in the treatment of atopic dermatitis in infants and children: the effects of ethnic origin and baseline disease severity on treatment outcome. Int J Dermatol. 2005;44(1):70–5. https://doi.org/10.1111/j.1365-4632.2004.02234.x.

107. Kim KH, Kono T. Overview of efficacy and safety of tacrolimus ointment in patients with atopic dermatitis in Asia and other areas. Int J Dermatol. 2011;50(9):1153–61. https://doi.org/10.1111/j.1365-4632.2011.04881.x.

108. Meduri NB, Vandergriff T, Rasmussen H, Jacobe H. Phototherapy in the management of atopic dermatitis: a systematic review. Photodermatol Photoimmunol Photomed. 2007;23(4):106–12. https://doi.org/10.1111/j.1600-0781.2007.00291.x.

109. Syed ZU, Hamzavi IH. Role of phototherapy in patients with skin of color. Semin Cutan Med Surg. 2011;30(4):184–9. https://doi.org/10.1016/j.sder.2011.08.007.

110. Syed ZU, Hamzavi IH. Photomedicine and phototherapy considerations for patients with skin of color. Photodermatol Photoimmunol Photomed. 2011;27(1):10–6. https://doi.org/10.1111/j.1600-0781.2010.00554.x.

111. Jacobe HT, Cayce R, Nguyen J. UVA1 phototherapy is effective in darker skin: a review of 101 patients of Fitzpatrick skin types I-V. Br J Dermatol. 2008;159(3):691–6. https://doi.org/10.1111/j.1365-2133.2008.08672.x.

112. Mok ZR, Koh MJ, Chong WS. Is phototherapy useful in the treatment of atopic dermatitis in Asian children? A 5-year report from Singapore. Pediatr Dermatol. 2014;31(6):698–702. https://doi.org/10.1111/pde.12405.

113. Beck LA, Thaci D, Hamilton JD, Graham NM, Bieber T, Rocklin R, et al. Dupilumab treatment in adults with moderate-to-severe atopic dermatitis. N Engl J Med. 2014;371(2):130–9. https://doi.org/10.1056/NEJMoa1314768.

114. Blauvelt A, de Bruin-Weller M, Gooderham M, Cather JC, Weisman J, Pariser D, et al. Long-term management of moderate-to-severe atopic dermatitis with dupilumab and concomitant topical corticosteroids (LIBERTY AD CHRONOS): a 1-year, randomised, double-blinded, placebo-controlled, phase 3 trial. Lancet Lond Engl. 2017;389(10086):2287–303. https://doi.org/10.1016/s0140-6736(17)31191-1.

115. Simpson EL, Bieber T, Guttman-Yassky E, Beck LA, Blauvelt A, Cork MJ, et al. Two phase 3 trials of dupilumab versus placebo in atopic dermatitis. N Engl J Med. 2016;375(24):2335–48. https://doi.org/10.1056/NEJMoa1610020.

116. Clark S, Long AA, Gaeta TJ, Camargo CA Jr. Multicenter study of emergency department visits for insect sting allergies. J Allergy Clin Immunol. 2005;116(3):643–9. https://doi.org/10.1016/j.jaci.2005.06.026.

117. Golden DB, Demain J, Freeman T, Graft D, Tankersley M, Tracy J, et al. Stinging insect hypersensitivity: a practice parameter update 2016. Ann Allergy Asthma Immunol. 2017;118(1):28–54. https://doi.org/10.1016/j.anai.2016.10.031.

118. Golden DBK, Bernstein DI, Freeman TM, Tracy JM, Lang DM, Nicklas RA. AAAAI/ACAAI joint venom extract shortage task force report. J Allergy Clin Immunol Pract. 2017;5(2):330–2. https://doi.org/10.1016/j.jaip.2017.02.005.

119. Stoevesandt J, Trautmann A. Lessons from times of shortage: Interchangeability of venom preparations and dosing protocols. Allergy. 2019. https://doi.org/10.1111/all.13739.

Part II
Disparity on Allergic Conditions by Disease

Chapter 5
Disparity in Rhinitis and Rhinosinusitis

Alicia T. Widge and Anjeni Keswani

Nancy

Nancy is a 47-year-old white, single mother who is admitted to the medical intensive care unit (MICU) for significant respiratory distress and sepsis. Nancy lives in a small town in Pennsylvania with her four children where the closest hospital is almost 1 hour away. She has suffered from nasal polyps, asthma, and recurrent infections since she was 20 years old. For as long as she can remember, she has been unable to breathe well. It is almost impossible for her to breathe through her nose and she has no sense of smell. She suffers from recurrent sinus infections and recurrent "bronchitis." In the past year, her asthma was severely uncontrolled despite several courses of prednisone which she received from repeated ER visits. She saw an ear, nose, and throat (ENT) specialist 2 years ago who told her that she needed to undergo surgery for her nasal polyps and gave her two nasal sprays; however, it seemed nearly impossible to undergo the procedure, particularly because she would need almost five visits to the ENT office around that time and it is 65 minutes away from her work. She was also evaluated by an allergist/immunologist who ordered laboratory tests, as she suspected that there was something wrong with Nancy's immune system. However, she could not complete the blood work, as she had to head back home to her children. Her situation became more complicated when she lost her insurance coverage 1 month later. Nancy along with six other employees at the small supermarket where she worked was laid off when the supermarket went

A. T. Widge (✉)
National Institutes of Health, National Institute of Allergy and Infectious Diseases, Bethesda, MD, USA
e-mail: Alicia.Widge@NIH.gov

A. Keswani
GW School of Medicine & Health Sciences, Washington, DC, USA
e-mail: AKeswani@mfa.gwu.edu

© Springer Nature Switzerland AG 2020
M. Mahdavinia (ed.), *Health Disparities in Allergic Diseases*,
https://doi.org/10.1007/978-3-030-31222-0_5

out of business. Since then, she has worked two part-time jobs but does not have insurance and can hardly afford her medications. Yesterday, after a long day at work, while feeling feverish and suffering from headaches and shortness of breath, she drove herself to the ER. She was found to have severe pansinusitis, pneumonia, and low oxygen saturation. She was transferred to a tertiary care hospital in Pittsburgh and was admitted to the MICU.

Introduction

Rhinosinusitis is symptomatic inflammation of the paranasal sinuses and nasal cavity [1]. This condition is extremely common affecting one in eight adults in the United States with direct costs exceeding 11 billion dollars annually [1]. Socioeconomic, racial, and health insurance disparities are prevalent in the United States, and socioeconomic disparities are linked with higher mortality and worse health status [2]. Given the high prevalence and economic impact of rhinosinusitis, health disparities are likely to have a large effect on vulnerable populations. While disparities in patients with rhinosinusitis are underresearched and poorly understood, differences have been noted. Rhinosinusitis can be classified into acute versus chronic with etiologies including viruses, bacteria, environmental and seasonal allergens, and fungal triggers. The impact of health disparities on each will now be discussed.

Acute Rhinosinusitis

Acute rhinosinusitis (ARS) is defined as symptomatic inflammation of the nasal cavity and paranasal sinuses that lasts for less than 4 weeks [1]. ARS is extremely common in both adults and children with an estimated 20 million cases annually in the United States [3] and nearly a million pediatric visits in ambulatory and hospital settings [4]. ARS can be due to viral or bacterial etiologies, and differentiation has been the focus of recently renewed efforts to avoid overtreatment with antibiotics.

Complications including orbital or intracranial infection are rare, and most ARS visits are uncomplicated and can be managed in an outpatient setting with supportive care or oral antibiotics. Despite this, there are over 500,000 ED visits for ARS annually [5]. The prevalence of ED visits for ARS is associated with health insurance type and patient race independent of socioeconomic status. Both children and adults with Medicaid and self-pay utilize the ED more often than patients with private insurance [5, 6]. Multiple studies have shown an association between poor access to primary care and presentation to the ED for non-urgent conditions. Patients with lower socioeconomic status and those who are uninsured, underinsured, or have Medicaid tend to lack access to outpatient care, resulting in unnecessary ED utilization [7–9]. Medicaid and uninsured populations use overall less care for acute rhinosinusitis, but present disproportionately to the ED overnight and on weekends for uncomplicated ARS, indicating that barriers to healthcare access are likely to blame for ED overuse among these populations [10]. Using the ER for conditions that can be managed in the outpatient setting has an economic impact on overall healthcare spending and costs to individuals in terms of direct ER costs and indirect costs of lost time and productivity.

The reasons for differing ER utilization by insurance type for ARS is not clear; however, there is evidence to suggest that it is not related to disease severity. Medicaid patients have similar ARS symptomatology and levels of pain compared to privately insured patients; thus, symptomatology alone does not account for their disproportionate ED use. Furthermore, no difference was found in quality of care by insurance status to explain this increased ED utilization. Medicaid and self-insured patients received the same quality of care, and Medicaid patients spent more time with their doctor during visits for ARS than those with private insurance. Therefore, barriers to outpatient care are likely related to impaired access to primary care and after-hours outpatient care [11].

There are also differences in ER utilization for ARS by race. African American patients more likely present to the ED, even after adjustment for other socioeconomic variables [5]. There are racial differences in symptomatology. African American and Hispanic patients are more likely to have atypical symptoms with a lack of classic sinonasal symptoms than white patients. This may make it more difficult for these patients to accurately identify the source of their symptoms and result in their seeking ED care more commonly [12]. Symptomatology alone is unlikely to explain these racial differences, which are likely a combination of environmental differences, affordability, and access to care, genetic differences in disease progression, and cultural factors.

Complications of ARS are rare but can include preseptal or orbital cellulitis, orbital or subperiosteal abscesses, and intracranial complications like cavernous sinus thrombosis, intracranial abscesses, and meningitis. Children from higher socioeconomic status experience more frequent complications from acute bacterial sinusitis, but Medicaid and self-pay patients, markers of low socioeconomic status (SES), have higher intracranial complications, which are more severe [13]. Since patients with Medicaid and self-pay status are likely to have decreased access to primary care and timely preventative care [14, 15], they may be presenting with more severe manifestation of this disease. Children from low-income families with Medicaid or no health insurance are less likely to receive preventative care and therefore are more likely to present at advanced disease stages for a variety of conditions [16, 17]. Diagnostic imaging varies by SES with individuals from smaller metropolitan areas and lower median income significantly less likely to get a CT scan in the ED for sinusitis [18, 19].

There is some conflicting evidence regarding health disparities and ARS, and at least one study did not find a statistically significant association between acute sinusitis resource utilization and charges and insurance status or race [20] and another study which did not find differences in rates of surgical intervention in children based on SES or race [21].

Chronic Rhinosinusitis (CRS)

Chronic rhinosinusitis (CRS) is a common chronic disease affecting 2–16% of the population [22], and pediatric CRS affects 2.1% of children [23]. Symptoms include nasal obstruction, mucopurulent drainage, facial pain and pressure, and hyposmia lasting at least 12 weeks with evidence of nasal inflammation on examination or imaging [1]. CRS is most prevalent in adults between the age of 40 and 64 years and is more common in women (59%) than in men and in patients with asthma, chronic obstructive pulmonary disease, and allergic sensitization. Patients with CRS have significantly diminished quality of life with negative impacts on sleep quality, cognition, mood, and psychologic functioning [24]. Symptoms can be debilitating resulting in loss of productivity [25] and missed days of work and school with high individual and societal costs, particularly as CRS tends to affect patients within their most productive work years [24, 26]. There are geographic differences in CRS, which is more common in the Midwestern and Southern United States compared to the Northeastern and West [22]. The etiology of CRS is a combination of atopy, immune dysregulation, microbiome, and impaired mucociliary clearance with the end result of uncontrolled inflammation. As CRS is a common chronic medical condition that entails significant direct costs of medical visits, diagnostic expenses, medical therapy, and surgical costs in addition to indirect costs of lost productivity and work absenteeism, disparities may significantly impact racial minorities and socioeconomically disadvantaged populations.

Currently Existing Disparities in Rhinosinusitis

There are racial and ethnic differences in insurance status, specialist visits, and treatments for patients with CRS [27]. African American adults have the highest frequency of sinusitis (13.8%) and highest rates of work absenteeism (23%). More Hispanics and African Americans with CRS are uninsured and are more likely to delay medical care because of cost-related concerns compared with white and Asian adults [27]. White patients are more likely to have been seen by a specialist or received surgical treatment [27].

Social determinants of health are associated with utilization of tertiary care rhinology services. In children with CRS, white and privately insured patients are most likely to be seen by a tertiary care center otolaryngologist. Income, education level, insurance status, and white race were found to be associated with tertiary rhinology utilization, though the only independent predictor was education level [28]. White patients are more likely than African Americans to be seen by a specialist or receive surgery despite having similar rates of sinusitis [27]. These differences may be due to differences in access, perception of disease severity, or differences in the course and presentation of the disease [29].

In terms of differences in disease severity, lower SES is associated with higher subjective CRS symptomatology [30]. Hispanic patients report statistically significant worse baseline scores on the Rhinosinusitis Disability Instrument after controlling for socioeconomic factors; however, they did not report comparatively worse scores on the Chronic Sinus Survey (CSS) instrument, CT, or endoscopy [27]. Improvements in olfactory function and quality of life after surgical intervention also vary by SES with patients with the highest household income more than twice as likely to experience a clinically meaningful QOL improvement [31].

Similar to ARS, there are conflicting studies that do not show differences. One study did not find disparities in severity and previous medical management with regard to race/ethnicity, education status, or income level as determined by zip code; however, this was a disproportionately white population that self-referred to a tertiary care center in Massachusetts, a state which has higher than average insurance levels [32].

A recent systematic review concluded that there is a distinct association between CRS and low SES. This study also concluded that poor housing conditions with older housing, more environmental pollutants, and dampness are also associated with CRS prevalence and severity. The association between education level and CRS was less clear [33].

Overall, while data are limited, current evidence indicates that there are both racial and socioeconomic differences in the prevalence and treatment of CRS, and racial disparities are still seen even when controlling for socioeconomic variables.

Allergic Sensitization

Allergic sensitization is an important contributing factor to both chronic and acute rhinosinusitis. In CRS especially, there is a high prevalence of allergic sensitization to aeroallergens (50–85%) [34–38]. There are racial and socioeconomic differences in aeroallergen sensitization. A small number of studies have reported differing aeroallergen sensitization patterns with African American children and adults experiencing more sensitization to both food and aeroallergens than white patients; however, there is little consistency in which aeroallergens are most prevalent, and little is known about sensitization rates in other racial and ethnic minorities. One study done in Atlanta found that aeroallergen sensitization profiles differed between African American and white children after controlling for socioeconomic variables and geographic residential features by zip code. In white children, dust mite sensitization, pet sensitization, and a higher prevalence of indoor pet ownership predicted ED use, whereas in African American children, mold sensitization predicted ED use [39]. Another study of middle-class children in Suburban Detroit also found that African American children were more likely to be sensitized than white children to ragweed and bluegrass. This study compared children of similar socioeconomic status living in the same suburban city [40]. Another study found that in children with asthma, Puerto Rican ethnicity is associated with an increased risk of sensitization to indoor and outdoor allergens including cockroach, dust mite, mixed grass pollen, and mugwort/sage. They also found that African Americans have higher sensitization to outdoor allergens that included mixed tree and grass pollen, mugwort/sage, and ragweed [41].

African American women are more than twice as likely to be sensitized to at least three aeroallergens than white women. African American and Hispanic women were also found to be more likely to have asthma; however, they were less likely to have seasonal allergic rhinitis and eczema than white women [42]. Another study supported these findings that African American women were more likely than white woman to be sensitized to aeroallergens and have higher total IgE levels and a diagnosis of asthma, but are less likely to have seasonal allergic rhinitis and eczema than white women. These associations persisted after controlling for socioeconomic and environmental variables [43].

The etiology of these differences and the roles of genetics, socioeconomic, and other factors that contribute to these observed differences is not well understood, but current evidence and scientific reasoning do not indicate that genetics plays an overwhelming role in observed racial disparities [44]. Environmental exposure is a likely causal candidate; however, in many studies, differences persist even after adjusting for key environmental factors like allergen and endotoxin levels in home dust [44].

Allergic Fungal Rhinosinusitis (AFRS)

Several studies have found that allergic fungal rhinosinusitis (AFRS) is more common and more aggressive in African American males [45] with a higher incidence of AFRS in African American, uninsured, and Medicaid patients even after adjusting for socioeconomic factors such as insurance, education, and income [46]. Furthermore, African American adults have more severe symptoms from allergic fungal sinusitis, tend to present later in disease course, and have greater improvement after surgery than white patients [47]. However, other studies have not found an association with bone erosion and low SES [48]. A more recent study in a larger cohort found that disease severity was associated with lower SES by county level, but not by race, indicating that there are likely contributions of poor-quality housing and access to healthcare [49].

Conclusion and Final Remarks

There are many limitations to the current evidence on rhinosinusitis and health disparities. Only a small number of studies have been longitudinal, and there is a lack of standardized definitions, databases, and methods used to identify trends [33]. National administration databases, for example, the Nationwide Emergency

Department Sample database, Kids' Inpatient Database, and the National Hospital Ambulatory Medical Care Survey, do not report actual income level, but rather infer medical income level of the child's zip code. Much of the research to date utilizes ICD-9 coding, which can introduce biases due to incorrect coding. Most databases do not include data from all 50 states, and many are limited to a single city or geographic area, limiting generalizability [50]. There are significant differences in study methods, definitions, and measures used for SES and databases from which information was drawn, making it difficult to fully generalize findings [33].

Despite these limitations, the data still show important trends. Several studies have shown that there is a clear link between low SES and the prevalence and incidence of rhinosinusitis [33]. It is well known that economically advantaged patients have greater access to medical care and greater health literacy and that minorities and those with lower SES tend to delay medical care due to cost-related concerns, job security, and transportation concerns. Rhinosinusitis is an incredibly common condition with significant potential morbidity; therefore, health disparities are likely to have a large effect. The reasons behind these racial and SES differences are not completely clear. Controlling for socioeconomic factors like income, education, and insurance status will often account for some, but not all of, health differences by race [51]. Given the lack of true biological differences by race to account for this difference, there is likely residual confounding from undefined variables [27].

In case of our patient, Nancy, her disease poor outcome and significant morbidity could have been prevented by proper treatment and follow-up which were impacted by SES-related obstacles and low resources. Increasing our understanding of the existence of health disparities in the prevalence, treatment, and complications of rhinosinusitis can shape treatment decisions and affect patient outcomes.

References

1. Rosenfeld RM, Piccirillo JF, Chandrasekhar SS, Brook I, Kumar KA, Kramper M, et al. Clinical practice guideline (update): Adult Sinusitis Executive Summary. Otolaryngol Head Neck Surg. 2015;152(4):598–609.
2. Bor J, Cohen GH, Galea S. Population health in an era of rising income inequality: USA, 1980-2015. Lancet. 2017;389(10077):1475–90.
3. Anon JB, Jacobs MR, Poole MD, Ambrose PG, Benninger MS, Hadley JA, et al. Antimicrobial treatment guidelines for acute bacterial rhinosinusitis. Otolaryngol Head Neck Surg. 2004;130(1 Suppl):1–45.
4. Shapiro DJ, Gonzales R, Cabana MD, Hersh AL. National trends in visit rates and antibiotic prescribing for children with acute sinusitis. Pediatrics. 2011;127(1):28–34.
5. Scangas GA, Ishman SL, Bergmark RW, Cunningham MJ, Sedaghat AR. Emergency department presentation for uncomplicated acute rhinosinusitis is associated with poor access to healthcare. Laryngoscope. 2015;125(10):2253–8.
6. Bergmark RW, Ishman SL, Phillips KM, Cunningham MJ, Sedaghat AR. Emergency department use for acute rhinosinusitis: insurance dependent for children and adults. Laryngoscope. 2018;128(2):299–303.
7. Andrulis DP. Access to care is the centerpiece in the elimination of socioeconomic disparities in health. Ann Intern Med. 1998;129(5):412–6.

8. Kellermann AL, Weinick RM. Emergency departments, Medicaid costs, and access to primary care--understanding the link. N Engl J Med. 2012;366(23):2141–3.
9. Fiscella K, Franks P, Gold MR, Clancy CM. Inequality in quality: addressing socioeconomic, racial, and ethnic disparities in health care. JAMA. 2000;283(19):2579 84.
10. Bergmark RW, Ishman SL, Scangas GA, Cunningham MJ, Sedaghat AR. Socioeconomic determinants of overnight and weekend emergency department use for acute rhinosinusitis. Laryngoscope. 2015;125(11):2441–6.
11. Bergmark RW, Ishman SL, Scangas GA, Cunningham MJ, Sedaghat AR. Insurance status and quality of outpatient care for uncomplicated acute rhinosinusitis. JAMA Otolaryngol Head Neck Surg. 2015;141(6):505–11.
12. Bergmark RW, Sedaghat AR. Presentation to Emergency Departments for acute rhinosinusitis: disparities in symptoms by race and insurance status. Otolaryngol Head Neck Surg. 2016;155(5):790–6.
13. Sedaghat AR, Wilke CO, Cunningham MJ, Ishman SL. Socioeconomic disparities in the presentation of acute bacterial sinusitis complications in children. Laryngoscope. 2014;124(7):1700–6.
14. Feinberg E, Swartz K, Zaslavsky A, Gardner J, Walker DK. Family income and the impact of a children's health insurance program on reported need for health services and unmet health need. Pediatrics. 2002;109(2):E29.
15. Newacheck PW, Stoddard JJ, Hughes DC, Pearl M. Health insurance and access to primary care for children. N Engl J Med. 1998;338(8):513–9.
16. Skinner AC, Mayer ML. Effects of insurance status on children's access to specialty care: a systematic review of the literature. BMC Health Serv Res. 2007;7:194.
17. Todd J, Armon C, Griggs A, Poole S, Berman S. Increased rates of morbidity, mortality, and charges for hospitalized children with public or no health insurance as compared with children with private insurance in Colorado and the United States. Pediatrics. 2006;118(2):577–85.
18. Sethi RK, Kozin ED, Naunheim MR, Rosen M, Shrime MG, Sedaghat AR, et al. Variable utilization patterns of computed tomography for rhinosinusitis in emergency departments. Laryngoscope. 2017;127(3):537–43.
19. Sedaghat AR, Cunningham MJ, Ishman SL. Regional and socioeconomic disparities in emergency department use of radiographic imaging for acute pediatric sinusitis. Am J Rhinol Allergy. 2014;28(1):23–8.
20. Dugar DR, Lander L, Mahalingam-Dhingra A, Shah RK. Pediatric acute sinusitis: predictors of increased resource utilization. Laryngoscope. 2010;120(11):2313–21.
21. Mahalingam-Dhingra A, Lander L, Preciado DA, Taylormoore J, Shah RK. Orbital and periorbital infections: a national perspective. Arch Otolaryngol Head Neck Surg. 2011;137(8):769–73.
22. Halawi AM, Smith SS, Chandra RK. Chronic rhinosinusitis: epidemiology and cost. Allergy Asthma Proc. 2013;34(4):328–34.
23. Gilani S, Shin JJ. The burden and visit prevalence of pediatric chronic rhinosinusitis. Otolaryngol Head Neck Surg. 2017;157(6):1048–52.
24. DeConde AS, Soler ZM. Chronic rhinosinusitis: epidemiology and burden of disease. Am J Rhinol Allergy. 2016;30(2):134–9.
25. Rudmik L, Smith TL, Schlosser RJ, Hwang PH, Mace JC, Soler ZM. Productivity costs in patients with refractory chronic rhinosinusitis. Laryngoscope. 2014;124(9):2007–12.
26. Phillips KM, Hoehle LP, Bergmark RW, Caradonna DS, Gray ST, Sedaghat AR. Acute exacerbations mediate quality of life impairment in chronic rhinosinusitis. J Allergy Clin Immunol Pract. 2017;5(2):422–6.
27. Soler ZM, Mace JC, Litvack JR, Smith TL. Chronic rhinosinusitis, race, and ethnicity. Am J Rhinol Allergy. 2012;26(2):110–6.
28. Samuelson MB, Chandra RK, Turner JH, Russell PT, Francis DO. The relationship between social determinants of health and utilization of tertiary rhinology care. Am J Rhinol Allergy. 2017;31(6):376–81.

29. Smith DF, Ishman SL, Tunkel DE, Boss EF. Chronic rhinosinusitis in children: race and socio-economic status. Otolaryngol Head Neck Surg. 2013;149(4):639–44.
30. Kilty SJ, McDonald JT, Johnson S, Al-Mutairi D. Socioeconomic status: a disease modifier of chronic rhinosinusitis? Rhinology. 2011;49(5):533–7.
31. Beswick DM, Mace JC, Rudmik L, Soler ZM, Alt JA, Smith KA, et al. Socioeconomic factors impact quality of life outcomes and olfactory measures in chronic rhinosinusitis. Int Forum Allergy Rhinol. 2018;9:231.
32. Bergmark RW, Hoehle LP, Chyou D, Phillips KM, Caradonna DS, Gray ST, et al. Association of Socioeconomic Status, Race and Insurance Status with chronic rhinosinusitis patient-reported outcome measures. Otolaryngol Head Neck Surg. 2018;158(3):571–9.
33. Geramas I, Terzakis D, Hatzimanolis E, Georgalas C. Social factors in the development of chronic rhinosinusitis: a systematic review. Curr Allergy Asthma Rep. 2018;18(2):7.
34. Steinke JW, Borish L. Chronic rhinosinusitis phenotypes. Ann Allergy Asthma Immunol. 2016;117(3):234–40.
35. Sedaghat AR, Phipatanakul W, Cunningham MJ. Prevalence of and associations with allergic rhinitis in children with chronic rhinosinusitis. Int J Pediatr Otorhinolaryngol. 2014;78(2):343–7.
36. Gutman M, Torres A, Keen KJ, Houser SM. Prevalence of allergy in patients with chronic rhinosinusitis. Otolaryngol Head Neck Surg. 2004;130(5):545–52.
37. Tan BK, Zirkle W, Chandra RK, Lin D, Conley DB, Peters AT, et al. Atopic profile of patients failing medical therapy for chronic rhinosinusitis. Int Forum Allergy Rhinol. 2011;1(2):88–94.
38. Rosati MG, Peters AT. Relationships among allergic rhinitis, asthma, and chronic rhinosinusitis. Am J Rhinol Allergy. 2016;30(1):44–7.
39. Franklin JM, Grunwell JR, Bruce AC, Smith RC, Fitzpatrick AM. Predictors of emergency department use in children with persistent asthma in metropolitan Atlanta, Georgia. Ann Allergy Asthma Immunol. 2017;119(2):129–36.
40. Joseph CL, Peterson EL, Johnson CC, Ownby DR. Racial differences in allergen sensitivity. Chest. 2004;126(3):1004–5; author reply 5.
41. Celedon JC, Sredl D, Weiss ST, Pisarski M, Wakefield D, Cloutier M. Ethnicity and skin test reactivity to aeroallergens among asthmatic children in Connecticut. Chest. 2004;125(1):85–92.
42. Litonjua AA, Celedon JC, Hausmann J, Nikolov M, Sredl D, Ryan L, et al. Variation in total and specific IgE: effects of ethnicity and socioeconomic status. J Allergy Clin Immunol. 2005;115(4):751–7.
43. Wegienka G, Joseph CL, Havstad S, Zoratti E, Ownby D, Johnson CC. Sensitization and allergic histories differ between black and white pregnant women. J Allergy Clin Immunol. 2012;130(3):657–62.e2.
44. Wegienka G, Johnson CC, Zoratti E, Havstad S. Racial differences in allergic sensitization: recent findings and future directions. Curr Allergy Asthma Rep. 2013;13(3):255–61.
45. Wise SK, Venkatraman G, Wise JC, DelGaudio JM. Ethnic and gender differences in bone erosion in allergic fungal sinusitis. Am J Rhinol. 2004;18(6):397–404.
46. Wise SK, Ghegan MD, Gorham E, Schlosser RJ. Socioeconomic factors in the diagnosis of allergic fungal rhinosinusitis. Otolaryngol Head Neck Surg. 2008;138(1):38–42.
47. Champagne JP, Antisdel JL, Woodard TD, Kountakis SE. Epidemiologic factors affect surgical outcomes in allergic fungal sinusitis. Laryngoscope. 2010;120(11):2322–4.
48. Ghegan MD, Wise SK, Gorham E, Schlosser RJ. Socioeconomic factors in allergic fungal rhinosinusitis with bone erosion. Am J Rhinol. 2007;21(5):560–3.
49. Miller JD, Deal AM, McKinney KA, McClurg SW, Rodriguez KD, Thorp BD, et al. Markers of disease severity and socioeconomic factors in allergic fungal rhinosinusitis. Int Forum Allergy Rhinol. 2014;4(4):272–9.
50. Mehta VJ, Ling JD, Mawn LA. Socioeconomic disparities in the presentation of acute bacterial sinusitis complications in the pediatric population. Semin Ophthalmol. 2016;31(4):405–8.
51. Williams DR. The health of U.S. racial and ethnic populations. J Gerontol B Psychol Sci Soc Sci. 2005;60 Spec No 2:53–62.

Chapter 6
Disparities in Food Allergy

Ulyana Trytko, Hassan A. Ahmad, Leena Padhye, and Mary C. Tobin

Case History

Mike is a 6-year-old African American boy with moderate persistent asthma who presents to the emergency department with severe swelling of his face and tongue, shortness of breath, stridor, and hypotension. On arrival, his blood pressure is 90/40, heart rate is 98 beats per minute, respiratory rate is 25 breaths per minute, and oxygen saturation is 88% on room air. On physical exam, he appears lethargic and is unable to speak. He also has wheezing in all lung fields. Intramuscular epinephrine, diphenhydramine, and methylprednisolone are administered as anaphylaxis is suspected. Supplemental oxygen and intravenous fluids are also started. As he continues to appear lethargic with no improvement in oxygen saturation, he is emergently intubated and placed on mechanical ventilation. Once stabilized, you approach an anxious-appearing young woman standing near his bedside. You soon learn that this young woman is Mike's older sister, Kathia, who is 18 years old. She tells you that their mother is at work for another 5 hours and she has not been able to reach her. You learn that Mike has five siblings, all raised by a single mother, of whom Kathia is the oldest. Kathia informs you that Mike was diagnosed with peanut allergy several years ago but has been unable to follow up with his doctor. He has had multiple episodes of severe reactions since diagnosis due to accidental ingestion of different foods that possibly had peanuts in them. The older sister expresses frustration with herself, stating "I should have looked at the ingredients closer." You wonder how to prevent another episode of anaphylaxis, whether he will survive another severe reaction and if other undiagnosed food allergies may be present.

U. Trytko · H. A. Ahmad · L. Padhye · M. C. Tobin (✉)
Rush University Medical Center, Department of Internal Medicine,
Division of Allergy/Immunology, Chicago, IL, USA
e-mail: Ulyana_Trytko@rush.edu; Hassan_A_Ahmad@rush.edu;
Leena_Padhye@rush.edu; Mary_Tobin@rush.edu

© Springer Nature Switzerland AG 2020
M. Mahdavinia (ed.), *Health Disparities in Allergic Diseases*,
https://doi.org/10.1007/978-3-030-31222-0_6

Introduction

Food allergy is defined as an adverse health effect originating from a reproducible immune phenomenon on reexposure to a given food. The reaction typically occurs within minutes of ingesting the food due to recognition by food-specific IgE antibodies [2]. This adverse health event can range from very mild symptoms like pruritus and minimal swelling of the lips to a potential life-threatening event, anaphylaxis. When estimating the true prevalence of food allergy, it is important to recognize the difference between food allergy and food sensitization. According to the National Institute of Allergy and Infectious Disease, food sensitization occurs when an individual has made a specific IgE antibody to a food allergen but does not have clinical symptoms consistent with an allergic reaction after ingesting this food allergen [3]. Currently, the most common food allergens to cause food allergy include milk, egg, wheat, soy, peanut, tree nuts, shellfish, and fish [4]. While allergies to milk, egg, wheat, and soy may decrease with age, allergies to peanut, tree nuts, shellfish, and finfish typically persist into adulthood [4]. Increasing serum IgE to a specific food suggests a lower probability of outgrowing that food allergy over time, while decreasing levels imply a more likely resolution [4].

Currently Existing Disparities in Food Allergy

Prevalence

Food allergy prevalence has been increasing significantly over the last decade in the United States and worldwide. The prevalence appears to be related to multiple factors including geography. The current US data shows that the estimated patient-reported food allergy prevalence is about 8%, after excluding patients whose reaction history was inconsistent with an IgE-mediated reaction [1]. Keet et al. demonstrated that self-reported prevalence of food allergy in children increased 1.2 percentage points (95% CI 0.7–1.6) per 10-year period between 1988 and 2011 [5]. Prescott et al. launched a survey utilizing a standardized questionnaire via the World Allergy Organization including 89 countries in Europe, Asia, Oceania, the Americas, Africa, and the Middle East in an attempt to estimate the prevalence of FA worldwide. In infants and preschoolers, occurrence ranged from 2.5% to 5% in Sweden, France, Japan, and Taiwan to a high of 10% in Finland and Canada. In children older than 5 years, there was marked variation among countries with reports of 10–15% in Italy, Ghana, Columbia, Lithuania, Iceland, Tanzania, and Mozambique to less than 5% in Kenya, France, Estonia, Israel, and Australia [6]. There are many variables in these studies which can contribute to the wide range of FA prevalence. The HealthNuts study from Australia found an interesting correlation that might help explain the variation in FA prevalence. They demonstrated that high rates of food allergy were correlated to egg allergy in infancy [7]. It is thought that perhaps relating the specific food antigens commonly seen in a particular country to various geographic areas may provide additional insight for the FA differences [8].

Discrepancies in prevalence among various racial and ethnic groups have also been recognized. One report found the increase in self-reported food allergy prevalence in the last two decades varied by race: Non-Hispanic Blacks experienced 2.1% increase per decade compared to 1.2% among Hispanics and 1.0% in non-Hispanic Whites [5]. In a systematic review of multiple studies, Black children have been identified as more likely to have food allergy and sensitivity, but study limitations prohibited a definitive conclusion [2, 9]. Black patients do have a higher rate of self-reported food allergy as opposed to White patients [2, 5]. This finding suggests that genetic and environmental factors, including dietary influences and socioeconomic status, play a role in the immune-pathogenesis of food allergies. These influences may, in turn, play a role in the racial disparities reported in the literature. For instance, Taveras et al. showed a significant difference in breastfeeding rates and timing of introduction of solid foods among White, Black, and Hispanic children. Solid food introduction prior to 4 months of age was more common among Black and Hispanic children as opposed to White [10]. Environmental differences in exposure also appear to play a role in the expression of food allergy. Exposure to house dust mite and cockroach allergens, widespread in inner cities, appears to impact sensitization to shellfish and finfish [11, 12]. There is a high sequence homology identified between tropomyosin from fish and shellfish and house dust mites and cockroaches [12, 13]. This connection suggests that inhaled tropomyosin from cockroach and house dust mites act as sensitizers for fish and shellfish allergy which is often seen among minorities in inner cities. Exploring such dietary and environmental connections, in addition to genetics, can help us to better understand causes of food allergy and influence preventive strategies.

As mentioned earlier, understanding specific FA as it impacts multiple ethnic groups might give us clarity related to prevalence. In a retrospective review of a cohort of low-income minority patients from East Harlem, Taylor-Black and Wang reported peanut allergy prevalence was the highest at 1.6%, followed by allergies to shellfish (1.1%), tree nut (0.8%), egg (0.8%), milk (0.5%), fish (0.3%), fruit (0.3%), soy (0.2%), and wheat (0.06%) [14]. In this same study, anaphylaxis was seen in 15.1% of patients with peanut allergy, 12.5% with fish allergy, 11.1% with milk allergy, and 10.4% with tree nut allergy. The authors also found that Black children had significantly higher rates of allergy to peanut, shellfish, and tree nuts than Hispanic and multiracial children [14]. In a self-reported telephone survey, shellfish allergy was reported at a higher rate among Black than White individuals (3.1% vs 1.8%) [15]. Similarly, Branum et al. showed that non-Hispanic Black children had a significantly higher proportion of sensitization to shrimp, milk, and egg than non-Hispanic White children [16]. Mahdavinia et al., however, found that while peanut, egg, and milk allergy was similar among Black, Hispanic, and White children, rates of allergy to shellfish, corn, and fish were significantly higher in Hispanic and Black children [17]. These findings are crucial to explore further as the aforementioned foods are staples in these communities and thus difficult to avoid, particularly for low-income families. Furthermore, evaluation of these disparities in food allergy may lead to decreased accidental exposures and anaphylaxis rates in vulnerable groups [18].

Outcomes Related to Disparities in Food Allergy

Morbidity

The current approach to avoiding emergency room visits and hospitalizations is based on allergen avoidance and education on proper treatment of reactions [4]. Black and Hispanic patients have been found to have significantly higher odds of emergency room visits for food-induced reactions than White children [18]. A previous study found major discrepancies in injectable epinephrine dispersion rates among different races. White students were more likely to have been dispensed injectable epinephrine than non-Whites; this relation was also found for children with peanut, tree nut, and stinging insect allergy [19]. In another study, Medicaid-enrolled children presenting to the emergency room with food-induced anaphylaxis were less likely to receive epinephrine before the arrival to the emergency room than patients who were self-pay or had private insurance [12]. These findings are important as early treatment with epinephrine for food-induced anaphylaxis is associated with lower risk of hospitalization [20] which ultimately results in less patient morbidity and lower societal costs for treatment of food allergy.

Food Allergy-Related Anaphylaxis Hospitalizations for anaphylaxis have increased fourfold among young people in recent years [21]. Multiple studies have evaluated the risk of anaphylaxis among minorities and found increased risk among Black patients. Jeschow et al. showed that Black females are at a nearly twofold greater risk of food allergy-related anaphylaxis than Caucasian females and that males are at a threefold greater risk than their Caucasian counterparts [22]. This was also found in a study by Mahdavinia et al.: Black and Hispanic children had significantly higher rates of food-induced anaphylaxis than White children [17]. Further, a retrospective review of death certificates from the US National Mortality Database showed a higher rate of food-related anaphylaxis fatalities among Blacks compared to Caucasians [22]. Minority patients are at increased risk of food allergy-associated anaphylaxis compared to White patients. The exact cause of this observation is unclear. While it is plausible that minority patients may have increased exposure to accidental ingestions and thus greater chance for anaphylaxis to occur, it is also possible that there may be a distinct pathophysiology based on genetic factors that presents as a more severe phenotype. In addition, Taylor-Black and Wang found that while about 80% of food-allergic low-income minority patients have an epinephrine auto-injector prescription, only 40% had a food allergy emergency action plan [14]. This shows that while high-risk patients may have a lifesaving tool at their disposal, the educational component may be lacking and explain the higher rates of anaphylaxis reported. It appears that the absence of long-term allergy follow-up and the lack of food allergy action plans with instructions for the use of epinephrine auto-injectors may all contribute to the higher rate of anaphylaxis in low-income patients.

Cost

Due to the direct and indirect costs to families and the healthcare infrastructure, it is clear that food allergy is an important public health matter. In 2011–2012, food allergy prevention and treatment cost an estimated $25 billion dollars [18]. These costs fall disproportionately on lower-income families. Individuals living in many inner cities are predominantly Black and Hispanic, and these areas are known to have lower household median incomes compared to suburban and rural areas. The median urban household income in the United States with a householder under the age of 25 is $25,656 [23]. Children from lower-income homes have been shown to spend more on emergency department visits and hospitalizations related to food allergy and less on out-of-pocket costs when compared with children from higher-income households [18]. Moreover, families with lower median incomes often lack the financial means to access allergen-free foods to prevent allergic reactions [18]. The higher spending on acute visits, compared to preventative, as well as inability to afford allergen-free foods suggests that financial factors play a significant role in food allergy disparities [24].

On the other hand, it was noted that the odds of food allergy were significantly lower in households with an income less than $50,000 [24]. While this finding may seem surprising, it is important to take into account that it is from a cross-sectional survey which may include individuals with undiagnosed food allergy. Supporting this finding, McGowan et al. found that poverty was protective for perceived food allergy and food allergy had the lowest prevalence in urban neighborhoods when compared with suburban [25].

Reasons for Food Allergy Health Disparities

One may ask whether the hygiene hypothesis, access to the healthcare system, low recognition of disease importance, and underreporting of disease play a role in these findings. A study with Canadian patients suggests that underreporting of FA is occurring. The authors demonstrated that when reporting food allergies, 6.4% of patients without a college education reported food allergy [95% CI, 5.5–7.3%] versus 8.9% of those with a college education [95% CI, 7.7–10%] [26]. Additionally, inner city children tend to have earlier exposure to solid foods than recommended by the American Academy of Pediatrics; this early exposure could potentially be protective against food allergy development [27]. Protective factors versus underreporting of food allergy are important to study as these findings may impact delegation of resources to help prevent and treat food allergy. Moreover, low spending on out-of-pocket costs implies poor outpatient follow-up with subspecialists.

Access to the healthcare system may also be a factor contributing to disparities in food allergy. Taylor-Black and Wang found that the prevalence of food allergy among Black patients was significantly higher when compared with Hispanic and multiracial patients (4.7% vs 2.7%) [14]. Interestingly, Black, Asian, and Hispanic children have been shown to not only have a higher prevalence of food allergy but also lower odds of being diagnosed by a physician [21]. In more detailed studies, it was found that Black and Hispanic children have similar initial evaluations and referral rates to allergy specialists as White children [17]; however, they have shorter duration of follow-up with an allergist [17]. Patients with Medicaid also had significantly shorter duration of follow-up [17]. Less follow-up implies less visits where key tenants of food allergy management can be discussed and reinforced (i.e., food avoidance, use and storage of epinephrine auto-injector on the individual, etc.). Shorter follow-up has been shown to negatively affect food allergy outcomes and increase food allergy-related anaphylaxis and death [17]. Families who are not able to follow up frequently may have less healthcare literacy regarding new research findings as well as emerging treatments. As an example, the findings of the LEAP study have been adapted into a formal consensus statement issued by the NIH on prevention of peanut allergy in the United States. Those families who do not regularly follow up with an allergist or pediatrician may be unaware of these new recommendations to introduce peanut early in order to decrease the chance of peanut allergy. As we have already discussed previously, low-income minority children appear to have high rates of peanut allergy or sensitization; thus, early application of these guidelines for such children could be crucial in decreasing food allergy burden in both the individual and society. It is apparent that there is a crucial need for implementation of strategies to provide access to subspecialty care for all children with food allergy.

Several plausible explanations for these findings are worth exploring such as limited access to the healthcare system and lack of education about food allergies in certain communities. These become even more relevant when taking into consideration that almost 40% of children with food allergies have been shown to have a severe life-threatening reaction [21].

Comorbid Allergic Conditions

Food allergy is associated with multiple other atopic disorders, such as asthma and atopic dermatitis. Allergic reactions to food can result in life-threatening asthma attacks, leading to hospitalization, intubation, and death [28, 29]. Black and Hispanic children are known to be at higher risk for both atopic dermatitis and severe asthma, resulting in increased risk of emergency department visits [30]. A recent study investigating the relationship between food allergy and asthma in an urban school system showed that asthmatic children with food allergies have a higher risk of hospitalizations and use of controller medications [31]. Food allergic asthmatic children also had lower lung function including lower FEV1 percentage and FEV1/FVC ratio [31]. With regard to ethnic disparities, Mahdavinia et al. found that Black children with food allergies had significantly higher odds of comorbid asthma and atopic dermatitis [17]. These findings illustrate the importance of screening children with one atopic disorder for others in order to prevent morbidity and mortality in these children.

Disparities and Their Potential Impact on Future Directions: Prevention of Food Allergy

While no specific cause of food allergy has been identified, certain associations have been noted with subsequent hypotheses. It is thought that food allergies develop in infants when there is skin disruption, such as atopic dermatitis. This disruption allows allergens to enter the body and can lead to sensitization [32]. Although this is a plausible explanation, it does not explain development of food allergy in children and adults without disruption in the skin barrier.

The Learning Early about Peanut Allergy (LEAP) trial explored early introduction of peanut as a peanut allergy prevention strategy for infants at high risk of developing peanut allergy. High-risk infants were defined as those having severe eczema, egg allergy, or both. In LEAP, early introduction of peanut in these high-risk children significantly decreased the frequency of peanut allergy [33]. Since this trial, many healthcare providers promote introduction of allergenic foods at an earlier age in an effort to prevent the development of food allergy.

Timing of allergenic food introduction is unfortunately not the only factor impacting development of food allergy. Breastfeeding has also been associated with lower rates of food allergy development [34, 35]. Racial minorities, including Blacks and Hispanics, have lower rates of breastfeeding partially due to multiple socioeconomic and educational barriers. This may be one factor contributing to the increased allergic prevalence in this population [36]. Another interesting caveat to explore is that sensitization or elevated level of serum-specific IgE to a particular allergen does not equate to clinical food allergy, as mentioned previously. The National Institute of Allergy and Infectious Disease states that once a specific IgE (sIgE) is made to a particular food, an individual is considered sensitized to that food, but he or she may not have clinical symptoms consistent with an allergic reaction after an ingestion of this particular food [3]. Several studies mentioned previously determined the prevalence of food allergy based on sIgE levels. For example, Kumar et al. examined food sensitization using allergen sIgE in the Boston Birth Cohort, a predominantly minority cohort. Self-identified Black race and African ancestry were associated with food sensitization (Black race OR 2.22 [95% CI 1.20–4.11]; African ancestry OR 1.07 [95% CI 1.02–1.13]) [37]. Specifically, African ancestry but not self-identified Black race was found to be associated with peanut sensitization with peanut sIgE ≥ 5 [37]. Furthermore, self-identified Black race was associated with OR of 2.03 (95% CI 1.01–4.10) for sensitization to 1 or 2 foods and 3.76 (95% CI 1.09–12.97) for sensitization to 3 or more foods [37]. We have previously discussed that most research indicates food allergy is more common in Blacks as opposed to Whites and Hispanics. The aforementioned findings raise an interesting question: Are there racial differences in food sensitization vs. food allergy, and what may this mean? This question remains to be answered.

Conclusion and Final Remarks

It is clear that food allergy has increased over the last 30 years in westernized, industrialized areas of the world including the United States. Disparities in food allergy affect subsequent care and outcomes. As we have discussed, most of the underlying reasons behind these inequalities are unclear. Given the substantial societal impact of food allergy, further understanding of the relationship between food allergy, race/ethnicity, geography, genetics, and socioeconomics will encourage individualized, cost-effective utilization of healthcare resources. This will include greater access to specialty care and diagnostic testing, patient-specific counseling, and culturally sensitive prevention practices especially for those at greatest risk in the lower socioeconomic strata.

Other key interventions include education of primary care physicians and allergists to understand that these disparities exist and to use available resources in assisting both minorities and low-income families suffering from food allergy. This involves ensuring that food allergic patients are appropriately diagnosed and have access to injectable epinephrine. A written food allergy action plan should be provided to educate children and their families about how to recognize food allergy reactions and provide proper treatment. As many inner city children are often cared for by multiple caregivers, it is important to prescribe adequate numbers of injectable epinephrine devices and to educate all caregivers on the use of these devices. Further, the importance of carrying injectable epinephrine devices with the child at all times should be stressed.

Finally, we return to the case of our patient, Mike, who suffered from a severe anaphylactic occurrence after accidentally consuming peanut. In this case, Mike had multiple risk factors for severe anaphylaxis including history of peanut allergy and asthma. It has been shown that minorities with comorbid asthma and food allergy have increased risk of hospitalization. Also, his history is significant for multiple prior accidental exposures and his sister noted that ingredients may not have been carefully read prior to consumption of the food. Here, we have discussed the importance of regular follow-up with an allergy specialist, and in Mike's case, the education reinforced at each follow-up may have prevented his life-threatening reaction. Further, Mike was being cared for by his older sister and not his mother who presumably may have had knowledge of correct injectable epinephrine administration (although not necessarily). Perhaps Mike's reaction may have been far less severe if there had been injectable epinephrine readily available at a known location in the house and if his sister had been trained on appropriate administration. Thus, while we continue to promote research aimed toward further elucidating food allergy disparities and cures, the emphasis on food allergy education and proper administration of epinephrine through regular follow-up with an allergist or pediatrician is paramount.

References

1. Gupta RS, Warren CM, Smith BM, Blumenstock JA, Jiang J, Davis MM, et al. The public health impact of parent-reported childhood food allergies in the United States. Pediatrics. 2018;142(6).
2. Sicherer SH, Sampson HA. Food allergy: a review and update on epidemiology, pathogenesis, diagnosis, prevention, and management. J Allergy Clin Immunol. 2018;141(1):41–58.
3. Disease NIoAaI. Guidelines for the diagnosis and management of food allergy in the United States. 2011;11–7699.
4. Sicherer SH, Sampson HA. Food allergy: epidemiology, pathogenesis, diagnosis, and treatment. J Allergy Clin Immunol. 2014;133(2):291–307; quiz 8.
5. Keet CA, Savage JH, Seopaul S, Peng RD, Wood RA, Matsui EC. Temporal trends and racial/ethnic disparity in self-reported pediatric food allergy in the United States. Ann Allergy Asthma Immunol. 2014;112(3):222–9 e3.
6. Prescott SL, Pawankar R, Allen KJ, Campbell DE, Sinn J, Fiocchi A, et al. A global survey of changing patterns of food allergy burden in children. World Allergy Organ J. 2013;6(1):21.
7. Osborne NJ, Koplin JJ, Martin PE, Gurrin LC, Lowe AJ, Matheson MC, et al. Prevalence of challenge-proven IgE-mediated food allergy using population-based sampling and predetermined challenge criteria in infants. J Allergy Clin Immunol. 2011;127(3):668-76 e1-2.
8. Sicherer SH. Epidemiology of food allergy. J Allergy Clin Immunol. 2011;127(3):594–602.
9. Greenhawt M, Weiss C, Conte ML, Doucet M, Engler A, Camargo CA Jr. Racial and ethnic disparity in food allergy in the United States: a systematic review. J Allergy Clin Immunol Pract. 2013;1(4):378–86.
10. Taveras EM, Gillman MW, Kleinman KP, Rich-Edwards JW, Rifas-Shiman SL. Reducing racial/ethnic disparities in childhood obesity: the role of early life risk factors. JAMA Pediatr. 2013;167(8):731–8.
11. Call RS, Smith TF, Morris E, Chapman MD, Platts-Mills TA. Risk factors for asthma in inner city children. J Pediatr. 1992;121(6):862–6.
12. Huang F, Chawla K, Jarvinen KM, Nowak-Wegrzyn A. Anaphylaxis in a New York City pediatric emergency department: triggers, treatments, and outcomes. J Allergy Clin Immunol. 2012;129(1):162-8 e1-3.
13. Wong L, Huang CH, Lee BW. Shellfish and house dust mite allergies: is the link tropomyosin? Allergy Asthma Immunol Res. 2016;8(2):101–6.
14. Taylor-Black S, Wang J. The prevalence and characteristics of food allergy in urban minority children. Ann Allergy Asthma Immunol. 2012;109(6):431–7.
15. Sicherer SH, Munoz-Furlong A, Sampson HA. Prevalence of seafood allergy in the United States determined by a random telephone survey. J Allergy Clin Immunol. 2004;114(1):159–65.
16. Branum AM, Lukacs SL. Food allergy among children in the United States. Pediatrics. 2009;124(6):1549–55.
17. Mahdavinia M, Fox SR, Smith BM, James C, Palmisano EL, Mohammed A, et al. Racial differences in food allergy phenotype and health care utilization among US children. J Allergy Clin Immunol Pract. 2017;5(2):352-7 e1.

18. Bilaver LA, Kester KM, Smith BM, Gupta RS. Socioeconomic disparities in the economic impact of childhood food allergy. Pediatrics. 2016;137(5).
19. Hannaway PJ, Connelly ME, Cobbett RM, Dobrow PJ. Differences in race, ethnicity, and socioeconomic status in schoolchildren dispensed injectable epinephrine in 3 Massachusetts school districts. Ann Allergy Asthma Immunol. 2005;95(2):143–8.
20. Fleming JT, Clark S, Camargo CA Jr, Rudders SA. Early treatment of food-induced anaphylaxis with epinephrine is associated with a lower risk of hospitalization. J Allergy Clin Immunol Pract. 2015;3(1):57–62.
21. Gupta RS, Springston EE, Warrier MR, Smith B, Kumar R, Pongracic J, et al. The prevalence, severity, and distribution of childhood food allergy in the United States. Pediatrics. 2011;128(1):e9–17.
22. Jerschow E, Lin RY, Scaperotti MM, McGinn AP. Fatal anaphylaxis in the United States, 1999-2010: temporal patterns and demographic associations. J Allergy Clin Immunol. 2014;134(6):1318–28 e7.
23. Bishaw A. A comparison of rural and urban America: household income and poverty. US Census, 2016.
24. Gupta R, Holdford D, Bilaver L, Dyer A, Holl JL, Meltzer D. The economic impact of childhood food allergy in the United States. JAMA Pediatr. 2013;167(11):1026–31.
25. McGowan EC, Matsui EC, McCormack MC, Pollack CE, Peng R, Keet CA. Effect of poverty, urbanization, and race/ethnicity on perceived food allergy in the United States. Ann Allergy Asthma Immunol. 2015;115(1):85–6 e2.
26. Soller L, Ben-Shoshan M, Harrington DW, Knoll M, Fragapane J, Joseph L, et al. Prevalence and predictors of food allergy in Canada: a focus on vulnerable populations. J Allergy Clin Immunol Pract. 2015;3(1):42–9.
27. Bronner YL, Gross SM, Caulfield L, Bentley ME, Kessler L, Jensen J, et al. Early introduction of solid foods among urban African-American participants in WIC. J Am Diet Assoc. 1999;99(4):457–61.
28. Wang J, Visness CM, Sampson HA. Food allergen sensitization in inner-city children with asthma. J Allergy Clin Immunol. 2005;115(5):1076–80.
29. Roberts G, Patel N, Levi-Schaffer F, Habibi P, Lack G. Food allergy as a risk factor for life-threatening asthma in childhood: a case-controlled study. J Allergy Clin Immunol. 2003;112(1):168–74.
30. Mehta NK, Lee H, Ylitalo KR. Child health in the United States: recent trends in racial/ethnic disparities. Soc Sci Med. 2013;95:6–15.
31. Friedlander JL, Sheehan WJ, Baxi SN, Kopel LS, Gaffin JM, Ozonoff A, et al. Food allergy and increased asthma morbidity in a school-based Inner-City asthma study. J Allergy Clin Immunol Pract. 2013;1(5):479–84.
32. Asai Y, Greenwood C, Hull PR, Alizadehfar R, Ben-Shoshan M, Brown SJ, et al. Filaggrin gene mutation associations with peanut allergy persist despite variations in peanut allergy diagnostic criteria or asthma status. J Allergy Clin Immunol. 2013;132(1):239–42.
33. Du Toit G, Roberts G, Sayre PH, Bahnson HT, Radulovic S, Santos AF, et al. Randomized trial of peanut consumption in infants at risk for peanut allergy. N Engl J Med. 2015;372(9):803–13.
34. Lopez-Exposito I, Song Y, Jarvinen KM, Srivastava K, Li XM. Maternal peanut exposure during pregnancy and lactation reduces peanut allergy risk in offspring. J Allergy Clin Immunol. 2009;124(5):1039–46.
35. Sardecka I, Los-Rycharska E, Ludwig H, Gawryjolek J, Krogulska A. Early risk factors for cow's milk allergy in children in the first year of life. Allergy Asthma Proc. 2018;39(6):e44–54.
36. Jones KM, Power ML, Queenan JT, Schulkin J. Racial and ethnic disparities in breastfeeding. Breastfeed Med. 2015;10(4):186–96.
37. Kumar R, Tsai HJ, Hong X, Liu X, Wang G, Pearson C, et al. Race, ancestry, and development of food-allergen sensitization in early childhood. Pediatrics. 2011;128(4):e821–9.

Chapter 7
Asthma Health Disparities

Andrea A. Pappalardo and Molly A. Martin

Jayden

Jayden, a 17-year-old African American male living on the south side of Chicago, presented to the emergency room intubated and in septic shock. The last time he accessed the healthcare system was as an outpatient to a primary care physician at the age of 15. His chart indicated nonadherence to inhaled corticosteroids throughout his childhood, six hospitalizations, and no asthma subspecialist consultation. Spirometry from several years ago revealed severe obstruction that was fixed (unresponsive to albuterol). He had been intubated twice for asthma, at age 9 (when he had influenza) and age 13. He dropped out of high school this year because he missed too many school days. He started smoking cigarettes at 12 years of age and was smoking one pack per day at the time of admission. His nasal swab tested positive for influenza A. His mother revealed that he did not get the influenza vaccine because she had heard that the influenza vaccine makes you sick. He had been using his brother's albuterol over the last week, but Jayden's mother thinks the pump is empty now. Upon arrival, Jayden was immediately transferred to the pediatric intensive care unit. Unfortunately, he could not maintain oxygenation despite mechanical ventilation. He was placed on an oscillator, and the intensivists were preparing for extracorporeal membrane oxygenation when he coded and died.

A. A. Pappalardo (✉)
Department of Pediatrics, University of Illinois at Chicago, Chicago, IL, USA

Department of Medicine, University of Illinois at Chicago, Chicago, IL, USA
e-mail: apappa2@uic.edu

M. A. Martin
Department of Pediatrics, University of Illinois at Chicago, Chicago, IL, USA
e-mail: mollyma@uic.edu

© Springer Nature Switzerland AG 2020
M. Mahdavinia (ed.), *Health Disparities in Allergic Diseases*,
https://doi.org/10.1007/978-3-030-31222-0_7

Introduction

Asthma is a common disease of varying severity. When left untreated or inade quately treated, asthma can be fatal. Asthma deaths, in many cases, are considered preventable. In this case presentation, a child on the verge of adulthood died of a communicable disease called influenza that in the setting of asthma has increased risk of secondary bacterial infections and adverse outcomes [1–3]. Jayden's death was preventable. Health disparities contributed to his poor asthma management, lack of medicine, refusal of the influenza vaccine, tobacco addiction, and late presentation for emergency care. This chapter will discuss how asthma health disparities relate to asthma prevalence, risk, outcomes, and management. Ways to mitigate these disparities will also be described, using Chicago as an example.

Existing Health Disparities in Asthma

Asthma is common in both adults and children, and its prevalence, morbidity, and mortality are not experienced equally in the United States. For decades, these asthma health disparities have been known and yet they continue. We will now review the current epidemiologic evidence of asthma health disparities.

Prevalence

Asthma prevalence for both children and adults increased steadily from 1980 to 1996 and then plateaued [4, 5]. The results of the National Health Interview Survey (NHIS) completed in 2016 through the Centers for Disease Control (CDC) reported an overall prevalence of current asthma as 8.3% [6]. The highest prevalence age group was in young adolescents aged 12–14 years (11.2%) [6]. Asthma was overall more common in females (9.7%) compared to males (6.9%), but in school-aged children, boys had more current asthma (9.2%) than girls (7.4%) [6]. Disparities in prevalence by race/ethnicity documented in the 1980s in both adults and children remain today [4, 6]. The highest prevalence of current asthma in 2016 by race was in non-Hispanic black (15.7%) and Puerto Rican (14.3%) children. Current asthma prevalence for non-Hispanic white children was 7.1% [6]. Asthma prevalence also varies by income level with an asthma prevalence of 11.8% in persons 100% below the poverty level, compared to 7.1% in those 450% of the poverty level or higher [6].

Asthma disparities are even more dramatic in certain urban areas. Data from the Medical Expenditure Panel Survey (MEPS) 2000–2014 database showed that low-income urban children throughout the country had some of the highest rates of asthma attacks and were less likely to use controller medicines. However, NHIS data from 2009 to 2011 suggested that non-Hispanic black race, Puerto Rican ethnicity, and low-income status were more powerful predictors of asthma prevalence than urban status [7]. In a school-based survey conducted in Chicago, asthma prevalence for children in non-Hispanic black neighborhoods was 19.9% compared to 11.4% in non-Hispanic white neighborhoods and 12.1% in Hispanic neighborhoods [8] (Fig. 7.1). While age, gender, family medical history of asthma, and neighborhood socioeconomic status were associated with asthma prevalence, they could not explain the differences seen between neighborhoods [8]. Race did explain a large portion of the variation between neighborhoods [8]. A population-based survey of asthma in Chicago reported that more than a third of Puerto Rican children had likely asthma. Non-Hispanic black children followed closely behind at 25% with likely asthma [9]. This is in comparison to 20% with likely asthma in non-Hispanic white children [9]. Cities like New York and Miami share similar statistics [10, 11].

Disparities also exist in rural areas where access issues are magnified, especially in the setting of poverty [12]. Most published literature and interventions focus on urban populations, leaving a gap in our understanding of asthma in rural populations. Although some studies report a lower prevalence of asthma in rural population [13] (others have shown similar prevalence) [14], there are significant access to care issues including location of clinics and potential problems related to quality of care [14]. In Arkansas, Pesek et al. reported that rural children were more likely to

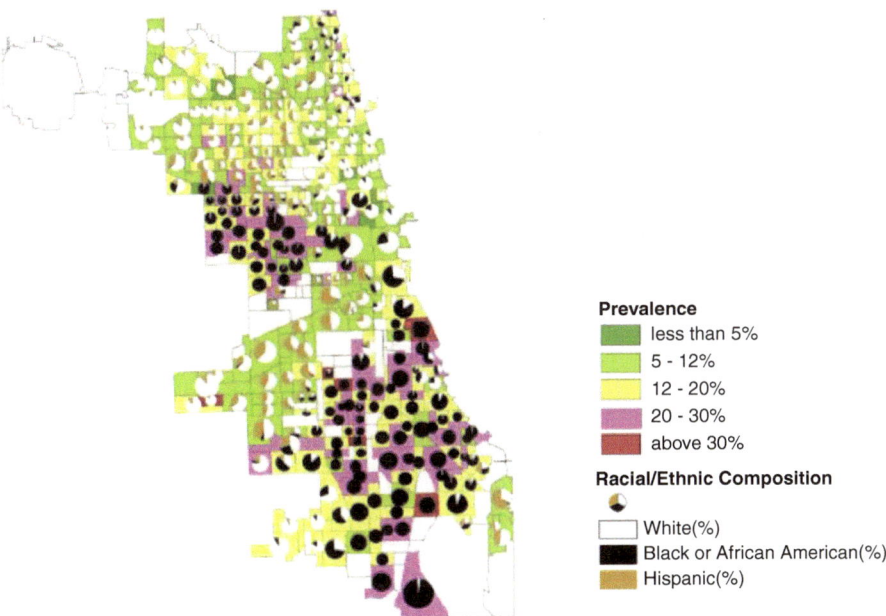

Fig. 7.1 Child asthma prevalence and race/ethnicity in Chicago. (Gupta et al. J Allergy Clin Immunol 2008)

be labeled as having "chronic bronchitis" instead of asthma; this misdiagnosis has implications for their asthma management and surveillance [14]. Rural populations are more likely to have lower income and governmental insurance, compared to urban populations [13] and a higher risk of death [15]. Probst et al. attributed rural asthma disparities to these differences in income, education, and insurance coverage [15]. Limited access to asthma care extends to the school setting, where children spend a lot of time. School nurses in rural communities have been shown to have less access to asthma educational resources and to provide less asthma education to students [16, 17]. They also provide less asthma assessments and management, provide fewer referrals for asthma, and have reduced access to asthma specialists in comparison to urban communities [16, 17].

Environmental exposures are different in rural and urban areas, likely contributing to some of the differences in asthma prevalence. Nonatopic asthma, which has a different presentation and treatment approach than atopic asthma, may be more common in rural areas when certain exposures are present [18]. The hygiene hypothesis speculates a potential protective effect of farm and rural exposures related to the development of atopic asthma [19]. Additionally, rural areas' reliance on biomass fuels constitutes another potential negative exposure; however, further studies need to be done to better understand these exposures [20].

Outcomes Related to Disparities in Asthma

Asthma health disparities are not limited to prevalence; certain population groups suffer worse asthma morbidity than others. This is demonstrated by differences in hospitalizations, emergency department (ED) visits, health status, asthma severity, and quality of life. National data demonstrated that ED use for non-Hispanic black adults and children was over two times greater than for non-Hispanic white adults and children; separating out for age did not modify these results [21]. These trends apply to a lower likelihood of outpatient asthma management as well, even for those with severe asthma [21]. Urban, minority children have been shown to have more daily asthma symptoms, exacerbations, ED visits, hospitalizations, less asthma action care plans, and less access to specialists [6, 22]. Inpatient asthma management also varies by race/ethnicity. Chandra et al. showed that 37% of Hispanic children compared to 60% of non-Hispanic white children and 63% of non-Hispanic black children received an asthma action plan at discharge [23].

Morbidity

Data from the Centers for Disease Control's 2015 Behavioral Risk Factor Surveillance System (BRFSS) showed that adults with asthma were more likely to self-describe their health status as fair to poor opposed to the other options of good, very good, or excellent [24]. Specifically, individuals with asthma described their health as fair to poor 33.1% of the time compared to fair to poor health 15.9% of the time in those without asthma [24]. For school-aged children with asthma in Chicago, non-Hispanic white children had better quality of life and less severe asthma attacks compared to non-Hispanic black and Hispanic children; this difference could not be fully attributed to income differences [25]. In Chicago adults with asthma, Hispanic adults described a lower quality of life, and non-Hispanic black and Hispanic adults did worse compared to their non-Hispanic white counterparts in all outcomes related to asthma [26]. While socioeconomic status and health literacy partially explained these findings, nothing other than difference in race explained the higher hospitalization rates in non-Hispanic black adults [26].

Poorly controlled asthma can interfere with school attendance for children, affect academic performance, and cause parents to miss work. The number of reported missed school days among children with asthma from Centers for Disease Control data varies annually, from 12.4 million in 2003 to 13.8 million in 2013 [27]. Since the number of children with asthma has changed over time, another way to consider school attendance is the actual percentage of children with asthma who reported one or more asthma-related missed school days; these rates were 61.4% in 2003, 59.6% in 2008, and 49% in 2013 (49.0%) [27]. The reported missed school days in each year did not differ by age, sex, race or ethnicity, and poverty level [27]. However, data from state insurers and other sources suggest there is a disparity in missed school days for children with asthma and workdays for parents. For example, Lieu et al. reported more missed school days for non-Hispanic black and Hispanic children compared to non-Hispanic white children in their analysis of Medicaid-insured children [28]. Another study showed that urban minority children missed more school, experienced more asthma-related symptoms and healthcare utilization, and caregivers missed more work when compared to non-Hispanic white peers [22].

Mortality

National data shows that non-Hispanic black individuals with asthma are 2.8 times more likely to die from asthma than non-Hispanic white individuals [29]. Urban areas make up a disproportionate number of these deaths. In 1985, Cook County (Chicago area) and New York City accounted for 21.1% of all asthma deaths for 5–34-year-olds with asthma in the United States [30, 31]. The rate of asthma deaths decreased from 15 per million in 2001 ($n = 4269$) to 10 per million ($n = 3518$) in 2016 but this improvement is not experienced equally [32]. Non-Hispanic black adults and children remain much more likely to die from asthma [32]. The death rate for non-Hispanic black adults and children from 2016 was 22.3 per million compared to 8.2 per million in non-Hispanic whites [32]. Overall mortality rates for those of Hispanic ethnicity appear lower than non-Hispanic whites but when Hispanic subgroups are examined, Puerto Ricans have a higher mortality rate [33, 34].

Costs

If not swayed by the ethical dilemma surrounding disparate asthma outcomes, society must at least acknowledge the financial costs of asthma health disparities. Medical costs for asthma from 2008 to 2013 totaled $50.3 billion/year, with the average cost per person with asthma estimated to be $3266 per year [35]. The medical costs for those living under the poverty line were higher, at $3581 per person annually. Asthma-related mortality (which is largely preventable) cost another $29 billion/year [35]. Missing school and work also has a cost, reported as $3 billion/year [35]. These estimates do not include the long-term consequences of missed school such as future potential earnings.

Reasons for Asthma Health Disparities

Models for Examining the Etiology of Health Disparities

Before effective treatments can be developed and delivered, we need to understand two main things about asthma: (1) Why do some people develop asthma? and (2) What contributes to asthma morbidity and mortality? When considering health disparities, these questions become modified: Why are some population groups differentially affected in the development of asthma? Why do some population groups suffer worse asthma outcomes than others? Is it genetic? Environmental? Or a mixture of both, such as epigenetics?

We can begin to understand these questions by looking at asthma health disparities from the lens of the socioeconomic model (Fig. 7.2). At the individual level,

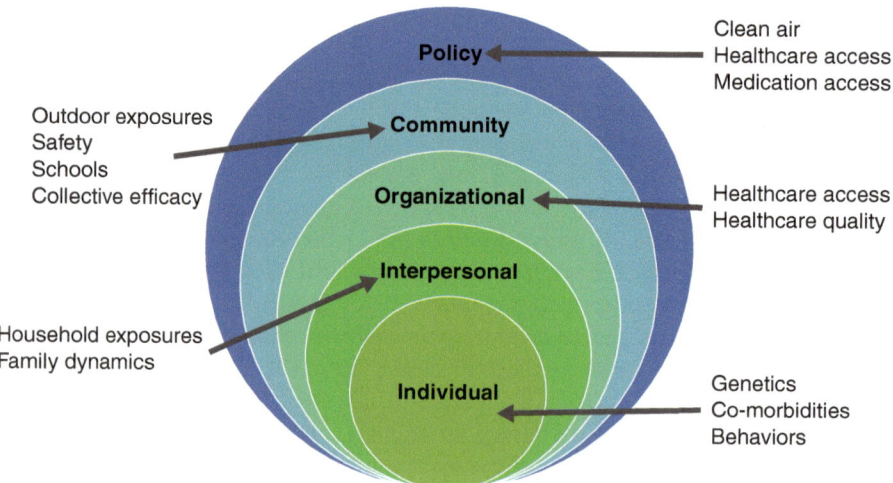

Fig. 7.2 Asthma Disparities Applied to the Socioecological Model

factors such as genetics, comorbidities, and asthma management behaviors drive development of asthma and its outcomes. Household exposures and family dynamics contribute. At the organizational level, families receive varying degrees of guidelines-based asthma care depending on their healthcare access and quality. Community settings bring challenges of environmental exposures, violence, school factors, and issues such as collective efficacy. Finally, policy influences air quality and access to healthcare resources and medications.

Even though many of the causes and influences of asthma fall outside the individual domain, children experiencing asthma health disparities bear a disproportionate burden. Children live in homes, under the care and influence of families. Modifiable factors such as beliefs, behaviors, and psychological stress come to play in homes. Homes are located in communities that may be prone to environmental factors like outdoor allergens, pollutions, and neighborhood stress. Children then interact with the healthcare system and providers, where operations and practices may not always be supportive of best care for the children. Finally, children also spend a huge portion of their time in schools which have a whole other set of modifiable and environmental factors. These different settings all impact the child and each other, but they do not communicate with each other except through the child/caregiver. For some families with low resources or skills, this burden is intolerable; they cannot bridge the settings (Fig. 7.3) [36, 37]. Primary care providers do not always know about ED visits. Parents sometimes do not get or give medicines.

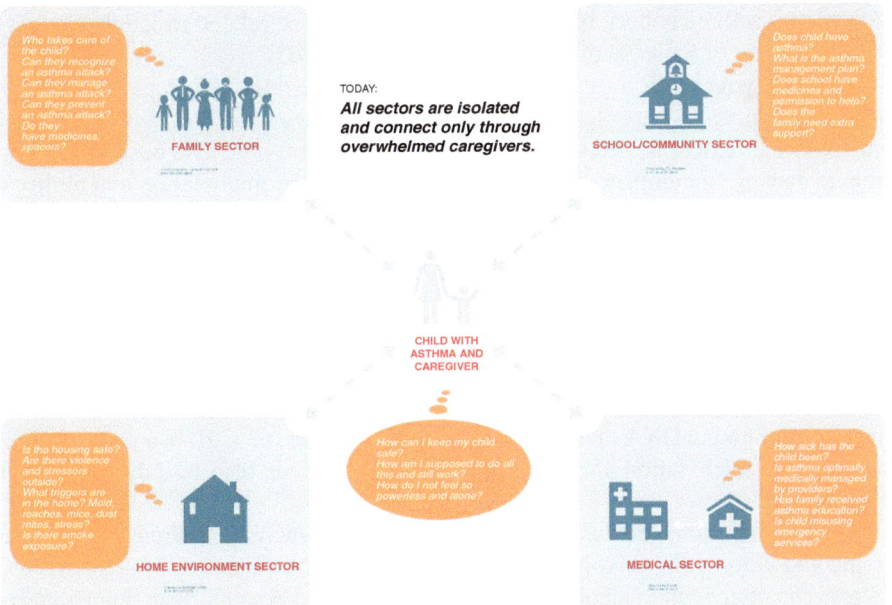

Fig. 7.3 The current burden of asthma on children and families. (Martin MA, et al. J Allergy Clin Immunol 2016)

Next, we will summarize some of the primary evidence of contributing factors to asthma. This is not an exhaustive review. These factors can have influences on the individual with asthma, as well as effects on offspring, household members, and communities.

Genetics and Epigenetics

Genetics are a known contributor to the development of asthma and also influence early respiratory infection severity which may contribute to future asthma persistence [38–40]. Overall, there are several distinct possible genetic predispositions to asthma that are hypothesized or correlated with the future development of asthma [39, 41–52], some specific to Hispanic populations [53]. No ethnic-specific asthma susceptibility gene has yet been defined in Hispanic subgroups [33, 54–57], making the genetic link likely more complex. There have been differences in single nucleotide polymorphisms that differentiate certain individuals with asthma to be more or less steroid responsive [58]. Some variants in the 17q21 locus seem to have the greatest effect on the pathogenesis of asthma in Puerto Ricans, but this still needs to be further validated [39, 55]. A review of genetic variants on the asthma susceptibility 17q21 locus showed possible, but inconsistent, connections to genetic polymorphisms seen in non-Hispanic black individuals [59]. Genetic variants in the Native American population are similar to the overall population in terms of common genetic variants associated with an increased risk of asthma [60]. In a severe asthma cohort, biologic factors seemed to be related to asthma severity, but the nature of these factors was not entirely clear [61].

Not everyone with a genetic predisposition for asthma develops asthma, and some have more severe or less severe asthma for reasons we do not understand. This suggests that external factors might alter asthma expression. The best evidence of this to date are the impact of stress and trauma on DNA methylation and ability to respond to steroids [62, 63]. DNA methylation is the change of genetic expression based on exposure to various factors [63, 64]. Even in children with an identical twin with exactly the same DNA, the gene expression can be different based on the DNA methylation patterns [64]. In asthma, one example of this is the demonstrated links between genetic expression changes and airway epithelial cells [65–72], leading to airway cells that are more vulnerable to stress and skew toward a proinflammatory cytokine and expression milieu [73–78]. Environmental factors have been implicated in DNA methylation patterns in asthma [63, 79]. In a mouse model, these DNA methylation changes to gene expression can also be inherited to offspring [80].

Chronic stressors modulate lung development, airway epithelium, neuroendocrine and autonomic nervous system responses, and the immune system [81–87]. Stress can change the response to the adrenal axis and potentially create enhanced airway hyperactivity and obstruction to triggers [58, 88]. Even prenatally, cord blood mononuclear cells have been shown to produce a skewed Th2 cytokine milieu with increased IL13 production after dust mite stimulation [88, 89]. Prenatal psychosocial stressors in parents in two birth cohorts found an association with future diagnosis of childhood asthma [90, 91]. Postnatal stress induces both a pro-inflammatory Th1 response and Th2 via increased total IgE at 2 years of age [92, 93]. Stress has been shown to decrease expression of steroid-responsiveness genes, which may contribute toward reduced inhaled corticosteroid and/or oral glucocorticoid effectiveness in treatment of asthma [94, 95]. Additional stressors to the body including particulate matter have also been shown to change expression and lead to pro-inflammation markers increasing regardless of asthma status [96].

Minorities in the USA and those living in poverty are exposed to more stressors, which affect health negatively [97]. These stressors have been linked to both asthma development and worse asthma morbidity [86]. This has been shown in the setting of survivors of physical and sexual abuse in both minority women and children [98, 99]. Exposure to violence in the urban, minority community also affects wheeze in children [91, 100]. The everyday stressors that minority families living in poverty have to deal with can affect asthma control in children [101]. There is some evidence to believe that stressors may be modulated depending on coping mechanisms and resilience that an individual with asthma may have [102], further complicating this relationship between stress and asthma, but also offering a glimmer of hope in perhaps finding a target for potential intervention.

Comorbidities

Allergic Diseases

Allergic disease is a significant and common comorbidity in the setting of asthma. Allergies are often thought to be the precursor to asthma in the theory of the atopic march [103–114]. There are significant health disparities seen in other allergic diseases which can directly influence asthma. We will not expand on these in this chapter, as they will be extensively covered in other chapters in this book.

Obesity

Health disparities related to obesity exist, with more non-Hispanic black children being obese than non-Hispanic white children; these disparities are independent of asthma risk [115]. Obesity is a risk factor for asthma. Asthma prevalence is higher in overweight and obese children and adults, and epidemiologic data suggest that obesity precedes asthma development [116–124]. The mechanisms proposed to explain this association include reduced lung volume and tidal volume with obesity, low-grade systemic inflammation from obesity, obesity-related changes in adipose-derived hormones such as leptin and adiponectin, common genetics, common in utero conditions, common predisposing dietary factors, and comorbidities of obesity such as dyslipidemia, gastroesophageal reflux, sleep-disordered breathing, type 2 diabetes, and hypertension [121, 122]. Obesity also seems to contribute to greater asthma morbidity. A multicenter study by Belamarich et al. reported that inner-city children with asthma who were obese used more medicine, wheezed more, and had more unscheduled emergency department visits than children with asthma who were not obese [116]. Being overweight has been associated with more severe asthma in a cohort of inner-city non-Hispanic black and Hispanic children in New York [125]. Obese children with asthma exacerbations in an intensive care unit had longer hospital stays and required more medications than nonobese children [126].

Mental Health

Stress and mental health issues are worse in populations where health disparities exist. Depression and anxiety symptoms predict worse asthma outcomes, including increased functional impairment, severity of asthma, rescue medication use, and frequency of emotional triggers [127–133]. Mothers of children with asthma have been reported to have higher rates of depression and anxiety, and caregiver depression has been repeatedly associated with worse asthma severity [133–141]. A large cross-sectional analysis of the National Health and Nutrition Examination Survey (NHANES) demonstrated that adults with asthma who also have depression are two times more likely to have poor asthma outcomes for several indicators [142]. These findings have been shown in other studies as well [143, 144]. Non-Hispanic black women are at greater risk than other groups; this may be linked to the experience of racism [145]. Stress and depression distort perceptions of access and can serve as a barrier to seeking care, especially in urban, low-income communities [146, 147].

Behaviors

Non-Hispanic white populations have been shown to use inhaled corticosteroids, which are proven to help control asthma in most individuals, more frequently than other groups [148–153]. Despite the efficacy of inhaled corticosteroids, there is a low adherence to inhaled corticosteroids in all age and race/ethnic minority groups with persistent asthma [154, 155]. This includes never starting the medication at all, only filling the first month of the inhaler, or using the inhaler sub-optimally [154–161]. Studies show that minority groups are less likely to take offered daily controller inhalers prescribed to control asthma across all age groups [28, 136, 162–167]. When reviewing interventions to improve adherence in minority populations, many approaches have not been associated with improvements in study participants [168]. This is compounded by the episodic nature of asthma symptoms, perpetuating the beliefs that many have that asthma disappears and there is no need to take medication in periods of wellness [169].

Multiple factors likely contribute to worse adherence to controller medications in disadvantaged, minority populations; however, a primary marker seems to be race/ethnic minority status coupled with low socioeconomic status [162, 163]. Fear of inhaled steroid medications as well as beliefs such as inevitable dependence on the medications contribute to low adherence to inhaled controller medications in asthma [157, 170, 171]. These beliefs have been documented in both non-Hispanic black and Hispanic populations [167, 172–174]. Depression in caregivers and in patients with asthma of all ages can affect adherence to controller medications [136, 175–177].

Perceived discrimination has been linked with worse asthma outcomes. In the United States, our prior history of misconduct in research fuels this legitimate concern in minority populations [178]. In an analysis that combined two large datasets of predominantly minority youth, perceived discrimination was found to increase the likelihood of having poor asthma control in non-Hispanic black youth [179]. Race and discrimination can affect healthcare outcomes through conscious or unconscious bias, and through social or environmental stressors which can affect chronic disease outcomes, such as asthma [180]. Racial discrimination has been linked to a significant change in bronchodilator response in non-Hispanic black and Hispanic children with asthma which correlated with higher TNF-alpha, a pro-inflammatory cytokine [181].

Tobacco exposure is a risk factor for the development of asthma both in utero and postnatally [182–184], and worse asthma-related health outcomes [185]. The National Heart, Lung, and Blood Institute Expert Panel Report 3 guidelines cite B-level evidence for avoidance in pregnant women and in household contacts of children with asthma [186–189], and a grade A recommendation is made by the US Preventative Task Force [190]. The effects of smoking tobacco for adults and youth are well known, leading to worsened asthma, lung cancer, chronic obstructive pulmonary disease (COPD), and heart disease, among other factors [187, 190–195]. Tobacco use is not equal. Overall tobacco smoking rates are highest nationally for Puerto Ricans (28.5%), followed by non-Hispanic white adults (24.9%) [196]. The Centers for Disease Control published slightly lower rates by ethnicity: non-Hispanic white (15.2%), non-Hispanic black (14.9%), Native American (24.0%), and Hispanic (9.9%, without division of Latino subgroups). The CDC classifies a prevalence of 20.6% for "multi-race." [197]

Exposure to secondhand smoke in the United States has been declining from 1988 to 2014, from 87.5% to 25.2% [198]. Secondhand smoke exposure is likely higher than what is self-reported. A review of the National Health and Nutrition Examination Survey (NHANES) data from 1999 to 2010 reported 6% exposure to tobacco in the home and 14% in the workplace; however, serum cotinine was detected in 40% of these individuals [199]. Those in lower socioeconomic brackets were found to be more likely to have secondhand smoke exposure [199]. Despite these reductions, non-Hispanic black and Hispanic children are disproportionately exposed to secondhand tobacco smoke compared to non-Hispanic white children [200–203]. Recent data links nicotine aerosols that may be delivered in an alternate device distinct from classic cigarettes with worsened asthma morbidity, so recent trends of these devices also carry significant risk to children [204].

These data indicate that secondhand smoke – despite decreasing smoking prevalence in the population – is common in both adults and children and more common in the same populations that have the worst asthma outcomes.

Influenza vaccination is important for adults and children with asthma. The Centers for Disease Control report that 46.7% of adults over the age of 18 with asthma are vaccinated compared to 39% of adults without asthma [205]. In children, these rates are higher with 63.7% of children with asthma receiving an influenza vaccination [205]. In adults, influenza vaccine rates are significantly different between non-Hispanic black and white adults [206].

Environmental Exposures

Environmental exposures and their control are essential to asthma care [187]. Some hypothesize that a key distinction in health disparities in asthma can be explained in large part by disproportionate amount of environmental exposures that minorities and those with low socioeconomic statuses are exposed to [207], many of which are unavoidable. In this section, we will describe modifiable and nonmodifiable exposures which are disproportionately affecting minorities in the United States.

Allergens

Allergen exposure can affect everyone who has atopic or allergic asthma, and avoidance or mitigation of triggers is a key part of guideline-based asthma care [187]. There is a relationship between exposure of allergens and sensitization to the allergens in children living in the inner-city [208], especially when allergens are present in the bedroom at home. The Childhood Asthma Management Program verified this for both cockroach and dust mite allergen [209]. Indoor allergen sensitization, especially cockroach, has been shown to be higher in non-Hispanic black and Mexican American children compared to non-Hispanic white children [209–211]. Further, those with the highest-risk asthma in a predominantly African American inner-city cohort were found to be more sensitized to mouse allergen as well as overuse of albuterol [212]. Other indoor allergens have also been associated with asthma in minority populations [213]. Pest and indoor allergen reduction strategies may be helpful in these cases [214], depending on the approach and the control the individuals have over the home environment. Studies have attributed much of the unavoidable indoor allergen exposure, such as cockroach, to dilapidated housing infrastructure [215, 216]. Some have proposed that interventions would need to be community-wide in order to make a meaningful impact on allergen exposure in asthma [217]. This phenomenon is best understood in children; the relationships between allergen exposure and health disparities are less studied in adults [218, 219].

Allergen exposure is not limited to homes. In the School Inner-City Asthma Study, exposure to mouse allergen in the school building was found to be associated with increased asthma symptom days and decreased Forced Expiratory Volume in one second or FEV1 [220, 221]. What was particularly interesting is that this effect was seen regardless of the allergen sensitization status, suggesting that those without mouse sensitization and that also had asthma were also negatively affected by the exposure [220]. A similar phenomenon is seen in high schools in regard to mouse and cockroach [222]. Newer studies are also suggesting that fungal spore exposure is another possible allergen in schools that can affect asthma morbidity [223, 224].

Allergen exposure and sensitization are important, as they relate to severity of asthma and asthma morbidity [225]. Sensitization is associated with increased risk of atopic diseases such as asthma, especially when skin tests demonstrate sensitization to multiple allergens [226–228]. For example, the quantity of air-borne mouse allergen levels in inner-city homes has been shown to be directly correlated with asthma symptoms and worse asthma outcomes [229]. Mouse allergen exposure has also been connected to asthma severity in minorities [229–231]. Those children who were most atopic with asthma in the inner-city were shown to require greater amounts of medications, severity scores, and worse lung function [225]. In "difficult-to-control" asthma, asthma severity did not improve and remained difficult to control in those inner-city groups who had worse atopy and rhinitis scores [232]. These data demonstrate that allergen exposures in the inner-city directly affect asthma and remain a significant public health concern.

Air Quality and Pollution

Poor air quality and pollution influence asthma in many ways including the development of asthma [213, 233–239]. In inner-city schools reviewed for air quality, researchers found that fine particulate matter, nitric dioxide, carbon monoxide, and physical dilapidation of school buildings contributed to poor air quality in many inner-city schools [240, 241]. This was not an isolated incident – inner-city children and minority children with asthma across the country are exposed to significant pollution [242, 243]. Pollution increases asthma morbidity and mortality [244, 245], as well as affects lung function [234, 246]. One study in the Bronx reported that children with asthma exposed to higher pollution levels were 66% more likely to be hospitalized for their asthma [247].

The poor air quality that minorities are exposed to, coupled with other environmental exposures, can be directly linked to community housing infrastructure [248]. The National Institutes of Health recognized this threat and recently published a workgroup report on suggested areas of further research to better measure, understand, and intervene on quality concerns throughout the country, especially in the most vulnerable populations [249]. The American Thoracic Society also urges collaboration with public health efforts to combat the concept of "respiratory health equality" [250]. Segregation may play a role in how individuals react to pollution exposures [251]. It is possible that how one responds to air pollution may be dependent on psychosocial and genetic factors [243].

Occupational hazards also lead to poor respiratory health by either worsening asthma control or by contributing to the development of occupational asthma [252]. The risk of occupational hazard exposure is higher in minority populations [253, 254]. A recent review details significant work-related exposure experienced by adult immigrants within the United States, and in some cases, their children that can lead to adverse allergic and respiratory disease effects [255]. In Michigan, workers from minority racial/ethnic backgrounds were overrepresented in lower-paid jobs with greater occupational risks, with an increase in work-related asthma seen in non-Hispanic black adults along with silicosis and pesticide injury in Hispanic adults [256]. Increased efforts to protect minorities in the workplace are necessary to protect from exposures that can affect respiratory health and the overall health and well-being [257].

Healthcare Access and Quality

Insurance-related barriers are significant in minority populations, especially those individuals on public insurance [163, 258, 259]. Many clinics do not accept state insurance plans. In one study that looked at multiple clinics' willingness to schedule patients with either state or private insurance, there was a 66% denial rate with state insurance compared to 11% for private insurance [258]. Minority status was associated with absence of referrals and chronic disease diagnosis [258]. Improving access and insurance coverage does improve healthcare disparities and should be more aggressively targeted for intervention [260].

Access to care issues directly affects asthma control [261]. In the inner-city, access to care is less and this disproportionately affects minorities. Non-Hispanic black children with asthma use more emergency services, and less use of ambulatory and asthma specialty services than non-Hispanic white children [262]. This is a missed opportunity for prevention. Inner-city minority children also lack asthma care plans, are less likely to be referred to an asthma specialist, and are more likely to utilize emergency services overall [22]. Looking at parental perspectives, these barriers are so prominent that parents believe that seeking emergency services for asthma is usual care [263].

Access to medications is affected by insurance status [264, 265]. The patient costs related to prescriptions create a barrier [266, 267]. Inner-city children with asthma are less likely to be prescribed the medications they require for their asthma [268]. When research assistants looked into the medications available in the home of Puerto Rican youth in Chicago with persistent asthma, 74.9% had a quick reliever and 48.6% had a controller [269]. This means that one in four children was without a potentially life-saving reliever medication available to them in their home. Further, only 35.6% of children were able to properly identify >70% of steps in how to take their inhaler [269]. There is a clear disconnect at every level in the treatment of asthma, which emphasizes the need to target interventions to consider the many facets of health disparities in asthma.

Guideline-based asthma care [187] is often not routinely followed by practitioners in the United States for multiple reasons; some studies suggest that this is worse in minority populations [268, 270–273]. Despite difficulty in implementing guidelines, their implementation works to improve asthma control and therefore should be the standard of care for all. Care may also be influenced by the homogeneity of providers, racism, and implicit bias toward racial minorities [274–276]. Language barriers between providers and patients can also influence adherence to medications and affect asthma management, especially in elderly Hispanic populations [277, 278]. Educating providers on guideline-based asthma care has been shown to increase inhaled corticosteroid prescription rates, but not to address the other barriers to adherence [279]. Coordinated efforts to improve access to care and remove system-level barriers can improve systematic health disparities in asthma and have the potential to improve health in minorities [280].

Lastly, adolescents as a group pose a slightly different challenge to asthma care. Adolescents are less likely to seek healthcare, thus compromising access further [281]. In asthma, there is significant stigma against the use of inhalers, which further complicates this issue [282, 283]. Adherence in adolescents with asthma to controllers is particularly low [283]. Minority teens are more likely to die and have significant morbidity from asthma than other age groups [262]. Beliefs may affect adherence to medications, access to care, and asthma perception [284]. Adolescent perception of asthma symptoms may not be accurate or congruent with parent's perception [285]. Transition to adult care may also be an area that may be difficult to gauge in adolescents with asthma, with some adolescents demonstrating readiness more than others [286].

Potential Solutions to Asthma Disparities: Community-Driven Intervention Development in Chicago

The multifactorial nature of asthma and asthma disparities require innovative solutions that target problems at multiple levels and engage all stakeholders. Chicago serves as an example of this type of approach. Termed "Asthma's Ground Zero," Chicago is an example of how to leverage community organization and data to drive research and policy initiatives aimed at improving asthma outcomes for all and eliminating asthma disparities.

Defining Asthma in Chicago

Chicago's asthma epidemic was highlighted early, through detailed analyses of mortality data [30]. From 1980 to 2002, non-Hispanic black adults were nearly eight times more likely to die from asthma than non-Hispanic white adults [287]. The Illinois Department of Public Health funded numerous surveillance initiatives to monitor asthma in EDs throughout Chicago and the State. Data from 2011 showed that while 74% of adults in the EDs had moderate/severe asthma, only 46% were taking an inhaled corticosteroid [288]. Thirty-nine percent used more than one canister/month of albuterol and 27% had three or more ED visits in the past 12 months [288]. Data for children were similar. Adults and children were not receiving optimal guideline-based asthma care.

At the same time, several large research studies aimed to better characterize asthma disparities. One study conducted from 2003 to 2005 followed 353 adults and 561 children with asthma recruited from 105 Chicago schools [289]. The diagnosed asthma rate was 21.2% for non-Hispanic black children, compared to 9.7% for non-Hispanic white and 11.8% for Hispanic children [290]. Non-Hispanic black children were more than twice as likely and Hispanic children were 1.57 times more likely than non-Hispanic children to have diagnosed asthma [290]. This persisted at all school district income levels even when controlling for other household members with asthma, type of school, age of the child, gender, and language preference [290]. Non-Hispanic white children and adults had better asthma-specific quality of life and fewer severe asthma exacerbations compared to non-Hispanic black and Hispanic children and adults [25]. While non-Hispanic white children also had fewer days with asthma symptoms, no ethnic differences in the frequency of asthma symptoms were seen among adults [25]. Socioeconomic status was shown to mediate race/ethnic disparities in asthma outcomes [291]. Asthma prevalence was also associated with neighborhood race/ethnicity, demonstrating the importance of neighborhood factors but raising questions about what neighborhood race/ethnicity actually represents [8].

A separate study screened for asthma in six diverse Chicago neighborhoods from 2002 to 2003. Data were gathered from 1699 adults and 811 children (ages 0–12 years). Rates of physician-diagnosed asthma for adults were 18–19% in three of the neighborhoods, compared to 11% nationally [9]. These three neighborhoods were low-income and primary non-Hispanic black and Puerto Rican ethnicity. In two neighborhoods, almost half of adults with asthma reported poor asthma control [9]. Rates were even higher for children. Twenty-one percent of Puerto Rican children and 16% of non-Hispanic black children had physician-diagnosed asthma [9]. When children with probable asthma (due to report of significant asthma symptoms) were added, 33% of Puerto Rican children and 25% of non-Hispanic black children had likely asthma [9]. Over half of children with potential asthma had been to the ED in the past year with asthma-related symptoms. In three neighborhoods, 48–59% of children with diagnosed asthma lived with a smoker [9, 292].

The Chicago Department of Public Health analyzed city-level data from 2011 on asthma. The overall Chicago rate of asthma-related ED visits for children was 147 per 10,000 but the rate for non-Hispanic black children was double [293]. Asthma prevalence was concentrated in certain zip codes, mainly on the west and south side where the majority of residents are non-Hispanic black and Hispanic [293]. The map of child asthma ED visits mirrors almost exactly the map of child "low opportunity index" [293]. Analysts calculated the low opportunity index using measures of relative opportunity that include access to daycare centers, parks, and schools [294]. Nearly one in two children living in a low opportunity index was non-Hispanic black or Hispanic, compared to 1 in 50 non-Hispanic white children [293].

Intervention Development and Testing

One of the main interventions developed to combat the asthma crisis in Chicago involved asthma community health workers (CHWs). CHWs are frontline public health workers who are trusted members of and/or have an unusually close understanding of the community served [295]. The Sinai Urban Health Institute (the research arm of the Sinai Health System) began testing CHW asthma interventions in 2001. They trained laypeople to deliver home and hospital-based asthma education and support services for high-risk families. Their programs for both adults and children showed a reduction in asthma ED visits and hospitalizations by 50–80%, decreased symptom frequency, improved quality of life, and a cost saving of $3–8 for every dollar spent [296]. Other child-focused CHW studies using rigorous designs determined that CHW programs need to be community-wide, not targeted at just one population group [297]. Four home visits were not adequate to achieve improved asthma control [297]. CHWs needed to be formally connected with clinical partners, and mental health issues were impacting asthma control significantly [297, 298].

School-based asthma management programs are also being developed to address the high burden of asthma reported in schools. For over 100 years, the Respiratory Health Association has been educating and advocating in the Chicago area regarding asthma and other lung health issues. They created a program called Fight Asthma Now©, which is an evidence-based curriculum delivered to youth in schools [299]. The Respiratory Health Association also developed the Asthma Management program for adults interacting with children with asthma. This is delivered to parents, school staff, childcare providers, and park district staff.

Collaboration to Challenge Asthma

Chicago has a long history of health advocacy and collaboration. The epidemiologic data from the 1990s were so concerning that leaders in asthma research and advocacy founded the Chicago Asthma Consortium in 1996 to specifically address asthma disparities [300]. In 2003, the Chicago Emergency Department Asthma Collaborative began citywide quality improvement initiatives at 28 local hospitals. This effort expanded statewide into the Illinois Emergency Department Asthma Surveillance Project, monitoring 70 EDs throughout Illinois. Researchers at multiple institutions coordinated asthma interventions to maximize the community and scientific impacts [301]. But disparities persisted. In May of 2012, the Academic

Chicago EMED Collaborative to Improve Public Health: Focus on Asthma was convened in Chicago. Attendees represented academic, governmental, and social service institutions from throughout the Chicago area. After reviewing data and discussion, the Collaborative expressed interest in moving forward to seek additional funding. The Coordinated Healthcare Interventions for Childhood Asthma Gaps in Outcomes (CHICAGO) Plan idea was formed.

With funding from a Patient-Centered Outcomes Research Institute (PCORI) award, the CHICAGO Plan moved forward an initiative to develop and test interventions to improve asthma outcomes for high-risk children presenting to EDs. This began in June of 2014 with a public stakeholder meeting on the emergency management of asthma led by the Chicago Asthma Consortium. A formative assessment was then conducted that involved focus groups, interviews, and observations with families and healthcare providers and nurses in EDs, outpatient settings, and homes [302]. In the EDs, patient education was found to be positioned at the weakest moment and the discharge experience was often fragmented. In homes, families had a lot of challenges getting and using medicines properly. They could not get or attend follow-up appointments. Families did not have good ways to coordinate care and share information within the families. Discharge information was stored out of sight. Finally, caregivers had an incomplete understanding of asthma [302]. These data led to the creation of a new ED discharge tool called the CHICAGO Action Plan after ED discharge (CAPE) [303].

The CHICAGO Plan then conducted a three-arm randomized controlled trial. All groups received routine ED care and basic inhaler instruction. Group 1 served as the comparison arm. Group 2 also received the CAPE. Group 3 received the CAPE and five home CHW visits [304]. Despite involvement of six clinical centers, recruitment from the ED was difficult and retention at 6 months was 63%. Of the 373 children enrolled, no difference was seen in asthma outcomes at 6 months. However, families in the arms receiving the CAPE were more likely to receive guideline-based asthma care in the ED [305].

As this trial was being conducted in EDs, investigators and partners explored opportunities to expand asthma care. The CHICAGO Plan II study was funded by an award from the National Institutes of Health (U34HL130787). Led by a team of five principal investigators from two health systems, Respiratory Health Association, and the Chicago Asthma Consortium, the group set out to conduct a community-based needs assessment for childhood asthma. Using a mixed-methods approach, 162 different stakeholders were engaged, 9 citywide project meetings were held, and 31 small meetings were conducted. Stakeholders came not only from individual patients/families and hospital and healthcare systems but also from schools, the Chicago Department of Public Health, the Chicago Housing Authority, the Illinois Institute of Technology Institute of Design, multiple advocacy organizations, and health insurance payers. The results showed the lines of communication and collaboration between stakeholders (hospitals, EDs, clinics, families, and schools) were weak; caregivers were the only consistent force and could not always manage this burden [37]. Recommendations for interventions and how to implement them were generated. The main interventions needed were CHWs that were based outside the healthcare setting, to maintain their skills and support, and to be able to follow families wherever they go. An electronic version of the CAPE was recommended, to allow families to communicate their children's asthma plan with other family, schools, and healthcare providers. School-based asthma education was also identified as a need [37].

Because of the close collaboration with the Chicago Department of Public Health on the CHICAGO Plan II, these interventions are now part of Chicago's strategic plan for asthma. Asthma CHW programs are being implemented and tested in a variety of formats and settings to determine integration protocols, dosing, and reimbursement opportunities. A digital version of the CAPE was created and is ready for testing. Asthma education continues in schools throughout Chicago. Researchers and schools are also working closely together to identify strategies for expanding asthma services [306, 307]. These will include identification of high-risk schools and school-specific asthma needs assessments and supports provided by CHWs. Clinical asthma services continue to be provided in partnership with schools in mobile asthma clinics from Mobile Care Chicago.

Asthma Policy Efforts

While efforts to improve asthma for individuals usually constitute the main discussion of asthma interventions, policy efforts deserve attention as well. Changes on a policy level can have drastic impacts on many. As shown in Fig. 7.4, asthma has been supported by a range of policy efforts over the last two decades. Much of these policies are related to schools. First, school code was modified to allow children to self-administer and carry asthma medication. The asthma emergency response protocol in 2016 gave schools more ability to care for children in emergencies. As of 2018, schools now have a policy allowing the use of stock albuterol which is critical

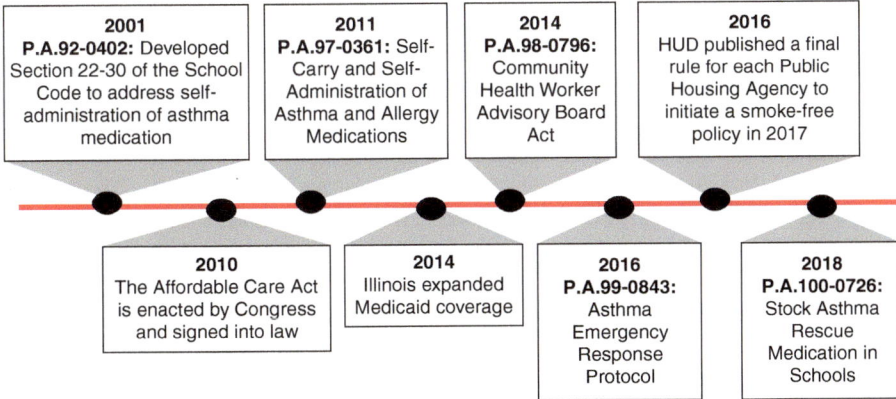

Fig. 7.4 Asthma-related policy achievements in Chicago

for ensuring non-expired medication is available and used when needed. These policies were supported by expansions in health insurance and Medicaid that provided more access to healthcare coverage and medications for children and their families.

Conclusion and Final Remarks

Jayden's death, like the deaths of many others with asthma, was preventable. Multiple systematic failures contributed to his death. Despite having severe, persistent asthma with fixed obstruction from years of chronic inflammation, he had not successfully been seen by an asthma subspecialist. Perhaps, he had been referred and never went. If that was the reason, he may not have gone because of insurance barriers. Perhaps, the asthma subspecialist was very far away and his family could not take the time off work to bring him or afford the transportation and parking costs. Very likely, he was not referred, which happens frequently in urban minority populations [22, 258]. A primary care provider could have managed his asthma with additional medications according to guideline-based asthma care [187]. Unfortunately, young males are the least likely to seek healthcare [281] and not all primary care providers follow evidence-based asthma guidelines [271, 272]; this is more common in low-income neighborhoods [266, 267]. He might not have been adherent to those medications even if they were prescribed; he did not have his own albuterol inhaler at the time of his admission to the hospital. Asthma medications can be very expensive, confusing to use, and are felt to be socially unacceptable by adolescents [269, 282, 308, 309]. He did not receive an influenza vaccination. Influenza vaccine adherence is low overall and even lower in African American communities [206]. He may have been offered it and refused, but it also may not have been available to him if he did not go to a clinic. He and his family did not fully comprehend his asthma symptoms or the severity of his illness, as they waited too long to seek emergency care. Blame for Jayden's death cannot be assigned to one person or component of the system. Many factors conspired to create an environment that led to the worst possible outcome.

Models of health disparities in asthma cite multiple factors related to the health disparities that work in parallel to negatively impact asthma management [162]. To combat health disparities, we need to take into consideration these multiple factors and realize that systematic change requires complex partnerships, collaboration, and multilevel interventions. While much remains unknown about why asthma occurs, we do know how to treat asthma and prevent exacerbations. The goal of reducing health disparities is to ensure these treatments are accessed by all.

For individuals with asthma, we need to ensure they have healthy homes, families, and neighborhoods where their exposures to physical and emotional triggers are minimized. Children and adults with asthma need unrestricted access to the right medications and devices. They need education on asthma symptom and trigger recognition, and how to manage medication regimens. All with asthma deserve care from providers that practice guideline-based asthma care and are accessible. At schools and in the workplace, children and adults with asthma need an environmentally healthy environment with appropriate access to medications and communication with families and healthcare providers.

To move this agenda forward, health system reform and partnerships are essential. Partnerships include healthcare systems and families, and also public health departments, housing agencies, and school systems to support sustainable change. Implementation science is a field designed to bring about systematic changes and provides a structure for how to implement and evaluate these efforts.

Support of all with asthma to reach their potential by keeping them safe and healthy is a common goal. It should be our goal for both ethical and financial reasons to overcome asthma health disparities and ensure everyone can breathe and contribute to our society. While novel drug development and mechanistic bench research are important, ensuring equal access to known therapies and comparable outcomes for all should be prioritized at the same level, if not higher. The benefits to society would be many.

References

1. Nair HD, Brooks WA, Katz M, et al. Global burden of respiratory infections due to seasonal influenza in young children: a systematic review and meta-analysis. Lancet. 2011;378(9807):1917–30.
2. Wong KK, Jain S, Blanton L, et al. Influenza-associated pediatric deaths in the United States, 2004-2012. Pediatrics. 2013;132(5):796–804.
3. Centers for Disease Control and Prevention. The Flu Season. 2018; http://www.cdc.gov/flu/about/season/flu-season.htm. Accessed 18 April 2019.
4. Moorman JE, Rudd RA, Johnson CA, et al. National Surveillance for asthma — United States, 1980–2004. Morb Mortal Wkly Rep Surveill Summ. 2007;56(SS-8):1–54.
5. Moorman JE, Akinbami LJ, Bailey CM, et al. National surveillance of asthma: United States, 2001-2010. Vital Health Stat 3. 2012;(35):1–58.
6. Centers for Disease Control and Prevention. National Current Asthma Prevalence 2016. May 2018; https://www.cdc.gov/asthma/most_recent_national_asthma_data.htm. Accessed 18 April 2019.
7. Keet CA, McCormack MC, Pollack CE, Peng RD, McGowan E, Matsui EC. Neighborhood poverty, urban residence, race/ethnicity, and asthma: rethinking the inner-city asthma epidemic. J Allergy Clin Immunol. 2014;135(3):655–62.
8. Gupta RS, Zhang X, Sharp LK, Shannon JJ, Weiss KB. Geographic variability in childhood asthma prevalence in Chicago. J Allergy Clin Immunol. 2008;121(3):639–645.e631.
9. Whitman S, Williams C, Shah A. Sinai health system's community health survey: report 1. Sinai Health System: Chicago; 2004.
10. New York Health Department. 2017 health care disparities in New York State. New York State, 2017.
11. Beck-Sague CM, Arrieta A, Pinzon-Iregui MC, et al. Trends in racial and ethnic disparities in childhood asthma in Miami, Florida: 2005–2013. J Immigr Minor Health. 2018;20(6):1429–37.
12. Perry TTRM, Brown RH, Nick TG, Jones SM. Uncontrolled asthma and factors related to morbidity in an impoverished, rural environment. Ann Allergy Asthma Immunol. 2012;108(4):254–9.

13. Valet RS, Perry TT, Hartert TV. Rural health disparities in asthma care and outcomes. J Allergy Clin Immunol. 2009;123(6):1220–5.

14. Pesek RD, Vargas PA, Halterman JS, Jones SM, McCracken A, Perry TT. A comparison of asthma prevalence and morbidity between rural and urban schoolchildren in Arkansas. Ann Allergy Asthma Immunol. 2010;104(2):125–31.

15. Probst JC, Bellinger JD, Walsemann KM, Hardin J, Glover SH. Higher risk of death in rural blacks and whites than urbanites is related to lower incomes, education, and health coverage. Health Aff (Millwood). 2011;30(10):1872–9.

16. Huss K, Winkelstein M, Calabrese B, et al. Rural school nurses' asthma education needs. J Asthma. 2001;38(3):253–60.

17. Carpenter DMER, Robers CA, Elio A, Prendergast M, Durbin K, Jones GC, North S. Urban-rural differences in school nurses' asthma training needs and access to asthma resources. J Pediatr Nurs. 2017;36:157–62.

18. Lawson JA, Chu LM, Rennie DC, et al. Prevalence, risk factors, and clinical outcomes of atopic and nonatopic asthma among rural children. Ann Allergy Asthma Immunol. 2016;118(3):304–10.

19. Rönmark E, Lundbäck B, Jönsson E, Rönmark E, Lundbäck B, Platts-mills T. Different pattern of risk factors for atopic and nonatopic asthma among children – report from the obstructive lung disease in Northern Sweden Study. Allergy. 1999;54(9):926–35.

20. Jie Y, Isa ZM, Jie X, Ju ZL, Ismail NH. Urban vs. rural factors that affect adult asthma. Rev Environ Contam Toxicol. 2013;226:33.

21. Fitzpatrick AM, Gillespie SE, Mauger DT, et al. Racial disparities in asthma-related health care use in the National Heart, Lung, and Blood Institute's Severe Asthma Research Program. J Allergy Clin Immunol. 2019;143:2052.

22. Flores G, Snowden-Bridon C, Torres S, et al. Urban minority children with asthma: substantial morbidity, compromised quality and access to specialists, and the importance of poverty and specialty care. J Asthma. 2009;46(4):392–8.

23. Chandra D, Clark S, Camargo CA. Race/ethnicity differences in the inpatient management of acute asthma in the United States. Chest. 2009;135(6):1527–34.

24. Centers for Disease Control and Prevention. Asthma and Fair or Poor Health. 2017; https://www.cdc.gov/asthma/asthma_stats/default.htm. Accessed 18 April 2019.

25. Evans AT, Sadowski LS, VanderWeele TJ, et al. Ethnic disparities in asthma morbidity in Chicago. J Asthma. 2009;46(5):448–54.

26. Curtis LM, Wolf MS, Weiss KB, Grammer LC. The impact of health literacy and socioeconomic status on asthma disparities. J Asthma. 2012;49(2):178–83.

27. Centers for Disease Control and Prevention. Asthma-related missed school days among children aged 5–17 Years. 2015; https://www.cdc.gov/asthma/asthma_stats/missing_days.htm. Accessed 18 April 2019.

28. Lieu TA, Lozano P, Finkelstein JA, et al. Racial/ethnic variation in asthma status and management practices among children in managed Medicaid. Pediatrics. 2002;109(5):857–65.

29. Centers for Disease Control and Prevention. Current asthma prevalence precents by age, United States: national health interview survey, 2015. 2017; https://www.cdc.gov/asthma/nhis/2015/table4-1.htm. Accessed 18 April 2019.

30. Weiss KBWD. Changing patterns of asthma mortality. Identifying target populations at high risk. JAMA. 1990;264(13):1683–7.

31. Weiss KB. Geographic variations in US asthma mortality: small-area analyses of excess mortality, 1981-1985. Am J Epidemiol. 1990;132:S107–15.

32. Centers for Disease Control and Prevention. Asthma as the underlying cause of death. 2018; https://www.cdc.gov/asthma/asthma_stats/asthma_underlying_death.html. Accessed 18 April 2019.

33. Rosser FJ, Forno E, Cooper PJ, Celedón JC. Asthma in Hispanics. An 8-year update. Am J Respir Crit Care Med. 2014;189(11):1316–27.

34. Hunninghake GM, Celedon JC. Asthma in Hispanics. Am J Respir Crit Care Med. 2006;173(2):143–63.

35. Nurmagambetov T, Kuwahara R, Garbe P. The economic burden of asthma in the United States, 2008-2013. Ann Am Thorac Soc. 2018;15(3):348–56.

36. Martin MA, Press VG, Nyenhuis SM, et al. Care transition interventions for children with asthma in the emergency department. J Allergy Clin Immunol. 2016;138(6):1518–25.

37. Martin MA, Kapheim MG, Erwin K, et al. Childhood asthma disparities in Chicago: developing approaches to health inequities. Fam Community Health. 2018;41(3):135–45.

38. Taussig LM, Wright AL, Holberg CJ, Halonen M, Morgan WJ, Martinez FD. Tucson Children's respiratory study: 1980 to present. J Allergy Clin Immunol. 2003;111(4):661–75.

39. Moffatt MF, Kabesch M, Liang L, et al. Genetic variants regulating ORMDL3 expression contribute to the risk of childhood asthma. Nature. 2007;448(7152):470–3.

40. Matricardi PM, Illi S, Gruber C, et al. Wheezing in childhood: incidence, longitudinal patterns and factors predicting persistence. Eur Respir J. 2008;32(3):585–92.

41. Ober C. Perspectives on the past decade of asthma genetics. J Allergy Clin Immunol. 2005;116(2):274–8.

42. Ober C, Thompson EE. Rethinking genetic models of asthma: the role of environmental modifiers. Curr Opin Immunol. 2005;17(6):670–8.

43. Weiss ST, Raby BA, Rogers A. Asthma genetics and genomics 2009. Curr Opin Genet Dev. 2009;19(3):279–82.

44. Moffatt MF, Gut IG, Demenais F, et al. A large-scale, consortium-based genomewide association study of asthma. NEJM. 2010;363(13):1211–21.

45. Aoki T, Hirota T, Tamari M, et al. An association between asthma and TNF-308G/A polymorphism: meta-analysis. J Hum Genet. 2006;51(8):677–85.

46. Nishimura F, Shibasaki M, Ichikawa K, Arinami T, Noguchi E. Failure to find an association between CD14-159C/T polymorphism and asthma: a family-based association test and meta-analysis. Allergol Int. 2006;55(1):55–8.

47. Finkelstein Y, Bournissen FG, Hutson JR, Shannon M. Polymorphism of the ADRB2 gene and response to inhaled beta-agonists in children with asthma: a meta-analysis. J Asthma. 2009;46(9):900–5.

48. Hancock DB, Romieu I, Shi M, et al. Genome-wide association study implicates chromosome 9q21.31 as a susceptibility locus for asthma in mexican children. PLoS Genet. 2009;5(8):e1000623.

49. Himes BE, Hunninghake GM, Baurley JW, et al. Genome-wide association analysis identifies PDE4D as an asthma-susceptibility gene. Am Hum Genet. 2009;84(5):581–93.

50. Li X, Howard TD, Zheng SL, et al. Genome-wide association study of asthma identifies RAD50-IL13 and HLA-DR/DQ regions. J Allergy Clin Immunol. 2010;125(2):328–335. e311.

51. Mathias RA, Grant AV, Rafaels N, et al. A genome-wide association study on African-ancestry populations for asthma. J Allergy Clin Immunol. 2010;125(2):336–346.e334.

52. Sleiman PM, Flory J, Imielinski M, et al. Variants of DENND1B associated with asthma in children. NEJM. 2010;362(1):36–44.

53. Pino-Yanes M, Thakur N, Gignoux CR, et al. Genetic ancestry influences asthma susceptibility and lung function among Latinos. J Allergy Clin Immunol. 2014;135(1):228–35.

54. Gravel S, Zakharia F, Moreno-Estrada A, et al. Reconstructing native American migrations from whole-genome and whole-exome data. PLoS Genet. 2013;9(12):e1004023.

55. Galanter JM, Torgerson D, Gignoux CR, et al. Cosmopolitan and ethnic-specific replication of genetic risk factors for asthma in 2 Latino populations. J Allergy Clin Immunol. 2011;128(1):37–43.e12.

56. Yan Q, Brehm J, Pino-Yanes M, et al. A meta-analysis of genome-wide association studies of asthma in Puerto Ricans. Eur Respir J. 2017;49(5).

57. Szentpetery SE, Forno E, Canino G, Celedon JC. Asthma in Puerto Ricans: lessons from a high-risk population. J Allergy Clin Immunol. 2016;138(6):1556–8.

58. Chen E, Miller GE. Stress and inflammation in exacerbations of asthma. Brain Behav Immun. 2007;21(8):993–9.

59. Stein MM, Thompson EE, Schoettler N, et al. A decade of research on the 17q12-21 asthma locus: piecing together the puzzle. J Allergy Clin Immunol. 2018;142(3):749–764.e743.
60. Best LG, Azure C, Segarra A, et al. Genetic variants and risk of asthma in an American Indian population. Ann Allergy Asthma Immunol. 2017;119(1):31–36.e31.
61. Gamble CD, Talbott ED, Youk AP, et al. Racial differences in biologic predictors of severe asthma: data from the Severe Asthma Research Program. J Allergy Clin Immunol. 2010;126(6):1149–1156.e1141.
62. Stefanowicz D, Hackett T-L, Garmaroudi FS, et al. DNA methylation profiles of airway epithelial cells and PBMCs from healthy, atopic and asthmatic children. PLoS One. 2012;7(9):e44213.
63. Pascoe CD, Obeidat ME, Arsenault BA, et al. Gene expression analysis in asthma using a targeted multiplex array. BMC Pulm Med. 2017;17(1):189–14.
64. Fraga MF, Ballestar E, Paz MF, et al. Epigenetic differences Arise during the lifetime of monozygotic twins. Proc Natl Acad Sci U S A. 2005;102(30):10604–9.
65. Dunnill MS. The pathology of asthma, with special reference to changes in the bronchial mucosa. J Clin Pathol. 1960;13(1):27–33.
66. Amishima M, Munakata M, Nasuhara Y, et al. Expression of epidermal growth factor and epidermal growth factor receptor immunoreactivity in the asthmatic human airway. Am J Respir Crit Care Med. 1998;157(6 Pt 1):1907–12.
67. Trautmann A, Kruger K, Akdis M, et al. Apoptosis and loss of adhesion of bronchial epithelial cells in asthma. Int Arch Allergy Immunol. 2005;138(2):142–50.
68. Barbato A, Turato G, Baraldo S, et al. Epithelial damage and angiogenesis in the airways of children with asthma. Am J Respir Crit Care Med. 2006;174(9):975–81.
69. Fedorov IA, Wilson SJ, Davies DE, Holgate ST. Epithelial stress and structural remodelling in childhood asthma. Thorax. 2005;60(5):389–94.
70. de Boer WI, Sharma HS, Baelemans SM, Hoogsteden HC, Lambrecht BN, Braunstahl GJ. Altered expression of epithelial junctional proteins in atopic asthma: possible role in inflammation. Can J Physiol Pharmacol. 2008;86(3):105–12.
71. Hackett TL, Shaheen F, Johnson A, et al. Characterization of side population cells from human airway epithelium. Stem Cells. 2008;26(10):2576–85.
72. Hackett TL, Warner SM, Stefanowicz D, et al. Induction of epithelial-mesenchymal transition in primary airway epithelial cells from patients with asthma by transforming growth factor-beta1. Am J Respir Crit Care Med. 2009;180(2):122–33.
73. Hackett T-L, Singhera GK, Shaheen F, et al. Intrinsic phenotypic differences of asthmatic epithelium and its inflammatory responses to respiratory syncytial virus and air pollution. Am J Respir Cell Mol Biol. 2011;45(5):1090–100.
74. Kicic A, Sutanto EN, Stevens PT, Knight DA, Stick SM. Intrinsic biochemical and functional differences in bronchial epithelial cells of children with asthma. Am J Respir Crit Care Med. 2006;174(10):1110–8.
75. Mullings RE, Wilson SJ, Puddicombe SM, et al. Signal transducer and activator of transcription 6 (STAT-6) expression and function in asthmatic bronchial epithelium. J Allergy Clin Immunol. 2001;108(5):832–8.
76. Sampath D, Castro M, Look DC, Holtzman MJ. Constitutive activation of an epithelial signal transducer and activator of transcription (STAT) pathway in asthma. J Clin Investig. 1999;103(9):1353–61.
77. Holgate ST, Lackie P, Wilson S, Roche W, Davies D. Bronchial epithelium as a key regulator of airway allergen sensitization and remodeling in asthma. Am J Respir Crit Care Med. 2000;162(3 Pt 2):S113–7.
78. Lopez-Guisa J, Powers C, File D, Cochrane E, Jimenez N, Debley JS. Airway epithelial cells from asthmatic children differentially express proremodeling factors. J Allergy Clin Immunol. 2012;129(4):990–997.e996.
79. Esteller M. The necessity of a human epigenome project. Carcinogenesis. 2006;27(6):1121–5.

80. Hollingsworth JW, Maruoka S, Boon K, et al. In utero supplementation with methyl donors enhances allergic airway disease in mice. J Clin Investig. 2008;118(10):3462.
81. Forno E, Wang T, Qi C, et al. DNA methylation in nasal epithelium, atopy, and atopic asthma in children: a genome-wide study. Lancet Respir Med. 2019;7(4):336–46.
82. Rosenberg SL, Miller GE, Brehm JM, Celedón JC. Stress and asthma: novel insights on genetic, epigenetic, and immunologic mechanisms. J Allergy Clin Immunol. 2014;134(5):1009–15.
83. Yang IV, Pedersen BS, Liu A, et al. DNA methylation and childhood asthma in the inner city. J Allergy Clin Immunol. 2015;136(1):69–80.
84. Yang IV, Pedersen BS, Liu AH, et al. The nasal methylome and childhood atopic asthma. J Allergy Clin Immunol. 2017;139(5):1478–88.
85. Kang DH, Weaver MT. Airway cytokine responses to acute and repeated stress in a murine model of allergic asthma. Biol Psychol. 2010;84(1):66–73.
86. Yonas MA, Lange NE, Celedón JC. Psychosocial stress and asthma morbidity. Curr Opin Allergy Clin Immunol. 2012;12(2):202–10.
87. Bahreinian S, Ball GDC, Vander Leek TK, et al. Allostatic load biomarkers and asthma in adolescents. Am J Respir Crit Care Med. 2013;187(2):144–52.
88. Wright RJ, Cohen RT, Cohen S. The impact of stress on the development and expression of atopy. Curr Opin Allergy Clin Immunol. 2005;5(1):23–9.
89. Peters JL, Cohen S, Staudenmayer J, Hosen J, Platts-Mills TAE, Wright RJ. Prenatal negative life events increases cord blood IgE: interactions with dust mite allergen and maternal atopy. Allergy. 2012;67(4):545–51.
90. Klinnert MD, Nelson HS, Price MR, Adinoff AD, Leung DYM, Mrazek DA. Onset and persistence of childhood asthma: predictors from infancy. Pediatrics. 2001;108(4):e69.
91. Chiu Y-H, Coull BAP, Sternthal MJ, et al. Effects of prenatal community violence and ambient air pollution on childhood wheeze in an urban population. J Allergy Clin Immunol. 2013;133(3):713–722.e714.
92. Wright RO, Wright RJ, Finn P, et al. Chronic caregiver stress and IgE expression, allergen-induced proliferation, and cytokine profiles in a birth cohort predisposed to atopy. J Allergy Clin Immunol. 2004;113(6):1051–7.
93. Sternthal MJ, Coull BA, Chiu YH, Cohen S, Wright RJ. Associations among maternal childhood socioeconomic status, cord blood IgE levels, and repeated wheeze in urban children. J Allergy Clin Immunol. 2011;128(2):337–345.e331.
94. Miller GE, Chen E. Life stress and diminished expression of genes encoding glucocorticoid receptor and beta2-adrenergic receptor in children with asthma. Proc Natl Acad Sci U S A. 2006;103(14):5496–501.
95. Miller GE, Gaudin A, Zysk E, Chen E. Parental support and cytokine activity in childhood asthma: the role of glucocorticoid sensitivity. J Allergy Clin Immunol. 2009;123(4):824–30.
96. Iwanaga K, Elliott MS, Vedal S, Debley JS. Urban particulate matter induces pro-remodeling factors by airway epithelial cells from healthy and asthmatic children. Inhal Toxicol. 2013;25(12):653–60.
97. Matthews KA, Gallo LC. Psychological perspectives on pathways linking socioeconomic status and physical health. Annu Rev Psychol. 2011;62(1):501–30.
98. Cohen RT, Canino GJ, Bird HR, Celedon JC. Violence, abuse, and asthma in Puerto Rican children. Am J Respir Crit Care Med. 2008;178(5):453–9.
99. Coogan PF, Wise LA, O'Connor GT, Brown TA, Palmer JR, Rosenberg L. Abuse during childhood and adolescence and risk of adult-onset asthma in African American women. J Allergy Clin Immunol. 2013;131(4):1058–63.
100. Eldeirawi K, Kunzweiler C, Rosenberg N, et al. Association of neighborhood crime with asthma and asthma morbidity among Mexican American children in Chicago, Illinois. Ann Allergy Asthma Immunol. 2016;117(5):502–507.e501.
101. Bellin MH, Collins KS, Osteen P, et al. Characterization of stress in low-income, inner-city mothers of children with poorly controlled asthma. J Urban Health. 2017;94(6):814–23.

102. Chen EP, Strunk RC, Trethewey A, Schreier H, Maharaj N, Miller GE. Resilience in low-socioeconomic-status children with asthma: adaptations to stress. J Allergy Clin Immunol. 2011;128(5):970–6.
103. Guilbert TW, Morgan WJ, Zeiger RS, et al. Atopic characteristics of children with recurrent wheezing at high risk for the development of childhood asthma. J Allergy Clin Immunol. 2004;114(6):1282–7.
104. Gustafsson D, Sjoberg O, Foucard T. Development of allergies and asthma in infants and young children with atopic dermatitis a prospective follow-up to 7 years of age. Allergy. 2000;55(3):240–5.
105. Kapoor R, Menon CP, Hoffstad O, Bilker WP, Leclerc P, Margolis DJ. The prevalence of atopic triad in children with physician-confirmed atopic dermatitis. J Am Acad Dermatol. 2008;58(1):68–73.
106. Kulig M, Bergmann R, Klettke U, Wahn V, Wahn U, Tacke U. Natural course of sensitization to food and inhalant allergens during the first 6 years of life. J Allergy Clin Immunol. 1999;103(6):1173–9.
107. Martinez FD, Wright AL, Taussig LM, et al. Asthma and wheezing in the first six years of life. NEJM. 1995;332(3):133–8.
108. Novembre E, Cianferoni A, Lombardi E, Bernardini R, Pucci N, Vierucci A. Natural history of "intrinsic" atopic dermatitis. Allergy. 2001;56(5):452–3.
109. Ohshima Y, Yamada A, Hiraoka M, et al. Early sensitization to house dust mite is a major risk factor for subsequent development of bronchial asthma in Japanese infants with atopic dermatitis: results of a 4-year followup study. Ann Allergy Asthma Immunol. 2002;89(3):265–70.
110. Ricci G, Patrizi A, Baldi E, Menna G, Tabanelli M, Masi M. Long-term follow-up of atopic dermatitis: retrospective analysis of related risk factors and association with concomitant allergic diseases. J Am Acad Dermatol. 2006;55(5):765–71.
111. van der Hulst AE, Klip H, Brand PL. Risk of developing asthma in young children with atopic eczema: a systematic review. J Allergy Clin Immunol. 2007;120(3):565–9.
112. Wüthrich B, Schmid-Grendelmeier P. The atopic eczema/dermatitis syndrome: epidemiology, natural course, and immunology of the IgE-associated ("extrinsic") and the nonallergic ("intrinsic") AEDS. J Investig Allergol Clin Immunol. 2003;13(1):1–5.
113. Spergel JM, Paller AS. Atopic dermatitis and the atopic march. J Allergy Clin Immunol. 2003;112(6):S118–27.
114. Tham EH, Leung DY. Mechanisms by which atopic dermatitis predisposes to food allergy and the Atopic March. Allergy, Asthma Immunol Res. 2019;11(1):4–15.
115. Ogden CL, Carroll MD, Lawman HG, et al. Trends in obesity prevalence among children and adolescents in the United States, 1988-1994 through 2013-2014. JAMA. 2016;315(21):2292–9.
116. Belamarich PF, Luder E, Kattan M, et al. Do obese inner-city children with asthma have more symptoms than nonobese children with asthma? Pediatrics. 2000;106(6):1436–41.
117. Beuther DA, Weiss ST, Sutherland ER. Obesity and asthma. Am J Respir Crit Care Med. 2006;174(2):112–9.
118. Halfon N, Larson K, Slusser W. Associations between obesity and comorbid mental health, developmental, and physical health conditions in a nationally representative sample of US children aged 10 to 17. Acad Pediatr. 2013;13(1):6–13.
119. Dixon AE, Holguin F, Sood A, et al. An official American Thoracic Society workshop report: obesity and asthma. Proc Am Thorac Soc. 2010;7(5):325–35.
120. Chen YC, Dong GH, Lin KC, Lee YL. Gender difference of childhood overweight and obesity in predicting the risk of incident asthma: a systematic review and meta-analysis. Obes Rev. 2013;14(3):222–31.
121. Shore SA. Obesity and asthma: possible mechanisms. J Allergy Clin Immunol. 2008;121(5):1087–93; quiz 1094-1085.
122. Matricardi PM, Gruber C, Wahn U, Lau S. The asthma-obesity link in childhood: open questions, complex evidence, a few answers only. Clin Exp Allergy. 2007;37(4):476–84.

123. Castro-Rodriguez JA, Holberg CJ, Morgan WJ, Wright AL, Martinez FD. Increased incidence of asthmalike symptoms in girls who become overweight or obese during the school years. Am J Respir Crit Care Med. 2001;163(6):1344–9.
124. Gilliland FD, Berhane K, Islam T, et al. Obesity and the risk of newly diagnosed asthma in school-age children. Am J Epidemiol. 2003;158(5):406–15.
125. Luder E, Melnik TA, DiMaio M. Association of being overweight with greater asthma symptoms in inner city black and Hispanic children. J Pediatr. 1998;132(4):699–703.
126. Carroll CL, Bhandari A, Zucker AR, Schramm CM. Childhood obesity increases duration of therapy during severe asthma exacerbations. Pediatr Crit Care Med. 2006;7(6):527–31.
127. Kean EM, Kelsay K, Wamboldt F, Wamboldt MZ. Posttraumatic stress in adolescents with asthma and their parents. J Am Acad Child Adolesc Psychiatry. 2006;45(1):78–86.
128. McCauley E, Katon W, Russo J, Richardson L, Lozano P. Impact of anxiety and depression on functional impairment in adolescents with asthma. Gen Hosp Psychiatry. 2007;29(3):214–22.
129. Richardson LP, Lozano P, Russo J, McCauley E, Bush T, Katon W. Asthma symptom burden: relationship to asthma severity and anxiety and depression symptoms. Pediatrics. 2006;118(3):1042–51.
130. Weil CM, Wade SL, Bauman LJ, Lynn H, Mitchell H, Lavigne J. The relationship between psychosocial factors and asthma morbidity in inner-city children with asthma. Pediatrics. 1999;104(6):1274–80.
131. Wood BL, Lim J, Miller BD, et al. Family emotional climate, depression, emotional triggering of asthma, and disease severity in pediatric asthma: examination of pathways of effect. J Pediatr Psychol. 2007;32(5):542–51.
132. Feldman JM, Siddique MI, Morales E, Kaminski B, Lu SE, Lehrer PM. Psychiatric disorders and asthma outcomes among high-risk inner-city patients. Psychosom Med. 2005;67(6):989–96.
133. Feldman JM, Steinberg D, Kutner H, et al. Perception of pulmonary function and asthma control: the differential role of child versus caregiver anxiety and depression. J Pediatr Psychol. 2013;38(10):1091–100.
134. Easter G, Sharpe L, Hunt CJ. Systematic review and meta-analysis of anxious and depressive symptoms in caregivers of children with asthma. J Pediatr Psychol. 2015;40(7):623–32.
135. Ortega AN, Goodwin RD, McQuaid EL, Canino G. Parental mental health, childhood psychiatric disorders, and asthma attacks in island Puerto Rican youth. Ambul Pediatr. 2004;4(4):308–15.
136. Bartlett SJ, Krishnan JA, Riekert KA, Butz AM, Malveaux FJ, Rand CS. Maternal depressive symptoms and adherence to therapy in inner-city children with asthma. Pediatrics. 2004;113(2):229–37.
137. Kozyrskyj AL, Mai XM, McGrath P, Hayglass KT, Becker AB, Macneil B. Continued exposure to maternal distress in early life is associated with an increased risk of childhood asthma. Am J Respir Crit Care Med. 2008;177(2):142–7.
138. Cookson H, Granell R, Joinson C, Ben-Shlomo Y, Henderson AJ. Mothers' anxiety during pregnancy is associated with asthma in their children. J Allergy Clin Immunol. 2009;123(4):847–853.e811.
139. Lefevre F, Moreau D, Semon E, Kalaboka S, Annesi-Maesano I, Just J. Maternal depression related to infant's wheezing. Pediatr Allergy Immunol. 2011;22(6):608–13.
140. Wright RJ, Cohen S, Carey V, Weiss ST, Gold DR. Parental stress as a predictor of wheezing in infancy: a prospective birth-cohort study. Am J Respir Crit Care Med. 2002;165(3):358–65.
141. Bartlett SJ, Kolodner K, Butz AM, Eggleston P, Malveaux FJ, Rand CS. Maternal depressive symptoms and emergency department use among inner-city children with asthma. Arch Pediatr Adolesc Med. 2001;155(3):347–53.
142. Patel PO, Patel MR, Baptist AP. Depression and asthma outcomes in older adults: results from the national health and nutrition examination survey. J Allergy Clin Immunol Pract. 2017;5(6):1691–1697.e1691.

143. Choi HG, Kim J-H, Park J-Y, Hwang YI, Jang SH, Jung K-S. Association between asthma and depression: a National Cohort Study. J Allergy Clin Immunol Pract. 2019;7(4):1239–1245.e1231.
144. Trojan TDMD, Khan DAMD, DeFina LFMD, Akpotaire ODS, Goodwin RDP, Brown ESMDP. Asthma and depression: the Cooper Center longitudinal study. Ann Allergy Asthma Immunol. 2014;112(5):432–6.
145. Coogan PFS, Yu JMPH, O'Connor GTMD, Brown TAP, Palmer JRS, Rosenberg LS. Depressive symptoms and the incidence of adult-onset asthma in African American women. Ann Allergy Asthma Immunol. 2014;112(4):333–338.e331.
146. Laster N, Holsey CN, Shendell DG, McCarty FA, Celano M. Barriers to asthma management among urban families: caregiver and child perspectives. J Asthma. 2009;46(7):731–9.
147. Welkom JS, Hilliard ME, Rand CS, Eakin MN, Riekert KA. Caregiver depression and perceptions of primary care predict clinic attendance in head start children with asthma. J Asthma. 2015;52(2):176–82.
148. Davidson AE, Klein DE, Settipane GA, Alario AJ. Access to care among children visiting the emergency room with acute exacerbations of asthma. Ann Allergy. 1994;72(5):469–73.
149. Rand CS, Butz AM, Kolodner K, Huss K, Eggleston P, Malveaux F. Emergency department visits by urban African American children with asthma. J Allergy Clin Immunol. 2000;105(1):83–90.
150. Warman KL, Silver EJ, McCourt MP, Stein RE. How does home management of asthma exacerbations by parents of inner-city children differ from NHLBI guideline recommendations? National Heart, Lung, and Blood Institute. Pediatrics. 1999;103(2):422–7.
151. Ortega AN, Gergen PJ, Paltiel AD, Bauchner H, Belanger KD, Leaderer BP. Impact of site of care, race, and Hispanic ethnicity on medication use for childhood asthma. Pediatrics. 2002;109(1):E1.
152. Diaz T, Sturm T, Matte T, et al. Medication use among children with asthma in East Harlem. Pediatrics. 2000;105(6):1188–93.
153. Halterman JS, Yoos HL, Kaczorowski JM, et al. Providers underestimate symptom severity among urban children with asthma. Arch Pediatr Adolesc Med. 2002;156(2):141–6.
154. Rust G, Zhang S, Reynolds J. Inhaled corticosteroid adherence and emergency department utilization among Medicaid-enrolled children with asthma. J Asthma. 2013;50(7):769–75.
155. Bender BG, Pedan A, Varasteh LT. Adherence and persistence with fluticasone propionate/salmeterol combination therapy. J Allergy Clin Immunol. 2006;118(4):899–904.
156. Corrao G, Arfe A, Nicotra F, et al. Persistence with inhaled corticosteroids reduces the risk of exacerbation among adults with asthma: a real-world investigation. Respirology. 2016;21(6):1034–40.
157. Apter AJ, Boston RC, George M, et al. Modifiable barriers to adherence to inhaled steroids among adults with asthma: It's not just black and white. J Allergy Clin Immunol. 2003;111(6):1219–26.
158. Morton RW, Everard ML, Elphick HE. Adherence in childhood asthma: the elephant in the room. Arch Dis Child. 2014;99(10):949–53.
159. Bollinger ME, Mudd KE, Boldt A, Hsu VD, Tsoukleris MG, Butz AM. Prescription fill patterns in underserved children with asthma receiving subspecialty care. Ann Allergy Asthma Immunol. 2013;111(3):185–9.
160. Wu AC, Butler MG, Li L, et al. Primary adherence to controller medications for asthma is poor. Ann Am Thorac Soc. 2015;12(2):161–6.
161. McNally KA, Rohan J, Schluchter M, et al. Adherence to combined montelukast and fluticasone treatment in economically disadvantaged african american youth with asthma. J Asthma. 2009;46(9):921–7.
162. Canino G, McQuaid EL, Rand CS. Addressing asthma health disparities: a multilevel challenge. J Allergy Clin Immunol. 2009;123(6):1209–17; quiz 1218-1209.
163. McQuaid EL. Barriers to medication adherence in asthma the importance of culture and context. Ann Allergy Asthma Immunol. 2018;121(1):37–42.

164. Kharat AA, Borrego ME, Raisch DW, Roberts MH, Blanchette CM, Petersen H. Assessing disparities in the receipt of inhaled corticosteroid prescriptions for asthma by Hispanic and non-Hispanic white patients. Ann Am Thorac Soc. 2015;12(2):174–83.

165. Lintzenich A, Teufel RJ, Basco WT Jr. Under-utilization of controller medications and poor follow-up rates among hospitalized asthma patients. Hosp Pediatr. 2011;1(1):8–14.

166. Mosnaim G, Li H, Martin M, et al. Factors associated with levels of adherence to inhaled corticosteroids in minority adolescents with asthma. Ann Allergy Asthma Immunol. 2014;112(2):116–20.

167. McQuaid EL, Vasquez J, Canino G, et al. Beliefs and barriers to medication use in parents of Latino children with asthma. Pediatr Pulmonol. 2009;44(9):892–8.

168. Riley WT, Pilkonis P, Cella D. Application of the National Institutes of Health Patient-reported Outcome Measurement Information System (PROMIS) to mental health research. J Ment Health Policy Econ. 2011;14(4):201–8.

169. Halm EA, Mora P, Leventhal H. No symptoms, no asthma - the acute episodic disease belief is associated with poor self-management among inner-city adults with persistent asthma. Chest. 2006;129(3):573–80.

170. Conn KM, Halterman JS, Lynch K, Cabana MD. The impact of Parents' medication beliefs on asthma management. Pediatrics. 2007;120(3):e521–6.

171. Peterson-Sweeney K, McMullen A, Yoos HL, Kitzman H. Parental perceptions of their child's asthma: management and medication use. J Pediatr Health Care. 2003;17(3):118–25.

172. Koinis-Mitchell D, McQuaid EL, Friedman D, et al. Latino Caregivers' beliefs about asthma: causes, symptoms, and practices. J Asthma. 2008;45(3):205–10.

173. Sidora-Arcoleo K, Yoos HL, McMullen A, Kitzman H. Complementary and alternative medicine use in children with asthma: prevalence and sociodemographic profile of users. J Asthma. 2007;44(3):169–75.

174. George M, Birck K, Hufford DJ, Jemmott LS, Weaver TE. Beliefs about asthma and complementary and alternative medicine in low-income inner-city African-American adults. J Gen Intern Med. 2006;21(12):1317–24.

175. Bender B, Zhang L. Negative affect, medication adherence, and asthma control in children. J Allergy Clin Immunol. 2008;122(3):490–5.

176. Smith A, Krishnan JA, Bilderback A, Riekert KA, Rand CS, Bartlett SJ. Depressive symptoms and adherence to asthma therapy after hospital discharge. Chest. 2006;130(4):1034–8.

177. Krauskopf KA, Sofianou A, Goel MS, et al. Depressive symptoms, low adherence, and poor asthma outcomes in the elderly. J Asthma. 2013;50(3):260–6.

178. Shavers VL, Lynch CF, Burmeister LF. Racial differences in factors that influence the willingness to participate in medical research studies. Ann Epidemiol. 2002;12(4):248–56.

179. Thakur N, Barcelo NE, Borrell LN, et al. Perceived discrimination associated with asthma and related outcomes in minority youth the GALA II and SAGE II studies. Chest. 2017;151(4):804–12.

180. Williams DR. Race, socioeconomic status, and health the added effects of racism and discrimination. Ann N Y Acad Sci. 1999;896(1):173–88.

181. Carlson S, Borrell LN, Eng C, et al. Self-reported racial/ethnic discrimination and bronchodilator response in African American youth with asthma. PLoS One. 2017;12(6):e0179091.

182. Agabiti N, Mallone S, Forastiere F, et al. The impact of parental smoking on asthma and wheezing. SIDRIA Collaborative Group. Studi Italiani sui Disturbi Respiratori nell'Infanzia e l'Ambiente. Epidemiology. 1999;10(6):692.

183. Gergen PJ, Fowler JA, Maurer KR, Davis WW, Overpeck MD. The burden of environmental tobacco smoke exposure on the respiratory health of children 2 months through 5 years of age in the United States: third national health and nutrition examination survey, 1988 to 1994. Pediatrics. 1998;101(2):E81–6.

184. Gilliland FD, Li YF, Peters JM. Effects of maternal smoking during pregnancy and environmental tobacco smoke on asthma and wheezing in children. Am J Respir Crit Care Med. 2001;163(2):429–36.

185. Mannino DM, Moorman JE, Kingsley B, Rose D, Repace J. Health effects related to environmental tobacco smoke exposure in children in the United States: data from the third national health and nutrition examination survey. Arch Pediatr Adolesc Med. 2001;155(1):36–41.
186. McEvoy CT, Spindel ER. Pulmonary effects of maternal smoking on the fetus and child: effects on lung development, respiratory morbidities, and life long lung health. Paediatr Respir Rev. 2016;21:27–33.
187. National Asthma Education and Prevention Program, Third expert panel on the diagnosis and management of asthma. Expert panel report 3: guidelines for the diagnosis and management of asthma. In: National Heart L, and Blood Institute ed. Bethesda, 2007.
188. Hayatbakhsh MR, Sadasivam S, Mamun AA, Najman JM, Williams GM, O'Callaghan MJ. Maternal smoking during and after pregnancy and lung function in early adulthood: a prospective study. Thorax. 2009;64(9):810–4.
189. Stocks J, Hislop A, Sonnappa S. Early lung development: lifelong effect on respiratory health and disease. Lancet Respir Med. 2013;1(9):728–42.
190. Force USPST. Final recommendation statement: tobacco smoking cessation in adults, including pregnant women: behavioral and pharmacotherapy interventions 2017.
191. Khokhawalla SA, Rosenthal SR, Pearlman DN, Triche EW. Cigarette smoking and emergency care utilization among asthmatic adults in the 2011 asthma call-back survey. J Asthma. 2015;52(7):732–9.
192. Thomson NC, Chaudhuri R. Asthma in smokers: challenges and opportunities. Curr Opin Pulm Med. 2009;15(1):39–45.
193. Dockery DW, Speizer FE, Ferris BG Jr, Ware JH, Louis TA, Spiro A. Cumulative and reversible effects of lifetime smoking on simple tests of lung function in adults. Am Rev Respir Dis. 1988;137(2):286–92.
194. Troisi RJ, Speizer FE, Rosner B, Trichopoulos D, Willett WC. Cigarette smoking and incidence of chronic bronchitis and asthma in women. Chest. 1995;108(6):1557–61.
195. Strachan DP, Cook DG. Health effects of passive smoking. 6. Parental smoking and childhood asthma: longitudinal and case-control studies. Thorax. 1998;53(3):204–12.
196. Martell BN, Garrett BE, Caraballo RS. Disparities in adult cigarette smoking — United States, 2002-2005 and 2010-2013. Morb Mortal Wkly Rep. 2016;65(30):753–8.
197. Centers for Disease Control and Prevention. Current cigarette smoking among Adults in the United States. National Center for Chronic Disease Prevention and Health Promotion; 2019.
198. Tsai J, Homa DM, Gentzke AS, et al. Exposure to secondhand smoke among nonsmokers - United States, 1988-2014. MMWR Morb Mortal Wkly Rep. 2018;67(48):1342–6.
199. Gan WQ, Mannino DM, Jemal A. Socioeconomic disparities in secondhand smoke exposure among US never-smoking adults: the national health and nutrition examination survey 1988-2010. Tob Control. 2015;24(6):568–73.
200. Neophytou AM, Oh SS, White MJ, et al. Secondhand smoke exposure and asthma outcomes among African-American and Latino children with asthma. Thorax. 2018;73(11):1041–8.
201. Zhang X, Johnson N, Carrillo G, Xu X. Decreasing trend in passive tobacco smoke exposure and association with asthma in U.S. children. Environ Res. 2018;166:35–41.
202. Ciaccio CE, DiDonna A, Kennedy K, Barnes CS, Portnoy JM, Rosenwasser LJ. Secondhand tobacco smoke exposure in low-income children and its association with asthma. Allergy Asthma Proc. 2014;35(6):462–6.
203. Fedele DA, Tooley E, Busch A, McQuaid EL, Hammond SK, Borrelli B. Comparison of secondhand smoke exposure in minority and nonminority children with asthma. Health Psychol. 2016;35(2):115–22.
204. Bayly JE, Bernat D, Porter L, Choi K. Secondhand exposure to aerosols from electronic nicotine delivery systems and asthma exacerbations among youth with asthma. Chest. 2019;155(1):88–93.
205. Centers for Disesae Control and Prevention. Flu vaccination among children with current asthma. 2017; https://www.cdc.gov/asthma/asthma_stats/flu_vaccination_child.html. Accessed 18 April 2019.

206. Quinn SC, Jamison A, Freimuth VS, An J, Hancock GR, Musa D. Exploring racial influences on flu vaccine attitudes and behavior: results of a national survey of White and African American adults. Vaccine. 2017;35(8):1167–74.
207. Forno E, Celedón JC. Asthma and ethnic minorities: socioeconomic status and beyond. Curr Opin Allergy Clin Immunol. 2009;9(2):154–60.
208. Eggleston PA, Rosenstreich D, Lynn H, et al. Relationship of indoor allergen exposure to skin test sensitivity in inner-city children with asthma. J Allergy Clin Immunol. 1998;102(4):563–70.
209. Huss K, Adkinson NF, Eggleston PA, Dawson C, Van Natta ML, Hamilton RG. House dust mite and cockroach exposure are strong risk factors for positive allergy skin test responses in the childhood asthma management program. J Allergy Clin Immunol. 2001;107(1):48–54.
210. Pacheco CM, Ciaccio CE, Nazir N, et al. Homes of low-income minority families with asthmatic children have increased condition issues. Allergy Asthma Proc. 2014;35(6):467–74.
211. Kattan M, Mitchell H, Eggleston P, et al. Characteristics of inner-city children with asthma: the National Cooperative Inner-City Asthma Study. Pediatr Pulmonol. 1997;24(4):253–62.
212. Bollinger ME, Butz AS, Lewis-Land C, DiPaula F, Mudd S. Characteristics of inner city children with life-threatening asthma. J Allergy Clin Immunol. 2015;135(2):AB80.
213. Sharma HP, Hansel NN, Matsui E, Diette GB, Eggleston P, Breysse P. Indoor environmental influences on Children's asthma. Pediatr Clin N Am. 2007;54(1):103–20.
214. Ahluwalia SK, Matsui EC. Indoor environmental interventions for furry pet allergens, pest allergens, and mold: looking to the future. J Allergy Clin Immunol Pract. 2018;6(1):9–19.
215. Rauh VA, Chew GL, Garfinkel RS. Deteriorated housing contributes to high cockroach allergen levels in inner-city households. Environ Health Perspect. 2002;110(2):323–7.
216. Arruda LK, Ferriani VPL, Vailes LD, Pomés A, Chapman MD. Cockroach allergens: environmental distribution and relationship to disease. Curr Allergy Asthma Rep. 2001;1(5):466–73.
217. Peters JL, Levy JI, Rogers CA, Burge HA, Spengler JD. Determinants of allergen concentrations in apartments of asthmatic children living in public housing. J Urban Health. 2007;84(2):185–97.
218. Wisnivesky JP, Sampson H, Berns S, Kattan M, Halm EA. Lack of association between indoor allergen sensitization and asthma morbidity in inner-city adults. J Allergy Clin Immunol. 2007;120(1):113–20.
219. Busse PJ, Lurslurchachai L, Sampson HA, Halm EA, Wisnivesky J. Perennial allergen-specific immunoglobulin E levels among inner-city elderly asthmatics. J Asthma. 2010;47(7):781–5.
220. Sheehan WJ, Permaul P, Petty CR, et al. Association between allergen exposure in inner-city schools and asthma morbidity among students. JAMA Pediatr. 2017;171(1):31–8.
221. Permaul P, Hoffman E, Fu C, et al. Allergens in urban schools and homes of children with asthma. Pediatr Allergy Immunol. 2012;23(6):543–9.
222. Chew GL, Correa JC, Perzanowski MS. Mouse and cockroach allergens in the dust and air in northeastern United States inner-city public high schools. Indoor Air. 2005;15(4):228–34.
223. Baxi SN, Sheehan WJ, Sordillo JE, et al. Association between fungal spore exposure in inner-city schools and asthma morbidity. Ann Allergy Asthma Immunol. 2019;122:610.
224. Baxi SN, Muilenberg ML, Rogers CA, et al. Exposures to molds in school classrooms of children with asthma. Pediatr Allergy Immunol. 2013;24(7):697–703.
225. Lu KD, Phipatanakul W, Perzanowski MS, Balcer-Whaley S, Matsui EC. Atopy, but not obesity is associated with asthma severity among children with persistent asthma. J Asthma. 2016;53(10):1033–44.
226. Arshad SH, Tariq SM, Matthews S, Hakim E. Sensitization to common allergens and its association with allergic disorders at age 4 years: a whole population birth cohort study. Pediatrics. 2001;108(2):e33.
227. Sheehan WJ, Rangsithienchai PA, Wood RA, et al. Pest and allergen exposure and abatement in inner-city asthma: a work group report of the American Academy of Allergy, Asthma & Immunology indoor allergy/air pollution committee. J Allergy Clin Immunol. 2010;125(3):575–81.

228. Lynch SV, Wood RA, Boushey H, et al. Effects of early-life exposure to allergens and bacteria on recurrent wheeze and atopy in urban children. J Allergy Clin Immunol. 2014;134(3):593–601.e512.

229. Matsui EC, Simons E, Rand C, et al. Airborne mouse allergen in the homes of inner-city children with asthma. J Allergy Clin Immunol. 2005;115(2):358–63.

230. Grant T, Aloe C, Perzanowski M, et al. Mouse sensitization and exposure are associated with asthma severity in urban children. J Allergy Clin Immunol Pract. 2016;5(4):1008–1014. e1001.

231. Ahluwalia SK, Peng RD, Breysse PN, et al. Mouse allergen is the major allergen of public health relevance in Baltimore City. J Allergy Clin Immunol. 2013;132(4):830–835.e832.

232. Pongracic JA, Krouse RZ, Babineau DC, et al. Distinguishing characteristics of difficult-to-control asthma in inner-city children and adolescents. J Allergy Clin Immunol. 2016;138(4):1030–41.

233. Dockery DW, Pope Iii CA. Acute respiratory effects of particulate air pollution. Annu Rev Public Health. 1994;15(1):107–32.

234. Nishimura KK, Galanter JM, Roth LA, et al. Early-life air pollution and asthma risk in minority children the GALA II and SAGE II studies. Am J Respir Crit Care Med. 2013;188(3):309–18.

235. Dockery DW. Health effects of particulate air pollution. Ann Epidemiol. 2009;19(4):257–63.

236. Guarnieri M, Balmes JR. Outdoor air pollution and asthma. Lancet. 2014;383(9928):1581–92.

237. Liu L, Poon R, Chen L, et al. Acute effects of air pollution on pulmonary function, airway inflammation, and oxidative stress in asthmatic children. Environ Health Perspect. 2009;117(4):668–74.

238. Barraza-Villarreal A, Sunyer J, Hernandez-Cadena L, et al. Air pollution, airway inflammation, and lung function in a cohort study of Mexico City schoolchildren. Environ Health Perspect. 2008;116(6):832–8.

239. Khreis H, Kelly C, Tate J, Parslow R, Lucas K, Nieuwenhuijsen M. Exposure to traffic-related air pollution and risk of development of childhood asthma: a systematic review and meta-analysis. Environ Int. 2017;100:1–31.

240. Majd E, McCormack M, Davis M, et al. Indoor air quality in inner-city schools and its associations with building characteristics and environmental factors. Environ Res. 2019;170:83–91.

241. Kravitz-Wirtz N, Teixeira S, Hajat A, Woo B, Crowder K, Takeuchi D. Early-life air pollution exposure, neighborhood poverty, and childhood asthma in the United States, 1990-2014. Int J Environ Res Public Health. 2018;15(6):1114.

242. Kanchongkittiphon W, Gaffin JM, Phipatanakul W. The indoor environment and inner-city childhood asthma. Asian Pac J Allergy Immunol. 2014;32(2):103–10.

243. Nardone A, Neophytou AM, Balmes J, Thakur N. Ambient air pollution and asthma-related outcomes in children of color of the USA: a scoping review of literature published between 2013 and 2017. Curr Allergy Asthma Rep. 2018;18(5):1–12.

244. Eggleston PA. The environment and asthma in US inner cities. Chest. 2007;132(5):782S–8S.

245. Bryant-Stephens T. Asthma disparities in urban environments. J Allergy Clin Immunol. 2009;123(6):1199–206.

246. Neophytou AM, White MJ, Oh SS, et al. Air pollution and lung function in minority youth with asthma in the GALA II (Genesenvironments and admixture in Latino Americans) and SAGE II (study of African Americans, asthma, genes, and environments) studies. Am J Respir Crit Care Med. 2016;193(11):1271–80.

247. Maantay J. Asthma and air pollution in the Bronx: methodological and data considerations in using GIS for environmental justice and health research. Health Place. 2007;13(1):32–56.

248. Servadio JL, Lawal AS, Davis T, et al. Demographic inequities in health outcomes and air pollution exposure in the Atlanta area and its relationship to urban infrastructure. J Urban Health. 2019;96(2):219–34.

249. Gold DR, Adamkiewicz G, Arshad SH, et al. NIAID, NIEHS, NHLBI, and MCAN workshop report: the indoor environment and childhood asthma-implications for home envi-

ronmental intervention in asthma prevention and management. J Allergy Clin Immunol. 2017;140(4):933–49.

250. Celedón JC, Roman J, Schraufnagel DE, Thomas A, Samet J. Respiratory health equality in the United States: the American thoracic society perspective. Ann Am Thorac Soc. 2014;11(4):473–9.

251. Levy JI, Quiros-Alcala L, Fabian MP, Basra K, Hansel NN. Established and emerging environmental contributors to disparities in asthma and chronic obstructive pulmonary disease. Curr Epidemiol Rep. 2018;5(2):114–24.

252. Tarlo SM, Lemiere C. Occupational asthma. NEJM. 2014;370(7):640–9.

253. Steege AL, Baron SL, Marsh SM, Menéndez CC, Myers JR. Examining occupational health and safety disparities using national data: a cause for continuing concern. Am J Ind Med. 2014;57(5):527–38.

254. Gany F, Novo P, Dobslaw R, Leng J. Urban occupational health in the Mexican and Latino/Latina immigrant population: a literature review. J Immigr Minor Health. 2014;16(5):846–55.

255. Pappalardo AA, Mosnaim G. Immigrant respiratory health: a diverse perspective in environmental influences on respiratory health. Curr Allergy Asthma Rep. 2018;18(4):1–10.

256. Stanbury M, Rosenman KD. Occupational health disparities: a state public health-based approach: occupational health disparities. Am J Ind Med. 2014;57(5):596–604.

257. Smith CK, Bonauto DK. Improving occupational health disparity research: testing a method to estimate race and ethnicity in a working population. Am J Ind Med. 2018;61(8):640–8.

258. Bellinger JD, Hassan RM, Rivers PA, Cheng Q, Williams E, Glover SH. Specialty care use in US patients with chronic diseases. Int J Environ Res Public Health. 2010;7(3):975–90.

259. Shone LP, Dick AW, Brach C, et al. The role of race and ethnicity in the State Children's Health Insurance Program (SCHIP) in four states: are there baseline disparities, and what do they mean for SCHIP? Pediatrics. 2003;112(6):e521–E532.

260. Shone LP, Dick AW, Klein JD, Zwanziger J, Szilagyi PG. Reduction in racial and ethnic disparities after enrollment in the state Children's health insurance program. Pediatrics. 2005;115(6):e697–705.

261. Mansour ME, Lanphear BP, DeWitt TG. Barriers to asthma care in urban children: parent perspectives. Pediatrics. 2000;106(3):512–9.

262. Akinbami LJ, Moorman JE, Garbe PL, Sondik EJ. Status of childhood asthma in the United States, 1980-2007. Pediatrics. 2009;123(Supplement):S131–45.

263. Dinkevich EI, Cunningham SJ, Crain EF. Parental perceptions of access to care and quality of care for inner-city children with asthma. J Asthma. 1998;35(1):63–71.

264. Merrick NJ, Houchens R, Tillisch S, Berlow B, Landon C, Group M. Quality of hospital care of children with asthma: medicaid versus privately insured patients. J Health Care Poor Underserved. 2001;12(2):192–207.

265. Lantner R, Brennan RA, Gray L, McElroy D. Research, outcomes Committee of the Suburban Asthma C. Inpatient management of asthma in the Chicago suburbs: the Suburban Asthma Management Initiative (SAMI). J Asthma. 2005;42(1):55–63.

266. Frankenfield DL, Wei II, Anderson KK, Howell BL, Waldo DR, Sekscenski E. Prescription medication cost-related non-adherence among medicare CAHPS respondents: disparity by Hispanic ethnicity. J Health Care Poor Underserved. 2010;21(2):518–43.

267. Briesacher BA, Gurwitz JH, Soumerai SB. Patients at-risk for cost-related medication nonadherence: a review of the literature. J Gen Intern Med. 2007;22(6):864–71.

268. Riekert KA, Butz AM, Eggleston PA, Huss K, Winkelstein M, Rand CS. Caregiver-physician medication concordance and undertreatment of asthma among inner-city children. Pediatrics. 2003;111(3):e214–20.

269. Pappalardo AA, Karavolos K, Martin MA. What really happens in the home: the medication environment of urban, minority youth. J Allergy Clin Immunol Pract. 2017;5(3):764–70.

270. Hasegawa K, Stoll SJ, Ahn J, Kysia RF, Sullivan AF, Camargo CA. Association of insurance status with severity and management in ED patients with asthma exacerbation. West J Emerg Med. 2016;17(1):22–7.

271. Lingner H, Burger B, Kardos P, Criee CP, Worth H, Hummers-Pradier E. What patients really think about asthma guidelines: barriers to guideline implementation from the patients' perspective. BMC Pulm Med. 2017;17(1):13.
272. Fischer F, Lange K, Klose K, Greiner W, Kraemer A. Barriers and strategies in guideline implementation-a scoping review. Healthcare (Basel). 2016;4(3).
273. Finkelstein JA, Barton MB, Donahue JG, Algatt-Bergstrom P, Markson LE, Platt R. Comparing asthma care for Medicaid and non-Medicaid children in a health maintenance organization. Arch Pediatr Adolesc Med. 2000;154(6):563–8.
274. Paradies Y, Truong M, Priest N. A systematic review of the extent and measurement of healthcare provider racism. J Gen Intern Med. 2014;29(2):364–87.
275. Greenwald AG, McGhee DE, Schwartz JLK. Measuring individual differences in implicit cognition: the implicit association test. J Pers Soc Psychol. 1998;74(6):1464–80.
276. Sabin JA, Greenwald AG. The influence of implicit bias on treatment recommendations for 4 common pediatric conditions: pain, urinary tract infection, attention deficit hyperactivity disorder, and asthma. Am J Public Health. 2012;102(5):988–95.
277. Inkelas MP, Garro NMPH, McQuaid ELP, Ortega ANP. Race/ethnicity, language, and asthma care: findings from a 4-state survey. Ann Allergy Asthma Immunol. 2008;100(2):120–7.
278. Wisnivesky JP, Krauskopf KM, Wolf MS, et al. The association between language proficiency and outcomes of elderly patients with asthma. Ann Allergy Asthma Immunol. 2012;109(3):179–84.
279. Cloutier MM, Hall CB, Wakefield DB, Bailit H. Use of asthma guidelines by primary care providers to reduce hospitalizations and emergency department visits in poor, minority, urban children. J Pediatr. 2005;146(5):591–7.
280. Kercsmar CM, Beck AF, Sauers-Ford H, et al. Association of an asthma improvement collaborative with health care utilization in medicaid-insured pediatric patients in an urban community. JAMA Pediatr. 2017;171(11):1072–80.
281. Klein JD, McNulty M, Flatau CN. Adolescents' access to care: Teenagers' self-reported use of services and perceived access to confidential care. Arch Pediatr Adolesc Med. 1998;152(7):676–82.
282. Naman J, Press VG, Vaughn D, Hull A, Erwin K, Volerman A. Student perspectives on asthma management in schools: a mixed-methods study examining experiences, facilitators, and barriers to care. J Asthma. 2018:1–12.
283. KyngÄs HA, Kroll T, Duffy ME. Compliance in adolescents with chronic diseases: a review. J Adolesc Health. 2000;26(6):379–88.
284. Ahmad A, Sorensen K. Enabling and hindering factors influencing adherence to asthma treatment among adolescents: a systematic literature review. J Asthma. 2016;53(8):862–78.
285. Heyduck K, Bengel J, Farin-Glattacker E, Glattacker M. Adolescent and parental perceptions about asthma and asthma management: a dyadic qualitative analysis: adolescent and parental perceptions about asthma. Child Care Health Dev. 2015;41(6):1227–37.
286. Jones MR, Frey SM, Riekert K, Fagnano M, Halterman JS. Transition readiness for talking with providers in urban youth with asthma: associations with medication management. J Adolesc Health. 2019;64(2):265–71.
287. Naureckas E. Are we closing the disparities gap? Small-area analysis of asthma in Chicago. Chest. 2007;132(5 suppl):858S.
288. Health IDoP. Asthma burden update. 2013.
289. Weiss KB, Shannon JJ, Sadowski LS, et al. The burden of asthma in the Chicago community fifteen years after the availability of national asthma guidelines: the design and initial results from the CHIRAH study. Contemp Clin Trials. 2009;30(3):246–55.
290. Shalowitz MU, Sadowski LM, Kumar R, Weiss KB, Shannon JJ. Asthma burden in a citywide, diverse sample of elementary schoolchildren in Chicago. Ambul Pediatr. 2007;7(4):271–7.
291. Washington DM, Curtis LM, Waite K, Wolf MS, Paasche-Orlow MK. Sociodemographic factors mediate race and ethnicity-associated childhood asthma health disparities: a longitudinal analysis. J Racial Ethn Health Disparities. 2018;5(5):928–38.

292. Dell JL, Whitman S, Shah AM, Silva A, Ansell D. Smoking in 6 diverse Chicago communities--a population study. Am J Public Health. 2005;95(6):1036–42.
293. Dircksen JCPN, et al. Healthy Chicago 2.0: partnering to improve health equity. City of Chicago. In: Health CDoP, editor. . Chicago; 2016.
294. Management THSfSPa. Diversity Data kids. In. Waltham, MA: Brandeis University.
295. American Public Health Association Community Health Worker Section. http://www.dph. illinois.gov/sites/default/files/publications/healthy-smiles-09-050216.pdf. Accessed 15 April 2019.
296. Gutierrez Kapheim MCJ. Best practice guidelines for implementing and evaluating community health worker programs in health care settings: Sinai Urban Health Institute; 2014.
297. Martin MA, Mosnaim GS, Olson D, Swider S, Karavolos K, Rothschild S. Results from a community-based trial testing a community health worker asthma intervention in Puerto Rican youth in Chicago. J Asthma. 2015;52(1):59–70.
298. Martin MA, Floyd EC, Nixon SK, Villalpando S, Shalowitz M, Lynch E. Asthma in children with comorbid obesity: intervention development in a high-risk urban community. Health Promot Pract. 2016;17(6):880–90.
299. Mosnaim GS, Li H, Damitz M, et al. Evaluation of the Fight Asthma Now (FAN) program to improve asthma knowledge in urban youth and teenagers. Ann Allergy Asthma Immunol. 2011;107(4):310–6.
300. Naureckas ET, Wolf RL, Trubitt MJ, et al. The Chicago asthma consortium: a community coalition targeting reductions in asthma morbidity. Chest. 1999;116(4 Suppl 1):190s–3s.
301. Whitman S, Shah AM, Benjamins M. Urban health : combating disparities with local data. New York: Oxford University Press; 2011.
302. Martin MA, Press VG, Erwin K, et al. Engaging end-users in intervention research study design. J Asthma. 2017:1–9.
303. Erwin K, Martin MA, Flippin T, et al. Engaging stakeholders to design a comparative effectiveness trial in children with uncontrolled asthma. J Comp Eff Res. 2016;5(1):17–30.
304. Krishnan JA, Martin MA, Lohff C, et al. Design of a pragmatic trial in minority children presenting to the emergency department with uncontrolled asthma: the CHICAGO plan. Contemp Clin Trials. 2017;57:10–22.
305. Institute P-COR. Comparing three ways to prepare children and caregivers to manage asthma after an emergency room visit – the CHICAGO Trial. 2018; https://www.pcori.org/research-results/2013/comparing-three-ways-prepare-children-and-caregivers-manage-asthma-after. Accessed 18 April 2019.
306. Minier MHL, Ramahi R, Glassgow AE, Fox K, Martin M. An essential partnership for the effective care of children with chronic conditions. J School Health. 2017;88:699.
307. Pappalardo AA, Paulson A, Bruscato R, Thomas L, Minier M, Martin MA. Chicago public school nurses examine barriers to school asthma care coordination. Public Health Nurs. 2019;36(1):36–44.
308. Mahon J, Fitzgerald A, Glanville J, et al. Misuse and/or treatment delivery failure of inhalers among patients with asthma or COPD: a review and recommendations for the conduct of future research. Respir Med. 2017;129:98–116.
309. Volerman A, Toups MM, Hull A, Press VG. A feasibility study of a patient-centered educational strategy for rampant inhaler misuse among minority children with asthma. J Allergy Clin Immunol Pract. 2019;7:2028.

Chapter 8
Disparity in Atopic Dermatitis

Brandon E. Cohen, Nada Elbuluk, and Sindhura Bandi

Blake

Blake is a 13-year-old African American male. His mother works nights for a local chain restaurant and the patient lives in a shared home with his mother and grandparents. He presents as an acute visit to an urgent care center. Blake was diagnosed with atopic dermatitis by his pediatrician as an infant. His atopic dermatitis was previously well controlled with topical emollients and occasional topical steroids for exacerbations. However, the mother notes that since the patient started at a new middle school at age 11, his symptoms have significantly worsened. She also noted that this coincides with the patient taking on more responsibility with his own bathing, hygiene, and skin care in adolescence. Physical examination reveals erythematous papules and plaques on his bilateral arms, legs, trunk, and back. There are significant xerosis and excoriations of his skin diffusely, as well as lichenified plaques on his hands and bilateral popliteal fossa. There are also scattered areas of hypopigmentation on his cheeks and extensor forearms. The patient states that he is always up at night scratching his skin, often to the point of bleeding. He states that he is embarrassed by the physical appearance of his skin at school and also finds it difficult to concentrate. His performance at school has declined in the past year, and he attributes it to his tiredness, lack of self-esteem to contribute, and his pain and itching that make it impossible to concentrate. The mother states that she has tried to make appointments with the specialist, but because the appointments must be made so far in advance and her work schedule often changes, the patient has had multiple missed appointments. There is only one pediatric dermatologist in their

B. E. Cohen · N. Elbuluk
Dermatology, University of Southern California, Los Angeles, CA, USA

S. Bandi (✉)
Allergy and Immunology, Rush University Medical Center, Chicago, IL, USA
e-mail: sindhura_bandi@rush.edu

© Springer Nature Switzerland AG 2020
M. Mahdavinia (ed.), *Health Disparities in Allergic Diseases*,
https://doi.org/10.1007/978-3-030-31222-0_8

region who will accept their healthcare insurance. Both the mother and the patient express frustration with his current symptoms and request an "injection to make this go away."

Introduction

Atopic dermatitis (AD) is a chronic inflammatory condition of the skin that is associated with a personal or family history of other atopic diseases, namely, allergic rhinitis and asthma. AD is most prevalent among children, but may persist into adulthood in up to one-third of individuals [1]. AD is reported to affect up to 20% of children and 3% of adults worldwide [1]. In the United States (USA), according to the 2003 National Survey of Children's Health, the prevalence of AD in those younger than 18 years was 10.7% [2]. In adults, the reported prevalence in the USA ranges from 7.2% to 10.2% [2, 3]. Affected individuals may experience refractory pruritus, poor sleep quality, secondary infections, significant psychosocial distress, and restricted participation in activities [3–5]. AD imposes a significant burden not only on affected individuals and caretakers, but also on the larger healthcare system and society [4, 6]. In one study, when considering costs of medications, physician visits, and the indirect costs of lost productivity, the annual cost of AD in the USA was over 5.2 billion dollars [7].

While AD is closely associated with asthma and allergic rhinitis, there is growing evidence that AD exhibits distinct risk factors and involves complex interactions between genetic, environmental, and lifestyle factors. While underlying genetics are certainly an important determinant of AD prevalence and severity, there is an increasing appreciation for the importance of environmental and lifestyle factors. This is highlighted by reports that there is a lack of correlation between filaggrin mutations and severity of AD [8]. The notion that AD prevalence depends considerably on the surrounding environment highlights the potential for health disparities stemming from modifiable extrinsic factors. These factors contribute to potential disparities in prevalence, severity, and management between geographic locations, as well as across socioeconomic and racial groups.

Currently Existing Disparities in Atopic Dermatitis

Prevalence

The prevalence of atopy, including atopic dermatitis, has been increasing worldwide; however, the prevalence rates vary significantly among different geographic regions [9]. According to the Internal Study of Asthma and Allergies in Childhood, an international cross-sectional study of over 500,000 school-aged children, the prevalence of AD is significantly higher in Western and Northern Europe, Australia, South America, and urban regions of Africa and lower in Eastern Europe, the Middle

East, and China [10]. In another survey of schoolchildren in Oregon, USA, by Laughter et al., a higher prevalence of AD was reported in the USA, compared to estimates from Europe or Japan [6]. A number of other studies have similarly reported a higher prevalence of AD in more developed nations [6, 11, 12]. Hypothesized explanations for this trend include the effects of urbanization, climate, diet, and varying exposure to infections and airborne allergens [1, 10].

It has been further shown that the prevalence of AD can vary significantly within the same country. The 2003 National Survey of Children's Health reported higher rates of AD among states on the east coast, compared to other regions of the USA [2]. One proposed explanation is the greater number of metropolitan cities on the east coast, compared to other regions [2]. In this study, the examination of survey data revealed that living in an urban, compared to rural environment, was associated with an adjusted odds ratio of 1.67 for AD [2]. Similarly, Laughter et al. reported higher rates of AD among surveyed children living in urban versus rural areas in Oregon [6]. Proposed deleterious effects associated with urban living include exposure to a larger quantity or more varied allergens, decreased ultraviolet (UV) light exposure, and living in more modern insulated housing [3, 13, 14].

The impact of environmental factors is further highlighted when examining immigrant populations. Multiple studies have reported that Americans who were born outside of the USA have a lower prevalence of AD than those born in the USA [2, 3]. Nevertheless, over time, the rates of AD among immigrants living in the USA increase and exceed the rates of AD from their country of origin [14]. In the 2010 National Health Interview Survey, which examined AD in American adults, foreign-born Americans exhibited decreased rates of AD when compared to those born in the USA, but after living in the USA for at least 10 years, rates of AD among immigrant groups increased. The rate of eczema in immigrants living in the USA for less than 10 years was 4.3% versus 6.7% in those living in the USA for greater than 10 years [3]. Furthermore, Silverberg et al. reported a lower prevalence of AD in American children born and living outside the USA, compared to those born in the USA [3]. Similar trends have been observed when examining Asian children born in Australia, compared to Asian children who recently immigrated to Australia [13].

Impact of Socioeconomic Factors

Numerous studies worldwide have investigated potential association between the socioeconomic status and the prevalence or severity of AD. While socioeconomic factors have been shown to be determinants of AD, there is a lack of concordance between studies on whether AD prevalence and severity are associated with higher or lower socioeconomic status. For example, Williams and colleagues examined over 8000 children across the United Kingdom (UK), stratified participants into five socioeconomic classes, and reported a significant linear trend in AD prevalence with higher social class [12]. In this study, diagnosis of AD was confirmed by physical exam and analyses were adjusted for variables, such as gender, residence, family size, ethnic group, exposure to tobacco, and breastfeeding. Of note, no similar trend was observed when examining the prevalence of psoriasis or acne in the same cohort [12]. Furthermore, multiple separate studies, examining cohorts in the United States, Austria, Germany, and Japan, have reported an independent positive association between parental education level and AD prevalence, after adjusting for various confounding factors [3, 11, 13, 15]. Similarly, in a cross-sectional health survey conducted in Demark by Hammer-Helmich and colleagues, AD was significantly linked to higher parental education, while asthma and allergic rhinitis were associated with lower parental education [16]. Parental unemployment was also associated with a decrease in AD risk and severity [16].

Data-supported explanations for the associations between higher socioeconomic status and AD are lacking. One early hypothesis to explain the relationship between higher socioeconomic status and greater AD prevalence is the "hygiene hypothesis," or the proposed concept that increased exposure to various infectious agents confers a protective effect on the tendency to develop atopy. However, more recently, studies have reported no association between AD and factors related to the hygiene hypothesis such as larger family size and daycare attendance [15, 17]. Other explanations are that patients of higher socioeconomic class may be more likely to interact with the healthcare system and receive a diagnosis of AD, or be more likely to respond affirmatively to health surveys due to greater health literacy.

Notably, in the Danish study by Hammer-Helmich et al., while AD prevalence and severity was associated with higher parental education and parental employment, there was no association found between AD and household income, which the authors propose may relate to equivalent healthcare access in Denmark [16]. In the United States, where greater disparities in healthcare access exist, several large studies suggest that access to care may be contributing to observed trends in AD prevalence and severity. According to data from the 2010 National Health Interview Survey, the prevalence of AD was significantly associated with health insurance coverage and healthcare interaction in the past year; suggesting differences in prevalence may be related to differences in the rates of diagnosis [3]. In another study by Hanifin and Reed, an inverse relationship between household income and empirically defined AD was discovered, based on a health survey sent to a representative sample of the US population [18].

Racial and Ethnic Disparities in Atopic Dermatitis

There is a growing amount of research demonstrating that disparities in the prevalence and severity of AD exist between racial groups. Shaw and colleagues reported that based on data from the National Survey of Children's Health, African American race was associated with an increased prevalence of AD, compared to Caucasian race (15.9% vs. 9.7%, OR 1.7) [2]. In accordance, Fu et al. reported a higher prevalence of eczema in African American, compared to Caucasian children (19.3% vs. 16.1%), using 2005–2006 National Health and Nutrition Examination Survey

[20]. Williams and colleagues reported similar results in the UK in a study of nearly 700 London-born children, in which they reported a significantly higher rate of AD, diagnosed by a physician, in Black Caribbean, compared to White children (16.3% vs. 8.7%) [21]. Silverberg and Simpson also reported that based on the 2007 National Survey of Children's Health, eczema severity was reported to be associated with Hispanic or African American race in univariate analyses, although this association was no longer significant in multivariable models [8]. In a study of AD in adults using the 2010 National Health Interview Survey, a higher prevalence of AD was reported in those identifying as Hispanic or multiracial, compared to Caucasians, in multivariable models [3]. Furthermore, in a study using the National Ambulatory Medical Care Survey from 1990 to 1998, Janumpally et al. reported that the number of clinic visits for AD was significantly greater for African American (OR 3.4) and Asian/Pacific Islander (OR 6.7) patients, compared to Caucasians [14]. Of note, in this study, Caucasian individuals had a higher rate of medical visits overall, including visits for other dermatologic conditions, suggesting that the observed difference in visits for AD could not be attributed to differences in healthcare utilization in general [14].

Outcomes Related to Disparities in Food Allergy

Severity of Skin Disease

Lower socioeconomic status has been suggested to contribute to increased severity of AD. In a study by Silverberg et al., which examined data from the 2007 National Survey of Children's Health, greater AD severity, as determined from survey questions on three-point scale, was associated with lower parental education, lower household income, and poorer housing quality [8]. Proposed explanations for the relationship between greater AD severity and lower socioeconomic status include exposure to indoor pollutants in lower quality housing, greater exposure to cutaneous irritants, secondary infections, and reduced access to healthcare, resulting in poorer management and disease control [19].

Disparities among racial groups related to the severity of AD have also been identified. For example, in a study of pediatric patients with AD presenting to a tertiary care clinic, 75% of 60 African American patients qualified as having moderate–severe AD, compared to 40% among 100 Caucasian patients, based on Eczema Area and Severity Index and Investigator Global Assessment Scores [22]. In another study of 137 children with AD in the UK, the authors reported that Black children had nearly sixfold higher odds of having severe AD than White children [23]. Of note, in this study, the difference in AD severity persisted even after controlling for social class [23]. Possible causes for the differences in prevalence and severity of AD between racial groups include uneven access to care, differences in the presentation of AD in different skin types, and under-recognized differences between races in the underlying genetics and pathophysiology of AD.

Specific challenges associated with the management of AD in patients with skin of color have been described. For example, there is a higher risk of dyspigmentation associated with topical corticosteroid use in individuals with SOC. Furthermore, the dose or duration of certain treatments can depend on the race or skin type of the patient. For instance, it has been shown that the bioavailability of cyclosporine is significantly lower in African American compared to Caucasian individuals [36]. In addition, higher doses of phototherapy are required for patients with SOC [29].

Reasons for Atopic Dermatitis Health Disparities

Access to Healthcare

Access to dermatological specialty care has been suggested to be insufficient in general, stemming from a shortage of dermatologists nationally [24]. Furthermore, access to dermatology may be especially limited depending on insurance coverage, as highlighted by the results of a 2002 American Academy of Dermatology (AAD) survey reporting that only 40.8% and 51.3% of dermatologists accept new patients with Medicaid or no insurance, respectively [25]. In this report, patients receiving Medicaid comprised 5% of patients being seen at dermatology practices, significantly less than the 27% that would be predicted based on the percentage of patients receiving Medicaid in the population [25]. Differences by race in utilization of dermatological care have also been identified. In a study of the National Ambulatory Medical Care Survey, it was reported that in the USA over 90% of patients seen by dermatologists are Caucasian [26], which may reflect the inadequate treatment of AD among non-Caucasian patients. This discrepancy may relate to differences in insurance status, and in turn access to dermatology [14]. Previous studies have reported a higher rate of uninsured status among African Americans, compared to Caucasians, in the USA [14]. While this discrepancy has narrowed after healthcare reform, according to 2016 Center for Disease Control data, African American, as well as Hispanic individuals continue to demonstrate lower health insurance rates, compared to Caucasians [27].

The quality of care delivered by dermatologists for AD may also vary across racial groups due to differences in disease presentation and inadequate focus on these differences during physician training. In one survey of US dermatology chief residents, only 25.4% reported having had expert lectures on topics related to skin of color (SOC) and only 30.2% reported having a specific rotation during which experience in treating patients with SOC was obtained [28]. In another survey, 47% of dermatologists and dermatology residents reported feeling that their training was inadequate in conditions affecting individuals with SOC [24]. The lack of specialized training may contribute to disparities in diagnosis and management between patients of different racial groups and contribute to the observed differences in AD severity. In a study of 137 pediatric patients with AD in the UK by Ben-Gashir and colleagues, it was discovered that a lack of ability to appreciate erythema on the physical exam of Black patients resulted in an underestimate of AD severity [23]. In this study, AD severity was compared between Black and White children using the SCORAD scale, which relies on factors such as erythema, edema, excoriation, and lichenification. Initially, the authors discovered a nonsignificant greater severity among White patients; however, once erythema scores were omitted from the severity assessment tool, it was reported that Black children showed a significantly higher rate of severe AD than White children (OR 5.93, $p = 0.002$) [23]. After controlling for erythema scores, physician severity assessments became more aligned with parental severity scores. Adjustment of other factors, such as edema, excoriation, or lichenification, did not produce a difference in severity outcome. The authors emphasize that reliance on erythema, which is included in a number of severity measures, may result in a falsely low impression of AD severity in SOC [23]. Disparities in accurate diagnosis may further result from the potential for AD in SOC to present with more subtle lesions, different morphology, or with an atypical distribution. For example, AD in African Americans may present with follicular, papular, or lichenoid lesions, or with a greater involvement of extensor instead of flexural surfaces [1, 22, 29]. Consequently, these differences may result in delayed diagnosis, counseling, and appropriate management.

Genetic Beyond differences in the phenotypic expression of AD between skin types, there is emerging evidence that there may be racial differences in the underlying genes involved in AD. Several studies have reported that the prevalence of filaggrin null mutations is significantly lower in African American, compared to Caucasian, patients with AD [30, 31]. In one study of 857 children with AD by Margolis et al., at least one filaggrin null mutation was detected in 27.5% of Caucasian, compared to 5.8% of African Americans [31]. In another study, it was reported that two common FLG mutations in patients with European ancestry, namely, R501X and 2282del4, were absent in individuals of African or Asian ancestry [32]. These findings suggest that there are distinct genetic mechanisms underlying AD in different racial groups, which may contribute to differences in AD severity. A number of other physiologic differences important in AD differ by race. It has been reported that, compared to Caucasians, African Americans have higher serum levels of immunoglobulin E, larger mast cell granules, and polymorphisms in pruritus receptors [22, 29, 33, 34]. Further, African American patients may have a higher tendency toward xerosis, as it has been shown that African American skin at baseline demonstrates higher transepidermal water loss and a lower ratio of ceramide to cholesterol, compared to Caucasian or Asian skin [22].

Racial variations in the underlying immunologic phenotype for AD may exist as well, which may contribute to disparities in targeted treatments. In one study, lesional and nonlesional biopsies were performed on 30 patients with AD and reverse-transcriptase-polymerase chain reaction (RT-PCR) and immunochemistry were employed to make comparisons between Caucasian, African American, and control patients. Biopsy specimens from African American patients showed greater infiltration with dendritic cells with the high-affinity IgG receptor, compared to specimens from Caucasians [29]. In addition, while both European and African patients with chronic AD showed upregulation of Th2-related cytokines, African Americans demonstrated decreased expression of Th1- and Th17-related markers, suggesting that Th1 skewing in chronic AD may not occur uniformly across racial groups [29]. Nodal et al. analyzed biopsy samples of European American and Asian individuals with AD and reported that the immunologic phenotype of AD in Asian patients demonstrated a distinct profile, compared to European patients [35]. In this study, AD severity scores were equivalent between European and Asian patients. While both groups showed increased Th2 expression, Asian patients with AD demonstrated significantly greater Th17 activation, along with greater acanthosis, parakeratosis, and Ki67 counts. The authors suggest that racial differences in immune phenotypes require greater attention during the use and development of targeted therapies [35].

Conclusions

AD is complex in its etiology, challenging to treat, and significantly impacts the quality of life of those affected. Those individuals affected by the disparities in AD often do not achieve adequate control of their symptoms and treatment of their condition. It is important for health practitioners to recognize these disparities when evaluating and treating patients with atopic dermatitis. There is ongoing research on the identification of these unique patient factors and implementation of novel treatment modalities. This includes therapy targeted at the various immunologic mechanisms and phenotypes that exist in atopic dermatitis. The first such biologic therapy, Dupilumab, a monoclonal antibody that binds to interleukin-4 receptor subunit alpha (IL-4Rα) and subsequently blocks the Th2 immune response, has been approved in adults. Current studies are underway examining Il-31 as a molecular target to reduce the immune response associated with pruritus. The development of biomarkers, specific molecules which can identify the phenotype and clinical presentation of the disease, is the next step in creating targeted, individualized therapies in AD.

Going back to our case, severe AD has impacted this child's quality of life, performance at school, and potentially his future. His uncontrolled disease is impacted by lack of access to specialty care and inadequate treatments. The treatment of AD relies on daily care and use of multiple topical medications, which is only possible through education, close relation with healthcare providers, and teamwork. Furthermore, other factors, such as exposure to indoor pollutants, cutaneous irritants and allergens, and secondary infections, need to be assessed and addressed by specialist. As the pathogenesis of AD becomes better understood particularly among different populations and treatment options for AD evolve, efforts are also needed to develop programs for patients with limited resources. With the use of these programs along with novel treatment modalities, there is hope that the gap in AD disparities will narrow.

References

1. Mei-Yen Yong A, Tay YK. Atopic dermatitis: racial and ethnic differences. Dermatol Clin. 2017;35(3):395–402.
2. Shaw TE, Currie GP, Koudelka CW, Simpson EL. Eczema prevalence in the United States: data from the 2003 National Survey of Children's Health. J Invest Dermatol. 2011;131(1):67–73.
3. Silverberg JI, Hanifin JM. Adult eczema prevalence and associations with asthma and other health and demographic factors: a US population-based study. J Allergy Clin Immunol. 2013;132(5):1132–8.
4. Letourneau NL, Kozyrskyj AL, Cosic N, Ntanda HN, Anis L, Hart MJ, et al. Maternal sensitivity and social support protect against childhood atopic dermatitis. Allergy Asthma Clin Immunol. 2017;13:26.
5. Silverberg JI, Simpson EL. Association between severe eczema in children and multiple comorbid conditions and increased healthcare utilization. Pediatr Allergy Immunol. 2013;24(5):476–86.
6. Laughter D, Istvan JA, Tofte SJ, Hanifin JM. The prevalence of atopic dermatitis in Oregon schoolchildren. J Am Acad Dermatol. 2000;43(4):649–55.
7. Drucker AM, Wang AR, Li WQ, Sevetson E, Block JK, Qureshi AA. The burden of atopic dermatitis: summary of a report for the National Eczema Association. J Invest Dermatol. 2017;137(1):26–30.
8. Silverberg JI, Simpson EL. Associations of childhood eczema severity: a US population-based study. Dermatitis. 2014;25(3):107–14.
9. Beasley R. Worldwide variation in prevalence of symptoms of asthma, allergic rhinoconjunctivitis, and atopic eczema: ISAAC. The International Study of Asthma and Allergies in Childhood (ISAAC) Steering Committee. Lancet. 1998;351(9111):1225–32.
10. Odhiambo JA, Williams HC, Clayton TO, Robertson CF, Asher MI, Group IPTS. Global variations in prevalence of eczema symptoms in children from ISAAC Phase Three. J Allergy Clin Immunol. 2009;124(6):1251–8 e23.
11. Weber AS, Haidinger G. The prevalence of atopic dermatitis in children is influenced by their parents' education: results of two cross-sectional studies conducted in Upper Austria. Pediatr Allergy Immunol. 2010;21(7):1028–35.
12. Williams HC, Strachan DP, Hay RJ. Childhood eczema: disease of the advantaged? BMJ. 1994;308(6937):1132–5.
13. Diepgen TL. Atopic dermatitis: the role of environmental and social factors, the European experience. J Am Acad Dermatol. 2001;45(1 Suppl):S44–8.
14. Janumpally SR, Feldman SR, Gupta AK, Fleischer AB Jr. In the United States, blacks and Asian/Pacific Islanders are more likely than whites to seek medical care for atopic dermatitis. Arch Dermatol. 2002;138(5):634–7.
15. Miyake Y, Tanaka K, Sasaki S, Hirota Y. Parental employment, income, education and allergic disorders in children: a prebirth cohort study in Japan. Int J Tuberc Lung Dis. 2012;16(6):756–61.
16. Hammer-Helmich L, Linneberg A, Thomsen SF, Glumer C. Association between parental socioeconomic position and prevalence of asthma, atopic eczema and hay fever in children. Scand J Public Health. 2014;42(2):120–7.
17. Zutavern A, Hirsch T, Leupold W, Weiland S, Keil U, von Mutius E. Atopic dermatitis, extrinsic atopic dermatitis and the hygiene hypothesis: results from a cross-sectional study. Clin Exp Allergy. 2005;35(10):1301–8.
18. Hanifin JM, Reed ML, Eczema P, Impact Working G. A population-based survey of eczema prevalence in the United States. Dermatitis. 2007;18(2):82–91.
19. Mercer MJ, Joubert G, Ehrlich RI, Nelson H, Poyser MA, Puterman A, et al. Socioeconomic status and prevalence of allergic rhinitis and atopic eczema symptoms in young adolescents. Pediatr Allergy Immunol. 2004;15(3):234–41.

20. Fu T, Keiser E, Linos E, Rotatori RM, Sainani K, Lingala B, et al. Eczema and sensitization to common allergens in the United States: a multiethnic, population-based study. Pediatr Dermatol. 2014;31(1):21–6.
21. Williams HC, Pembroke AC, Forsdyke H, Boodoo G, Hay RJ, Burney PG. London-born black Caribbean children are at increased risk of atopic dermatitis. J Am Acad Dermatol. 1995;32(2 Pt 1):212–7.
22. Vachiramon V, Tey HL, Thompson AE, Yosipovitch G. Atopic dermatitis in African American children: addressing unmet needs of a common disease. Pediatr Dermatol. 2012;29(4):395–402.
23. Ben-Gashir MA, Hay RJ. Reliance on erythema scores may mask severe atopic dermatitis in black children compared with their white counterparts. Br J Dermatol. 2002;147(5):920–5.
24. Buster KJ, Stevens EI, Elmets CA. Dermatologic health disparities. Dermatol Clin. 2012;30(1):53–9, viii.
25. Resneck JS Jr, Isenstein A, Kimball AB. Few Medicaid and uninsured patients are accessing dermatologists. J Am Acad Dermatol. 2006;55(6):1084–8.
26. Stern RS. Dermatologists and office-based care of dermatologic disease in the 21st century. J Investig Dermatol Symp Proc. 2004;9(2):126–30.
27. Cohen RA, Zammitti EP, Martinez ME. Health insurance coverage: early release of estimates from the National Health Interview Survey, 2016: Center for Disease Control, National Center For Health Statistics; 2017.
28. Nijhawan RI, Jacob SE, Woolery-Lloyd H. Skin of color education in dermatology residency programs: does residency training reflect the changing demographics of the United States? J Am Acad Dermatol. 2008;59(4):615–8.
29. Sanyal RD, Pavel AB, Glickman J, Chan TC, Zheng X, Zhang N, et al. Atopic dermatitis in African American patients is TH2/TH22-skewed with TH1/TH17 attenuation. Ann Allergy Asthma Immunol. 2018;122:99.
30. Garrett JP, Hoffstad O, Apter AJ, Margolis DJ. Racial comparison of filaggrin null mutations in asthmatic patients with atopic dermatitis in a US population. J Allergy Clin Immunol. 2013;132(5):1232–4.
31. Margolis DJ, Apter AJ, Gupta J, Hoffstad O, Papadopoulos M, Campbell LE, et al. The persistence of atopic dermatitis and filaggrin (FLG) mutations in a US longitudinal cohort. J Allergy Clin Immunol. 2012;130(4):912–7.
32. Palmer CN, Irvine AD, Terron-Kwiatkowski A, Zhao Y, Liao H, Lee SP, et al. Common loss-of-function variants of the epidermal barrier protein filaggrin are a major predisposing factor for atopic dermatitis. Nat Genet. 2006;38(4):441–6.
33. Sueki H, Whitaker-Menezes D, Kligman AM. Structural diversity of mast cell granules in black and white skin. Br J Dermatol. 2001;144(1):85–93.
34. Wang H, Papoiu AD, Coghill RC, Patel T, Wang N, Yosipovitch G. Ethnic differences in pain, itch and thermal detection in response to topical capsaicin: African Americans display a notably limited hyperalgesia and neurogenic inflammation. Br J Dermatol. 2010;162(5):1023–9.
35. Noda S, Suarez-Farinas M, Ungar B, Kim SJ, de Guzman Strong C, Xu H, et al. The Asian atopic dermatitis phenotype combines features of atopic dermatitis and psoriasis with increased TH17 polarization. J Allergy Clin Immunol. 2015;136(5):1254–64.
36. Dirks NL, Huth B, Yates CR, Meibohm B. Pharmacokinetics of immunosuppressants: a perspective on ethnic differences. Int J Clin Pharmacol Ther. 2004;42(12):701–18.

Part III
Providing Solutions

Chapter 9
School-Based Educational Programs to Improve the Knowledge and Outcome in Allergic Conditions

Kylie N. Jungles and Roselyn M. Hicks

Introduction

Walk into an emergency department or pediatric intensive care unit on any given day, and you are likely to see at least one child being treated for an acute asthma exacerbation. Asthma is one of the most common chronic medical conditions among pediatric populations – with approximately 7 million children diagnosed with asthma in the United States alone [5]. Asthma impacts quality of life and daily productivity, including a child's general wellbeing and ability to participate in physical activity. Asthma exacerbations lead to direct and indirect costs of emergency department visits, hospital admissions, and school absenteeism. Recent studies suggest that 1 in 36,000 children and adolescents miss school each day due to asthma symptoms [5]. While these children should be in school learning, participating in sports, or playing with friends, they are instead spending countless hours within the healthcare system being treated for their chronic disease. Like many other chronic conditions, studies have found that asthma disproportionately impacts minority children and adolescents, as well as those living in low-income communities [12]. In fact, the prevalence of asthma is two times greater in African American children, and these children are twice as likely to be admitted to a hospital for an acute asthma exacerbation [5]. These trends are likely due to a myriad of patient factors including access to care, health literacy, and disease severity.

While the consequences of poorly controlled asthma can be severe, asthma control is possible with proper medication management, patient education, healthcare

K. N. Jungles (✉)
Department of Allergy and Immunology, Rush University Medical Center, Chicago, IL, USA
e-mail: kylie_n_jungles@rush.edu

R. M. Hicks
Satcher Health Leadership Institute, Division of Health Policy, Morehouse School
of Medicine, Atlanta, GA, USA

© Springer Nature Switzerland AG 2020
M. Mahdavinia (ed.), *Health Disparities in Allergic Diseases*,
https://doi.org/10.1007/978-3-030-31222-0_9

follow-up, and vigilant awareness of symptoms. Unfortunately, many of the patients who present to hospitals for acute exacerbations are often improperly managing their asthma, leading to frequent disease exacerbation. For parents and patients alike, asthma management seems like a tremendous feat. There are various inhaler medications to keep track of, not to mention spacer devices and asthma action plans. For many parents, this can all seem extremely overwhelming and can contribute to improper asthma management. Some of the most common mistakes that are seen in patients presenting with acute asthma exacerbations involve medication nonadherence, such as patients forgetting to take controller medications daily as prescribed or failing to use spacer devices to ensure proper delivery of inhaled medications [11]. Other common mistakes include failing to eliminate asthma triggers from the home – such as cigarette smoke, dust mites, and pets. Keeping medical appointments is another barrier to adequate care, which leads to missed opportunities for patient education and medication management. All of these factors can lead to improper asthma management and negatively impact disease control.

The idea of school-based asthma programs was initiated by analyzing many of the aforementioned shortcomings that typically impede proper asthma care [7]. Because students spend most of their day in school, having a school-based asthma education program in place helps to overcome the obstacle that parents face in bringing their child to regularly scheduled asthma-focused doctor's appointments. School-based programs can help to bridge the gap in healthcare, especially in low-income communities that lack access to quality primary care facilities and adequate public transportation [10]. Studies have found that school-based asthma education programs have established higher attendance rates compared to clinic-based programs, especially in urban settings. Additionally, many schools already possess the infrastructure necessary to carry out school-based asthma programs, with school nurses, support staff, and an organized teaching environment. Schools are equipped with school nurses who possess the appropriate training and medical background necessary to assist with education. Additionally, school nurses can be trained to perform asthma checks and assist with the continuity of care that is essential for students with chronic conditions, such as asthma. Studies have shown that in many cases, the school nurse is the only consistent healthcare provider that some students see – especially in low-income communities, which are disproportionately impacted by asthma. Finally, using a school environment, where students are already primed for learning, helps facilitate teaching students about asthma management [3].

In this chapter, we will discuss the background of school-based asthma programs, including the legislation that has paved the way for the development of many of the school-based asthma programs implemented in schools around the United States today. We will highlight the various frameworks used to develop school-based asthma programs. Then, we will discuss several of the school-based asthma programs that have been initiated in the USA, focusing on the implementation and outcomes associated with each program. Finally, we will touch on the overall benefits associated with these school-based programs and what the future of school-based asthma management may look like.

Background of School-Based Asthma Programs

Over the past several years, changes in legislation and health policy have paved the way for the implementation and growth of school-based asthma programs. In 2015, President Barack Obama signed the Every Student Succeeds Act, which served to replace the No Child Left Behind Act enacted by President George W. Bush [5]. This legislation shaped the federal government's role in education and funding for public education initiatives. The implementation of the Every Student Succeeds Act contributed to the success of many school-based asthma program initiatives because it allowed schools to apply for federal grants in order to fund asthma management in public schools [5]. Another influential policy statement was published in 2016 by the American Academy of Pediatrics Council on School Health. They released a policy revision regarding the role of school nurses in providing school health services. In their statement, they recommended a minimum of one school nurse in every school as well as additional medical oversight from a school physician [5]. They also outlined the importance of establishing a working relationship with school nurses in order to manage chronic conditions of students and highlighted the need for pediatricians to address school absenteeism at clinic appointments. While these all served as large steps forward in the evolution of school-based asthma programs, perhaps the largest feat was in 2016 with the creation of the School-Based Asthma Management Program (SAMPRO). SAMPRO is a school-based asthma program resource created by the American Academy of Allergy, Asthma, and Immunology and the National Association of School Nurses [5].

The role of SAMPRO is to provide resources and education for children, families, and clinicians alike for the development and implementation of school-based asthma programs. Their philosophy and resources are available for free online at http://wwww.aaai.org/SAMPRO [8]. The founders of SAMPRO created a workforce comprised of physicians, researchers, patient advocates, and policy makers to embark on their goals. Together, they created a model for the coordination of asthma care. SAMPRO's approach to asthma management is founded on a circle of support involving patients, families, and healthcare professionals [8]. They believe that a coordinated model of communication is essential in providing the best level of care for individuals with asthma, so they created various resources to aid in this process.

In their literature, the developers of SAMPRO outline four key components, which they feel are essential for the successful coordination of asthma care. The first is a circle of support, which is necessary to foster clear and open communication [8]. They encourage school-based asthma programs to establish a relationship between the child with asthma, their families, their primary care physician, and their school nurse. This helps to facilitate continuity of care both in the clinic and at school. SAMPRO encourages school nurses and families to work together to manage and track asthma symptoms at school. As part of SAMPRO's online toolbox, they offer checklists, which outline the roles of each member within the circle of support. SAMPRO's second component to success involves bidirectional communication between clinicians and schools [8]. This includes encouraging the use of asthma action plans and asthma emergency plans at home and school to guide *Step-Up* asthma management. They encourage clinicians and families to ensure that asthma medications are authorized for use at school and that children have extra medications that can be carried at school at all times. In order to foster a continuity of care, they also believe that periodic updates of the child's asthma status should be communicated between healthcare providers and school nurses. This can provide essential information about the child's asthma control status and need for medication adjustments. The third component to successful asthma management is the use of formal asthma education programs and care coordination programs [8]. They hope that the resources provided in their toolbox can be used nationwide to promote asthma education in resource-limited school districts. Finally, SAMPRO's fourth tenant is aimed at reducing asthma triggers within the school environment. They believe that school administrators, nurses, and personnel should work together to develop an indoor air quality management program, which has been established by the Environmental Protection Agency [8]. The toolkit they have developed provides a checklist that school systems can follow to assess air quality and ensure that their school is meeting the guidelines outlined by the Environmental Protection Agency.

While the implementation of SAMPRO is still in its early stages, the founders hope that the resources provided by SAMPRO online and within the toolkit can help resource-limited school districts address the needs of students with asthma [8]. While SAMPRO outlines the implementation of school-based asthma programs, it is not aimed at replacing programs that have already been established and have demonstrated efficacy. Currently, the American Academy of Allergy, Asthma, and Immunology lobbyists are working with national legislators to pass a congressional bill that will support funding for SAMPRO and school-based asthma programs. The School-Based Respiratory Health Management Act (H.R. 2285) was introduced to Congress as a bipartisan bill in May of 2017 [8]. The goal of the bill is to provide incentives to school systems that implement comprehensive school-based asthma programs. Although the bill failed to be passed by the 115th Congress, they hope to reintroduce the bill to the 116th Congress [8]. The future directions of SAMPRO include lobbying for this essential legislation and continuing to develop and implement the SAMPRO toolkit and other resources.

Framework for School-Based Asthma Programs

Over the years, school-based asthma programs have implemented various organizational frameworks. Some have aimed to enhance education, while others have focused on addressing the shortcomings of asthma care, such as medication adherence. First, we will review several ways school-based asthma programs have been implemented in recent years, followed by details of specific programs. Some studies have aimed to improve asthma screening in schools in order to address students with undiagnosed asthma. This is especially relevant in resource-limited areas, where students lack adequate primary care. The American Thoracic Society published a review, which analyzed the use of screening questionnaires in children with undiagnosed asthma. They found that a 2-item questionnaire had a 66% sensitivity and 96% specificity when validated against spirometry and a formal physician evaluation [1]. Similarly, a 4-item questionnaire developed by Head Start had a 73% sensitivity and 96% specificity in preschool-aged children [1]. These screening-based programs have found to be helpful in distinguishing students with severe asthma who may have never been diagnosed by a physician due to lack of resources.

Another approach used by school-based asthma programs focuses on medication management [1]. Medication nonadherence is often cited as a common reason for asthma exacerbations. Several programs have partnered with healthcare providers to ensure that students with asthma have rescue and controller medications available to them at school, while other school-based programs supervise the administration of controller inhalers to ensure that students are properly administering their daily controller medications [11]. Data from these studies suggest improvement in medication adherence and overall health outcomes in students participating in these medication-focused asthma programs [1].

Finally, some school-based asthma programs take a more holistic approach to the management of asthma. Some programs focus on care coordination among students, schools, and healthcare providers (refer to Fig. 9.1). These programs aim to identify students with asthma to ensure that they have an asthma action plan in place and adequate follow-up with a primary care provider to manage their asthma [1]. There have also been many programs which aim to improve asthma education via group workshops, computer games, web-based modules, peer education, and one-on-one teaching sessions. Many asthma education programs train school staff and nurses to recognize asthma symptoms and provide them with tools to teach students about asthma [1]. On the whole, many successful school-based asthma programs strike a balance between education and symptom management. All of these programs rely on a partnership between students, families, schools, and the healthcare system.

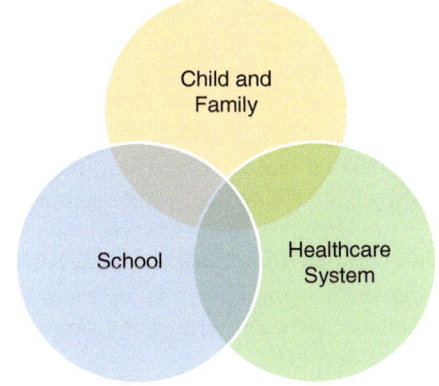

Fig. 9.1 The cornerstone of school-based asthma programs is developing a partnership between students, families, schools, and the healthcare system. Open and clear communication among these entities is essential for the success of any school-based asthma program

Examples of School-Based Asthma Programs

The School-Based Asthma Therapy (SBAT) program is an example of one medication-focused school-based asthma program. This program was launched in 2013 at an urban school district located in the Midwest [1]. The school district primarily served a socioeconomically disadvantaged and ethnically diverse population of young students. The main goal of this program was to increase compliance of inhaled corticosteroid (ICS) medications in children diagnosed with persistent asthma [1]. Children were enrolled in the study based on referrals from school nurses. Specifically, the nurses suggested that students with frequent asthma symptoms or the need for rescue inhaler use at school participate in this program. Other students were referred to the SBAT program by the physicians managing their asthma. Over the course of 3 years, 198 students from kindergarten to twelfth grade were enrolled via rolling admission into the research study [1]. Working together with each student's healthcare provider, the SBAT team developed asthma action plans for each student. The SBAT team also worked with both Medicaid and private insurance providers to ensure that each student was supplied with an ICS inhaler and spacer device for both home and school [1].

As part of the medication administration program, each student was administered their ICS inhaler in the morning prior to classes. The medication administration was observed and assisted by a school nurse or SBAT team member who was trained on the proper administration technique [1]. It was expected that each student received their ICS at home on days that school was not in session and in the evenings, if they required twice daily dosing. Each student's symptoms and asthma control were monitored based on Asthma Control Test forms, which were administered to parents every 2–3 months. These forms contained numerous questions about asthma symptoms, allowing for the quantification of disease severity [1]. If a student's Asthma Control Test score did not improve, an SBAT team member would contact the student's asthma care provider to discuss the findings and whether it was appropriate to step-up medication therapy.

The results of this study were very promising. The researchers found a statistically significant improvement in Asthma Control Test scores over the duration of the study [1]. They also observed a significant reduction in asthma-related emergency department visits and PICU admissions after 1-year post-enrollment of the study. The percentage of PICU care was noted to be 11% within the study population 2 years prior to study enrollment, which declined to just 1% 1 year after participation in SBAT [1]. Overall, the researchers found a tremendous improvement in medication compliance within the study group after participation in the program. They believe that one of the main reasons for the successful outcomes stems from improvement in medical knowledge and teaching of proper medication administration. They also felt that the success from the program was associated with facilitating open communication between physicians and school nurses to ensure that students were prescribed the proper medication regimen in order to target their symptoms [1].

Another example of a medication-focused school-based asthma program is the School-Based Telemedicine Enhanced Asthma Management (SB-TEAM) Program. This program was initiated in an ethnically diverse urban school district located in Rochester, New York, from 2012 to 2016 [6]. The goal of the program was to expand upon a preexisting school-based asthma supervised medication administration program by adding a telemedicine component. The researchers developed this randomized controlled clinical trial in order to assess whether adding the telemedicine component to the current medication administration program would improve overall outcomes. The study included 400 children from 3 to 10 years of age from 49 different schools within Rochester [6]. The majority of students within the school district were from racial/ethnic minority groups. The students enrolled were required to have either persistent asthma symptoms or poor asthma control based on National Heart, Lung, and Blood Institute Guidelines [6].

Prior to initiation of the study, the participants were screened for baseline asthma symptoms, caregiver depression, secondhand smoke exposure, and family medical history. For each patient, a saliva sample was collected to measure smoke exposure and a fractional exhaled nitric oxide measurement was used to measure airway inflammation [6]. Each child was then randomly assigned to either the SB-TEAM group or enhanced usual care (eUC) comparison group. Randomization of the groups was stratified based on the use of preventative medication at the patient's baseline asthma control level [6]. All families received educational packets on asthma, smoking cessation resources, and local asthma management resources. They were also given a journal and instructed to log asthma symptoms. The SB-TEAM cohort received a telemedicine visit at the beginning of the school year for an initial asthma assessment and to determine their asthma medication regimen. Follow-up telemedicine assessments were conducted at 4–6-week intervals [6]. The telemedicine follow-up visits allowed for necessary medication adjustments based on the patients' symptoms and asthma education. In addition to the telemedicine visits, these patients were also administered their inhalers at school. For most of the children, they received once daily dosing in order to improve compliance. For those who required more frequent dosing, additional inhaler treatments were administered at home by their parents [6]. The eUC group was screened with the baseline symptom assessment. However, no telemedicine or medication administration interventions were performed. They were given asthma education materials and a recommendation for preventative asthma medications. They were encouraged to follow up with their primary care physician regarding their asthma treatment and management [6].

Prior to the initiation of the SB-TEAM program, the children included in the study endorsed an average of 7.2 symptom-free days per 2 weeks with frequent daytime and nighttime symptoms [6]. The patients included in the study reported frequent use of rescue inhalers for symptom control. Almost half of patients also reported emergency department visits or hospitalizations for their asthma prior to initiation of the SB-TEAM program [6]. After completion of the SB-TEAM program, the researchers reported a significant improvement in asthma control in the SB-TEAM compared to the control group. Children in the SB-TEAM group, who were participating in the telemedicine visits, had more symptom-free days per 2 weeks (11.6 days) compared to the control group (10.97 days) [6]. These patients also reported fewer daytime and nighttime symptoms, hospitalizations, and activity limitations related to their asthma. Additionally, the SB-TEAM showed greater improvement in airway inflammation, which was quantified as a reduction in FeNO levels at the conclusion of the study [6]. The researchers attribute some of the success in symptom prevention to the medication management that was coordinated via the telemedicine visits. These visits allowed for physicians to better evaluate the patient's symptom control and adjust medication regimens as they deemed necessary. At the end of the study, more children in the SB-TEAM were prescribed controller medications as opposed to the control group, with 91% of patients in the SB-TEAM using a preventative asthma medication compared to only 67% of patients in the control group at the end of the study [6]. Parents whose children were a part of the SB-TEAM group felt as though the telemedicine visits helped improve their health literacy and better understand their child's asthma medication regimen. In both study groups, caregivers endorsed an improvement in the quality of life. Overall, this study demonstrated the benefits of incorporating telemedicine visits into a school-based asthma program to improve asthma control and symptom management in resource-poor areas. This unique model of care potentially highlights a new way to approach healthcare inequality and limitations in access in rural or underserved areas.

While the previously discussed programs focused primarily on the medication management of asthma symptoms, other programs focus entirely on educating children with asthma. The main goals are to help children better understand their chronic disease, symptoms, and how they can manage these symptoms throughout the course of their lives. Kickin' Asthma Program, which is an education-based program that was founded in California in 2002, aimed to develop an education-focused school-based asthma program primarily serving low-income and minority students. The program participants included seventh grade through twelfth grade students attending an urban school district in Oakland, California. The Oakland School District is a unique population to study because it is known for being one of the most diverse school systems in the country, with a student population consisting of 45% African American students, 31% Latino students, 17% Asian students, and 5% White students [10]. The school district also has very limited resources when compared to its student population, with a student-to-school nurse ratio of 1800:1 [10]. This limitation of resources poses a problem for managing the healthcare needs of the students within the school district.

Students were enrolled into the Kickin' Asthma Program during the beginning of the school year. Each student was asked to complete a pre-survey based on the International Study of Asthma and Allergies in Childhood questionnaire. Students who reported a physician's diagnosis of asthma, as well as either active asthma symptoms or a recent emergency visit for asthma were eligible for participation via an invitation sent to their teachers [10]. During the first 2 years of the program, students were given small incentives, such as $10 gift cards, for participation. The Kickin' It Asthma curriculum consisted of four educational sessions, which were developed by nurses, educators, and American Lung Association staff members [10]. Each session was 50 minutes in length and sessions were held weekly until the completion of the educational program. The sessions covered lessons on lung physiology, asthma symptoms and triggers, asthma warning signs, asthma medications, and asthma emergencies [10]. At the end of the educational program, students were given a post-program survey to complete. The pre- and post-program survey responses were then compared to assess the students' growth in knowledge. An individual morbidity score was also calculated for each student who completed both surveys. The program was continued at the Oakland School District for three consecutive school years, allowing for the creation of three study cohorts [10].

The results from the study indicated that the Kickin' Asthma Program was successful in improving student asthma education and symptom management. The researchers found that the number of asthma-related school absences was significantly reduced for each cohort. They also found that the incidence of asthma-related sleep disruption decreased significantly in two of the three cohorts [10]. The researchers reported that the frequency of daytime symptoms in these students declined for the first 3 years following completion of the educational program. Overall, the study found that this educational program assisted in decreasing the number of hospitalizations and overall utilization of the healthcare system by these students for disease exacerbation [10]. This program highlighted the power of health literacy and education on chronic disease management. The results of the Kickin' Asthma Program indicate that simply educating students about asthma may help to improve their symptoms and overall asthma management.

A similar education-focused school-based asthma program was initiated in Missouri, but took a slightly different approach with their curriculum. The Teaming Up for Asthma Control program was started in 2010 and targeted students aged 5 to 14 years enrolled in a Missouri School District [4]. The goal of the program was to improve asthma control in these youngsters, while improving the competency of school nurses in providing guideline-based asthma education. In order to participate in the program, students were required to have physician-diagnosed asthma, and their caregivers were required to speak and understand English. Students were excluded from the program if they had another concurrent respiratory condition [4]. Students who met the program requirements were sent informational packets and their parents were able to opt out of the entire program or specific components of the program. The Teaming Up for Asthma Control program also set standards for the school nurses involved in the program. The nurses were required to complete pretest and posttest educational comprehension assessments following the completion of an online training program [4]. Additionally, the nurses responsible for instructor-led group training sessions were required to demonstrate in-person assessment competency. With the leadership of school nurses, the students participating in the program were led through various educational workshops as well as instructional videos/ worksheets that were completed at home with their caregivers. Throughout the course of the educational program, the nurses conducted a series of three asthma assessments, which were performed at 1–2-week intervals [4]. The educational sessions and student assessments analyzed a breadth of asthma components and symptom management strategies. At each session, data was collected on the students' inhaler use and adherence, their inspiratory flow rate, and forced expiratory reserve volume (FEV_1), as well as their asthma symptoms. This data was used to assess each student's asthma control status [4]. Additional information was also collected such as exposure to tobacco smoke, environmental triggers, medication use, and each student's beliefs about asthma. The student's asthma control scores and assessment responses were then tracked throughout the duration of the program.

Throughout the course of the Teaming up for Asthma Control program, the program coordinators found a trend in improvement of health literacy and asthma symptoms. At the beginning of the program, 69.7% of the students enrolled in the study met the criteria for poorly controlled asthma. By the end of the educational program, then number of students with uncontrolled asthma decreased by 23.4% [4]. This translated into an overall decline of healthcare costs and utilization related to disease exacerbation. Throughout their participation in the program, students endorsed an improvement in knowledge regarding asthma medications and symptom control, which was reflected in their asthma control scores. The researchers suggest that between assessments one and three, the mean FEV_1 significantly increased from 82.9% to 92.1% of the predicted volume [4]. At the completion of the program, students also endorsed a significant improvement in their attitudes and beliefs about their asthma. This program highlights the benefits of a well-organized educational-based program as well as the important role school nurses play in implementing a school-based asthma program.

Finally, one of the most recognized school-based asthma programs is the *Step-Up* Asthma Program, which was launched in Denver, Colorado. The goal of this program was to create a sustainable model for asthma education in order to create an asthma-friendly school environment. The program included elementary and middle school students with asthma attending Denver public schools during the 2010–2012 school years [9]. Schools were selected to participate in the program based on their socioeconomic need, asthma prevalence, and percentage of minority students. Overall, the program included a total of 252 students who completed the program and were included in the data analysis. Of these participants, 49% had uncontrolled asthma prior to enrollment in the program and 94.5% represented racial/ethnic minorities [9]. The program was designed and directed by both a pediatric pulmonary/allergy specialist and a pediatric physician's assistant.

During the initial enrollment into the program, the primary care physician for each student was contacted in order to facilitate coordination of care. If a student did not have a primary care physician, one was established for the student. A measurement of baseline asthma control was assessed for each student using the Asthma Control Test, which is a validated tool used to assess asthma symptoms and disease control [9]. This test was repeated every 3 months throughout participation in the program in order to assess and track each student's asthma control. Students whose scores indicated suboptimal control were prompted to undergo additional steps to help improve their asthma control [9]. Bilingual asthma counselors assisted in the educational component of the program. These counselors were trained on patient navigation, motivational interviewing, and asthma self-management. The goal of these counselors was to facilitate communication with both the students and their parents. The counselors educated the students on proper asthma management, inhaler techniques, and instructed them on how to best manage their asthma at home [9]. The counselors also monitored each student's inhaler technique over time and scored their asthma technique in order to track their progress. Asthma counselors were responsible for communicating with families of the participants in person or via phone every 3 months in order to assess asthma control. They also served to reinforce the management plans that had been discussed with the students, as well as helping families overcome any barriers to care [5].

Over the course of the program, more than 90 Denver public school staff members received formal asthma education and 5 school nurses became certified asthma educators [9]. The program facilitators found a significant improvement in asthma control, health literacy, and individual asthma planning throughout the course of the program. Researchers cited a decreased number of asthma exacerbations, hospitalizations, school absences, and systemic corticosteroid use [9]. Program coordinators also found that through the guidance of the asthma counselors, the participant's inhaler technique scores improved during the course of the *Step-Up* program. Through implementation of the program, the *Step-Up* facilitators also found a significant increase in the number of asthma action plans and rescue medications in Denver public schools, paving the way for improved asthma control and planning for students in the future. The *Step-Up* Program generated many important learning points regarding the implementation of a large school-based asthma program. They stressed the key to any school-based program is open communication between students, schools, families, and healthcare providers. They also highlighted the importance of using a validated asthma assessment tool, such as the Asthma Control Test, to assess asthma control [9].

Final Thoughts and Future Directions

While this chapter was not meant to detail the myriad of school-based asthma programs that have been established in the United States over the past decade, the primary goal was to discuss some of the important milestones in the development of school-based asthma programs. These programs and studies have provided a foundation for the future development and implementation of school-based medical care programs. The aforementioned programs have highlighted numerous key learning points that are necessary to consider in future program development. They stress the importance of clear and open communication between all involved participants including students, parents, families, school nurses, teaching staff, and healthcare providers. The open line of communication is the foundation for excellent medical care coordination for these children. These programs stress the importance of improving health literacy through educational programs and individualized assessments. They also outline the role that medication adherence and inhaler technique play in proper asthma control. Overall, these school-based asthma programs provide a unique perspective to what may be the future of healthcare. These studies have shown that implementing a school-based approach to chronic disease management can significantly improve symptom control and health literacy, especially in underserved or resource-limited communities. These school-based asthma programs have demonstrated that by educating young students on their asthma, it can improve their asthma control, symptoms, and decrease the frequency of disease exacerbation. These studies have shown that these programs also contribute to an overall decline in the use of the healthcare system by reducing the number of emergency department, urgent care, and hospital visits due to asthma exacerbations. Ultimately, these studies have proven that school-based asthma programs help to improve the quality of life of children living with asthma and can better prepare them to manage their asthma symptoms in the future.

With the ever-changing healthcare system, public school funding, and healthcare guidelines, the future of school-based asthma programs remains unclear. However, many suggest that future directions for school-based asthma programs should focus on developing partnerships, solidifying funding support, and improving the implementation of these programs. Researchers stress the importance of continuing to foster partnerships between healthcare providers and schools in order to create a circle of support for school-based asthma programs [2]. Additionally, program administrators are urging for the implementation of streamlined asthma action plans that are consistent between healthcare providers and school districts. Facilitating the creation of a common asthma action plan can help curb confusion when it comes to implementation of asthma management at both school and home. Finally, generating financial support and securing federal grants are essential for the success of school-based asthma programs in the future. It is necessary to secure funding for more school nurses as the student-to-school nurse ratio continues to rise throughout the United States and secure funding for additional educational resources and asthma educators. Today, SAMPRO continues to urge the federal government to pass the School-Based Respiratory Health Management Act in order to create incentives for schools to implement school-based asthma programs. The passage of this legislation will also provide additional funding for the future development of these programs. Only time will tell how school-based asthma programs will continue to grow and evolve throughout the next decade.

In conclusion, school-based asthma programs provide a cutting-edge approach to management of chronic conditions in pediatric populations. These programs truly may be on the forefront of how we as a nation approach healthcare in the future. Aside from the health benefits associated with these programs, such as improvement in symptoms and decline in hospitalizations, these programs provide numerous personal benefits to these children. By creating these relationships among students, families, and program administrators, it facilitates important conversations between parents and their children regarding health promotion. If parents begin talking to their children about the importance of health and asthma management, it will pave the way for an open channel of communication in the future. School-based asthma programs also teach children that asthma is a serious health concern. This educational component can help to dispel the myths regarding asthma and even eliminate some of the shame and embarrassment children with asthma experience in school. Hopefully by improving health literacy regarding asthma in schools, it can also help to decrease the amount of bullying that children with asthma and other medical conditions face in school environments throughout their childhood. Perhaps most importantly, school-based asthma programs teach children how to be accountable for their own health. Through the help of these programs, children are learning how to manage their chronic disease and how to care for their own bodies, which is an essential skill for them to implement throughout the duration of their lives. These programs enforce responsibility and instill long-term strategies for managing asthma as these children progress from childhood to adulthood.

References

1. Allen ED, Arcoleo K, Rowe C, Long WW. Implementation of a "real world" school-Based asthma therapy program targeting urban children with poorly controlled asthma. J Asthma. 2018:55(10):1122–30.
2. Bruzzese J-M, Evans D, Kattan M. School-based asthma programs. J Allergy Clin Immunol. 2009;124:195–200.
3. Cicutto L, Gleason M, Szefler SJ. Establishing school-centered asthma programs. J Allergy Clin Immunol. 2014;134(6):1223–30.
4. Francisco B, Rood T, Nevel R, Foreman P, Homan S. Teaming up for asthma control: EPR-3 compliant school program in Missouri is effective and cost-efficient. Prev Chronic Dis. 2017;14(E40):170003.
5. Gleason M, Cicutto L, Haas-Howard C, Raleigh BM, Szefler SJ. Leveraging partnerships: families, schools, and providers working together to improve asthma management. Curr Allergy Asthma Rep. 2016;16:74.
6. Halterman JS, Fagnano M, Tajon RS, Tremblay P, Wang H, Butz A, et al. Effect of school-based telemedicine enhanced asthma management (SB-TEAM) Program on asthma morbidity: a randomized clinical trial. JAMA Pediatr. 2018;172(3):1–7.
7. Hollenbach JP, Cloutier MM. Implementing school asthma programs: lessons learned and recommendations. J Allergy Clin Immunol. 2014;134:1245–9.
8. Kakumanu S, Antos N, Szefler SJ, Lemanske RF Jr. Building school health partnerships to improve pediatric asthma care: the school-based asthma management program. Clin Opin Allergy Clin Immunol. 2017;17(2):160–6.
9. Liptzin DR, Gleason MC, Cicutto LC, Cleveland CL, Shocks DJ, White MK, et al. Developing, implementing, and evaluating a school-centered asthma progam: step-up asthma program. J Allergy Clin Immunol Pract. 2016;4(5):972–9.
10. Magzamen S, Patel B, Davis A, Edelstein J, Tager IB. Kickin' asthma: school-based asthma education in an urban community. J Sch Health. 2008;78(12):655–65.
11. Salazar G, Tarwala G, Reznik M. School-based educational programs to improve asthma outcomes: current perspectives. J Asthma Allergy. 2018;11:205–15.
12. Walter H, Sadeque-Iqbal F, Ulysse R, Castillo D, Fitzpatrick A, Singleton J. The effectiveness of school-based family asthma educational programs on the quality of life and number of asthma exacerbations of children aged five to 18 years diagnosed with asthma: a systematic review protocol. JBI Database System Rev Implement Rep. 2015;13(10):69–81.

Chapter 10
Providing Feasible Solutions
for an Asthmatic Impoverished Population

Arnaldo Capriles-Hulett and Mario Sánchez-Borges

Introduction

Allergic rhinitis and asthma, which are common inflammatory conditions of the airways, have been in rise during the past few decades globally. This is part of a phenomenon called the modern noninfectious epidemic [1–3]. The high morbidity, in the case of asthma, is directly associated with higher recurrence of exacerbations and hospitalizations. Furthermore, uncontrolled asthma is associated with significant school and work absenteeism. In this way, the high morbidity linked to asthma results in significant direct and indirect costs, not only to asthmatic patients themselves but also to the society [4–6].

Asthma is closely impacted by many social and economic complexities of "modern" life of populations living in poverty (i.e., not affording medications, low air quality, high tobacco exposure, violence, lack of access to medical care, obesity, and unhealthy environments/housing conditions) (Table 10.1) [7, 8]. These risk factors are linked not only to asthma but also to other respiratory noncommunicable diseases (NCD), and they are consequences of trends in increased low socioeconomic status in many urban populations around the world. Unlike the suburban life of many cities and urban centers in the developing countries, a "modern" living in underdeveloped countries often implies a stressful life in city dwellings [9], dealing

A. Capriles-Hulett (✉)
Hospital San Juan de Dios, Caracas, Venezuela

Centro Medico de Caracas, Centro Medico Docente La Trinidad, Caracas, Venezuela

M. Sánchez-Borges
Allergy and Clinical Immunology Department Centro Medico Docente La Trinidad, Caracas, Venezuela

Clinica El Avila, Caracas, Venezuela

© Springer Nature Switzerland AG 2020

M. Mahdavinia (ed.), *Health Disparities in Allergic Diseases*,
https://doi.org/10.1007/978-3-030-31222-0_10

Table 10.1 Environmental risk factors for asthma morbidity in socially deprived populations

Urban living
Poverty
Stressful daily life
Poor air quality
Unhealthy environments/housing conditions
Tobacco exposure
Social violence
Lack of access to medical care
Obesity

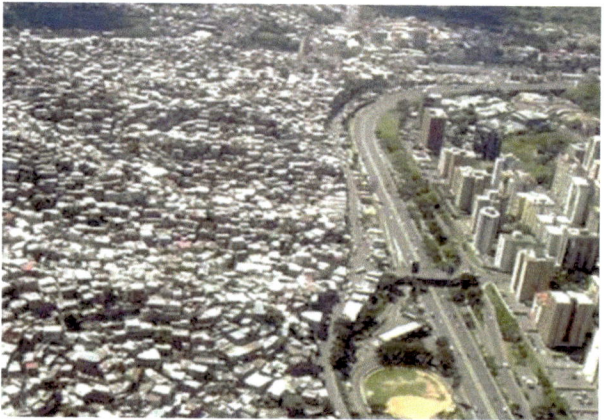

Fig. 10.1 A photo of an eastern segment of Caracas, capital city of Venezuela, where 80% or more of the population live in impoverished urban centers. A road (as shown above) separates the dwellings of the predominant living conditions of the population (left side of picture) from the socioeconomically affluent population (right side of picture). Eighty percent of inhabitants' living conditions are like the ones depicted on the left side of the photograph. (Reprinted [or adapted] with permission. Capriles-Hulett et al. [29])

with significant poverty and lack of access to necessities of life, such as safe housing and clean water or food (Fig. 10.1).

The recent Global Burden of Diseases Report (2013) estimated that asthma to be the fourteenth most impactful disorder in terms of disability in all ages [10]. The impacts on disability might be even more relevant in poor societies living in city dwellings. Urban living is a known environmental risk factor for allergies [11–13]. The loss of the protective effect of a farming/rural environment provided by the rich microbial exposures particularly in early life is a risk factor for allergic conditions in urban individuals. This has been proposed as the hygiene hypothesis [14, 15]. Violence, a more recently described risk factor [16–20], is also linked to living in poor and crowded urban dwellings. Venezuela registers more than 26,000 deaths per year, a quite significant toll affecting all of the population, and not just the socioeconomically deprived. This high rate of crime has made Venezuela the second most violent country in the world [21]. It is not surprising that the burden of asthma in this country is quite significant. It is noteworthy that the detrimental impact of violence and low socioeconomic on asthma is not exclusively seen in underdeveloped countries and can be seen in similar settings in some inner-city areas of developing countries as well. Living in extreme poverty results in adequate attention to medical conditions such as asthma all over the world [9]. This similarity between populations living in high-crime impoverished societies creates a link between the inner-city urban population of the developing countries [19] and crowded urban dwellings of the developing and underdeveloping countries in terms of difficulties in the management of asthma. Therefore, research on allergies and asthma management and development of individualized plans relevant to these inner-city populations are necessary and can be used in continuous expansion in any underserved society in developing or developing countries [19, 20].

What Is the Current Situation of Asthma in Venezuela?

Venezuela is located 10 degrees above the equator on the intertropical zone of Latin America. This country has a little over 30 million of mostly young and urban (>90% of the population live in crowded city dwellings) inhabitants with more than 80% of population living under poverty [22, 23] (Fig. 10.2). Asthma is a common condition in children (20% in preschoolers and 16% in adolescents) globally [1]. Unfortunately, a high number of children with asthma in Venezuela suffer from uncontrolled disease manifested by a large number of exacerbations. The asthma exacerbations rate is 4000 per 100,000 population per year. This is over five times of the exacerbations reported in the United States [24]. A public asthma control program was launched by the Ministry of Health (MoH), introducing the use of beclomethasone as the main controller drug in 1998. However, this plan was found to be ineffective in controlling the burden of asthma [25].

Fig. 10.2 This is a photo of the community where the study mentioned in reference [24] was carried out. Half of the people in Caracas live in conditions like the ones in the picture. Eighty percent of Venezuelans inhabit similar homes, in what is known as a *casa de barrio*. (Reprinted [or adapted] with permission. Capriles-Hulett et al. [29])

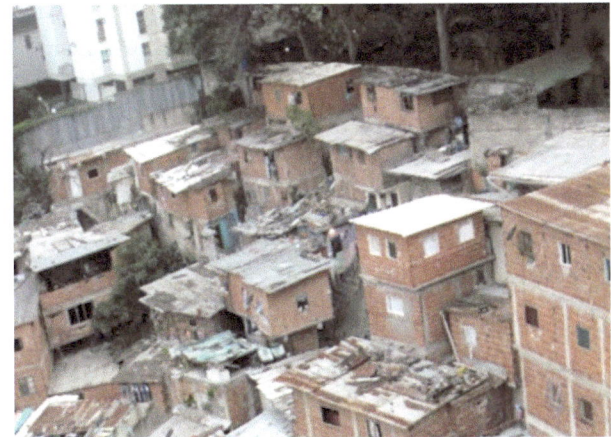

In the setting of the Ministry of Health (MoH) ambulatory care facilities, which serve more than two thirds of the population, acute asthma stands out as the most common reason for consultation among all respiratory diseases. Of note, asthma ranks second or third place when all conditions are considered; sometimes, it is positioned ahead of diarrheas [25]. The outlook of 15–20 nebulizers all running at the same time in an acute care health facilities is a common scene – evidence for the endemic nature and high impact of this illness in the country. In a study carried out in a poverty-stricken community in the capital city of Caracas, 60% of asthmatic adults and 70% of asthmatic children were found in the noncontrol status (based on asthma control test [ACT]) [25]. It is noteworthy that there is a significant out-of-pocket cost for asthma medications which many cannot simply afford. This results in poor compliance and more asthma exacerbations, further flooding the public acute healthcare facilities. On top of that, asthma attacks commonly occur at night, while healthcare services attended by these communities are closed [24].

Considering this commonly observed scenario [9], asthma is more than just a health condition affecting the patients, but it is a condition with strong impact on the whole society. For the individuals living in this condition of severe poverty and crime, asthma is a huge burden affecting their survival. In an essence, asthma is an illness with both social and health aspects [11].

As one can see the above living conditions are not amenable to the implementation of sophisticated treatment regimens for asthma, research is needed to identify feasible alternative treatment plans to optimize the outcomes by using cost-effective efficacious drugs for asthma [26]. In the following sections, we have detailed some of the recent approaches aiming to develop such simplified plans.

Proposed Strategies

Since 2006, considering the above conditions, a series of treatment proposals targeting the reality of life in these populations were designed and tested. This was a certain drift away from what is considered mainstream guidelines. As explained above, the mainstream guidelines for asthma treatment have proven to be too complicated and expensive for these populations. The intention was not to "force" one guideline approach into all contexts. Our goal was to look for the most feasible and appropriate approach specific to the urban poverty context we were dealing with. We also hoped to raise awareness about the severity of the condition and inform the public health establishment about possible alternatives and likely effective strategies that would work for asthma control in this environment.

We took few approaches to address this issue: (1) strategies for improvement of asthma control by designing simple and cost-effective medications regimen of inhaled and (2) oral medications, (3) strategies to decrease the burden of acute exacerbations on the public health facilitates by shortening the time that patients had to stay in an acute care facility for nebulized treatments, and (4) development of a cost-effective rapid immunotherapy method to decrease allergen response as a trigger for asthma. These approaches are detailed in the following:

Maintenance Treatment Plans for Asthma by Using Once-a-Day Dosing of Inhaled Corticosteroids

Inhaled corticosteroids are the most efficacious medications for asthma control. However, the compliance with these medications is less than optimal [27]. Basically, a large number of patients do not take them as prescribed, which is usually two to three times a day. Previous studies looking at the chronobiology of asthma and inhaled steroids have shown that a once-per-day administration of inhaled corticosteroids at the peak of its activity during the circadian rhythm could be as effective as the four times per day divided dosing in improving symptoms and pulmonary functions [27]. We performed a study to investigate the effect of inhaled budesonide 400 mcg on a once-a-day regimen at 5–6 pm in allergic asthmatic children attending an outpatient facility. These children were followed for 3.5 months. Budesonide was administered at 5–6 pm. This regimen had a significant impact in ameliorating symptoms (daytime, nighttime, exercise-induced symptoms, and use of rescue bronchodilators). However, there was only a nonsignificant trend toward improvement in peak flow measurements, which might have been due to the small number of patients studied [28]. Obviously, a once-a-day regimen will improve compliance, and as evidence by the study, it will result in better disease control.

Maintenance Treatment Plans for Asthma by Oral Medications

For the next step, an oral medication was investigated. Montelukast (MLK) is a medication with minimal side effects, and the bonus effect on allergic rhinitis appeared to be well suited for this task [29–31]. Furthermore, the beneficial effect of MLK is more pronounced in environments exposed to tobacco smoke [30], a feature commonly found in our low-income households [24]. It is noteworthy that MLK has been shown to be as effective as inhaled steroids in reducing the number of asthma exacerbations in children [32]. The simplicity of an oral once-a-day effective control medication makes it a more desirable option for control for asthmatic patients and their families. Of note, this cuts the need for education and repeated visits compared to more complex methods of drug delivery, such as inhaled medication. Thus, the medication could be easily started during the only contact an asthmatic patient might have with the health system, which usually occurs during an exacerbation. Additionally, an oral medication can overcome the compliance problem linked to existing worries and well-known cultural bias against inhaled medications in our population [29]. Of note, when questioned before the study, patients preferred an oral asthma control medication over an inhaled alternative counterpart.

A pilot study [29] was carried out over a year in a poverty-stricken district of Caracas. We performed a double-blind placebo-controlled study with the main outcome of "number of asthma exacerbations in need of bronchodilator nebulized treatment in an acute healthcare facility" to receive fenoterol + ipratropium bromide, as usually employed in our ambulatory health system. The acronym EESSO (**E**conomically feasible, **E**ffective, **S**ocial component, **S**afe, and **O**ral) was used to name this trial tailored to our population. The word "eso" in Spanish implies the imperative: "this is what it is." MLK use, dosed according to weight, achieved a compliance of >70%. This was estimated by counting the empty blisters used by patients. MLK was found to significantly improve the primary outcome during the first 6 months of treatment. Furthermore, a nonsignificant trend of improvement was observed during the next 6 months of the study. This observed lack of significant after 6 months of therapy was most likely due to the observed patients' attrition in our population. A one-page pictorial educational material complemented this strategy. Unfortunately, this population was not amenable to reading a written educational material. During the study, the compliance and periodic follow-up were done through monthly text messages and/or voice reminders via cell phone. Due to its simplicity, this approach could be used by nonphysician healthcare providers as effectively. It has been shown that simple medical approaches are used more efficaciously by nonphysician providers in the developing countries [33].

Another approach that was tested in our study and could be applied easily is for triage of patients. A simple rule of 2's would help identify patients in need of a controller asthma treatment, a useful simple concept that can be used by all providers in public health facilities. After starting the controlled medication if no improvement is detected (persistence of recurrent exacerbations) during the next acute visit, a referral to an asthma clinic would be needed. This allows for a better allocation of resources.

In theory, a combination of an oral antihistamine and MLK might be even more appropriate, by controlling the allergic trigger in upper and lower airways and hence enhancing the asthma control. Close to 60% of patients in this study had rhinitis and positive skin prick tests to *Dermatophagoides (Dp/Df)* and *Blomia tropicalis*.

Shortening the Time Spent in the Emergency Room

Another important obstacle in care of asthma patients is the overcrowded ambulatory and emergency settings that are flooded by acute asthma patients. Therefore, exploring alternative approaches tailored toward shortening the emergency room stay by decreasing the administration times of nebulized medications is needed. Formoterol, a long-acting β2-agonist bronchodilator with the additional short-acting effect, became a likely alternative to us. Randomly selected acute asthmatics (48 children) received either 2.5 mg of nebulized albuterol (every 20 minutes for 1 hour) or 24 mg of nebulized formoterol (two 12 mg plus 2-cc saline). Clinical parameters (asthma symptom score), oxygen saturations, and pulmonary functions were measured before and after treatments. Similar improvement in these parameters was shown for both modalities [34]. We concluded that one single nebulization of formoterol could shorten the time spent by patients in the emergency room settings. Furthermore, para-medical personnel's time will be saved in the delivering of medications, and they can help more patients and dedicate time to other acutely ill patients who are in line. Furthermore, prolonging the bronchodilator effect of this medication is an added significant benefit of a long-acting β-agonist.

Novel Rapid Approaches for Aeroallergen Immunotherapy

Immunotherapy (IT) is a highly effective method in reducing the allergic response, hence improving the outcome of allergic airways diseases. However, allergen immunotherapy is considered a luxury and infrequently accessed by low-income populations in the developing countries [35]. This is due to the high costs of the imported allergen extracts and other material, and multiple other factors linked to access to outpatient care. Another important consideration is that very small number of physicians are properly trained for preparation and administration of IT [34]. The process is very long taking 4–8 months of subcutaneous injections to reach the therapeutic concentrations and then another 4–5 years to maintain the tolerance. Intradermal route (ID) permits for lower major allergen concentrations to be employed and likely a more cost-effective treatment approach. Given the high immune response generated when allergens are applied through the intradermal (ID) route, its clinical effectiveness was assessed in a pilot study. Eight immunotherapy-naive children with allergic rhinitis were enrolled in the study [36]. A particular technique of weekly 0.05-ml ID injections in the arms (with 31 G-needle disposable syringes) was employed. The injections were repeated weekly for 3 months. Allergens employed were standardized mite mixtures; Dp/Df (10.000 AU/ml Dp/Df, Greer Labs) and Blomia tropicalis (Bial Labs, Zamudio, Bizkaia, Spain) were diluted at 5 ng per 0.05-ml ID injection/week, without weekly volume increments, thus bypassing a need for a build-up phase. This method is much faster than the approved weekly subcutaneous IT, resulting in significant cost savings. Assessment was carried out with measuring rhinitis symptom score, serial dilutions skin prick tests (SDSPT) and IgG4 measurements, before and after treatments. Results were encouraging, with significant symptom improvement starting at the fifth week of treatment. Furthermore, the rise in IgG4 for Dp/Df and SDSPT suggested the mounting of a significant protective immune response. No important side effects, except minor local injection site reactions, were noted. Mite allergens are the predominant allergens [37, 38] in the tropical environments. Our preliminary results are promising and warrant further investigation.

Concluding Remarks

All of the above approaches require confirmation in future studies, which are to be performed with larger number of patients. Notwithstanding, building of an asthma control culture is still a pending goal for practitioners and health system planners alike. This requires robust planning and investment in educational efforts at every level of care. An initial barrier to overcome is the absence of initiatives to move forward from a system focused on the acute asthma care to outpatient chronic care for improvement of control. Much is due to lack of information and knowledge. Patients believe that recurrent administration of bronchodilator treatments is an appropriate treatment plan for asthma, and, on the other hand, the health system is just focusing on treatment of these acute uncontrolled asthma exacerbations without investing in education and planning for controller maintenance modalities.

However, with regard to the extent of above-depicted burden of disease in the urban impoverished context and uncontrolled asthma's significant impact, an action that is customized to the needs and availabilities is highly in need. Obviously, a strong, ample, and easily accessible effective healthcare system, which is able to deliver highest quality care under proven established guidelines (i.e., GINA, in the case of asthma), is the best option. However, this might not be possible or even close to possible for certain areas in the developing countries [40]. Nonetheless, specially designed programs in the context of available resources have been tried and proven to be successful in some urban impoverished contexts. An example of that is the successful Pro-Air program [41] in Salvador de Bahia, Brazil. This exemplary program had educational components that with the help of international support resulted in consistent results. Some of the important characteristics of this program that resulted in its success include consistency over multiple years, international support (Wellcome Foundation), well-designed educational efforts (to over 500 health personnel), solid record keeping, use of primary healthcare settings, use of free high-dose inhaled corticosteroid + salmeterol combination for control, massive networking effort with main stakeholders, and, above all, engaging a young and enthusiastic group of people who have decided to move forward in tackling the asthma problem by creating a culture of disease control.

Nevertheless, a question arises: How many of the abovementioned characteristics can be easily reproduced in developing nations? This is a question that we as the healthcare providers, epidemiologist, and clinicians should think about.

Acknowledgments We thank Carolina Urdaneta Benítez, certified English public translator, for her thoughtful review of the manuscript and important contributions to the English syntax of this chapter.

References

1. Pearce N, Ait-Khaled N, Beasley R, et al. Worldwide trends in the prevalence of asthma symptoms: phase III of the International Study of Asthma and Allergies in Childhood (ISAAC). Thorax. 2007;62:758–66.
2. To T, Stanojevic S, Moores G, Gershon AS, Bateman ED, Cruz AA, Boulet LP. Global asthma prevalence in adults: findings from the cross-sectional world health survey. BMC Public Health. 2012;12:204.
3. Asher I, Pearce N. Global burden of asthma among children. Int J Tuberc Lung Dis. 2014;18(11):1269–78.

4. Luskin AT, Chipps BE, Rasouliyan L, Miller DP, Haselkorn T, Dorenbaum A. Impact of asthma exacerbations and asthma triggers on asthma-related quality of life in patients with severe or difficult-to-treat asthma. J Allergy Clin Immunol Pract. 2014;2(5):544–52.
5. Centers for Disease Control and Prevention, National Center for Environmental Health Asthma-related missed school days among children aged 5–17 years. Available from: https://www.cdc.gov/asthma/asthma_stats/missing_days.htm. Accessed on 11 March 2016.
6. Wang LY, Zhong Y, Wheeler L. Direct and indirect costs of asthma in school-aged children. Prev Chronic Dis. 2005:A11.
7. Murray CJ, Lopez AD. Measuring the global burden of disease. N Engl J Med. 2013;369(5):448–57.
8. Von Mutius E. Childhood origins of COPD. Lancet Respir Med. 2018. pii: S2213-2600(18)30141-3.
9. Sánchez-Borges M, Capriles-Hulett A, Caballero-Fonseca F. Asthma care in resource-poor settings. World Allergy Organ J. 2011;4:68–72.
10. Vos T, Flaxman AD, Naghavi M, et al. Years lived with disability (YLDs) for 1160 sequelae of 289 diseases and injuries 1990–2010: a systematic analysis for the Global Burden of Disease Study 2010. Lancet. 2013;380:2163–96.
11. Wright R, Suglia S, Levy J, Fortum K, Shields A, Subramaniam SV, Wright R. Transdisciplinary research strategies for understanding socially patterned diseases: the Asthma Coalition on Community, Environment, and Social Stress (ACCESSS) project as a case study. Cien Saude Colet. 2008;13(6):1729–42.
12. Haahtela T, Laatikainen T, Alenius H, Auvinen P, Fyhrquist N, Hanski I, von Hertzen L, Jousilahti P, Kosunen TU, Markelova O, Mäkelä MJ, Pantelejev V, Haahtela T, Laatikainen T, Alenius H, Auvinen P, Fyhrquist N, Hanski I, von Hertzen L, Jousilahti P, Kosunen TU, Markelova O, Mäkelä MJ, Pantelejev V, Uhanov M, Zilber E, Vartiainen E. Hunt for the origin of allergy-comparing the Finnish and Russian Karelia. Clin Exp Allergy. 2015;45(5):891–901.
13. Asher MI. Urbanisation, asthma and allergies. Thorax. 2011;66(12):1025–6.
14. Lim A, Asher MI, Ellwood E, Ellwood P, Exeter DJ. How are "urban" and "rural" defined in publications regarding asthma and related diseases? Allergol Immunopathol (Madr). 2014;42(2):157–61.
15. von Mutius E, Vercelli D. Farm living: effects on childhood asthma and allergy. Nat Rev Immunol. 2010;10:861–8.
16. Tabalipa F de O, Daitx RB, Traebert JL, Meyer AS, da Silva J. Indicators of violence and asthma: An ecological study. Allergol Int. 2015;64(4):344–50.
17. Yonas MA, Lange NE, Celedón JC. Psychosocial stress and asthma morbidity. Curr Opin Allergy Clin Immunol. 2012;12(2):202–10.
18. Bellin M, Osteen P, Collins K, Butz A, Land C, Kub J. The influence of community violence and protective factors on asthma morbidity and healthcare utilization in high-risk children. J Urban Health. 2014;91(4):677–89.
19. Wright RJ, Mitchell H, Visness CM, Cohen S, Stout J, Evans R, Gold DR. Community violence and asthma morbidity: the Inner-City Asthma Study. Am J Public Health. 2004;94(4):625–32.
20. Unger A. Children's health in slum settings. Arch Dis Child. 2013;98(10):799–805.
21. Observatorio Venezolano de la violencia (OVV). https://observatoriodeviolencia.org.ve/. Accessed on 5 April 2018.
22. www.worldbank.org/en/country/venezuela/overview.
23. www.elucabista.com/2018/.../resultados-encovi-2017-radiografia-la-crisis.
24. http://cdc.gov/nchs/data/ahcd/nhamc_emergency/2011_ed_web_tables.pdf. Accessed 12 Nov 2016.
25. Hulett AC, Yibirin MG, Brandt RB, García A, Hurtado D, Puigbó AP. Home/social environment and asthma profiles in a vulnerable community from Caracas: lessons for urban Venezuela? J Asthma. 2013;50(1):14–24.
26. McQuaid EL. Barriers to medication adherence in asthma: the importance of culture and context. Ann Allergy Asthma Immunol. 2018. pii: S1081-1206(18)30222-9.

27. Song JU, Park HK, Lee J. Impact of dosage timing of once-daily inhaled corticosteroids in asthma: a systematic review and meta-analysis. Ann Allergy Asthma Immunol. 2018. pii: S1081-1206(18)30222-9.
28. Capriles E, Du Campu A, Veide O, Pluchino S, Capriles Hulett A. Children's asthma and the third world: an approach. J Investig Allergol Clin Immunol. 2006;16(1):11–8.
29. Capriles Hulett A, Yibirin MG, Garcia A, Hurtado D. Montelukast for the high impact of asthma exacerbations in Venezuela: a practical and valid approach for Latin America? World Allergy Organ J. 2014;7(1):20, 29.
30. David Price, Todor A. Popov, Leif Bjermer, Susan Lu, Romana Petrovic, Kristel Vandormael, Anish Mehta, Jolanta D. Strus, Peter G. Polos, George Philip, (2013) Effect of montelukast for treatment of asthma in cigarette smokers. J Allergy Clin Immunol. 131;(3):763–71.e6.
31. Price D, Musgrave SD, Shepstone L, Hillyer EN, Sims EJ, Guilbert RF, Juniper EF, Ayres JG, Kemp L, Blyth A, Wilson EC, Wolfe S, Freeman D, Mugford HM, Murdoch J, Harvey I. Leukotrienes antagonists as first-line or add-on asthma controller therapy. N Engl J Med. 2011;364(18):1695–707.
32. Ducharme F, Noya FI, Allen-Rammey FC, Maisese EM, Gingres J, Blais L. Clinical effectiveness of inhaled corticosteroids versus montelukast in children with asthma: prescription patterns and patient adherence as key factors. Curr Med Res Opin. 2012;28(1):111–9.
33. Abegunde DO, Shengelia B, Luyten A, Cameron A, Celletti F, Nishtar S, Pandurangi V, Mendis S. Can non-physician health-care workers assess and manage cardiovascular risk in primary care? N Engl J Med. 2013;369(5):448–57.
34. Rodriguez E, Vera V, Perez-Puigbó A, Capriles-Hulett A, Ferro S, Manrique J, Abate J. Equivalence of a single saline nebulised dose of formoterol powder vs three doses of nebulised Albuterol every twenty minutes in acute asthma in children: a suitable cost effective approach for developing nations. Allergol Immunopathol (Madr). 2008;36(4):196–200.
35. Baena-Cagnani CE, Larenas Linnenman D, Gómez M, Díaz SG, Solé D, Borges MS, Bousquet J, Sisul JC, Canonica W. Immunotherapy Working Group Allergy training and immunotherapy in Latin America: results of a regional overview. Ann Allergy Asthma Immunol. 2013;111(5):415–9.
36. Viera J, Capriles-Hulett A, Sanchez-Borges M, Fabiano F, Albarran-Barrios C. Intradermal immunotherapy with low dose house dust mite allergies: a proof-of-concept study. Rev Alerg Mex. 2018;65(1):41–51.
37. Sánchez-Borges M, Fernández-Caldas E, Capriles-Hulett A, Caballero-Fonseca F. Mite hypersensitivity in patients with rhinitis and rhinosinusitis living in a tropical environment. Allergol Immunopathol (Madr). 2014;42(2):120–6.
38. Sánchez-Borges M, Capriles-Hulett A, Caballero-Fonseca F, Fernández-Caldas E. Mite and cockroach sensitization in allergic patients from Caracas, Venezuela. Ann Allergy Asthma Immunol. 2003;90(6):664–8.
39. Pearce N, Asher I, Billo N, Bissell K, Ellwood P, El Sony A, García-Marcos L, Chiang CY, Mallol J, Marks G, Strachan D. Asthma in the global NCD agenda: a neglected epidemic. Lancet Respir Med. 2013;1(2):96–8.
40. The Collapse of the Venezuelan Health System. The Lancet. Published on April 07, 2018.
41. Souza-Machado C, Souza-Machado A, Franco R, Ponte EV, Barreto MC, Rodrigues LC, Bousquet J, Cruz AA. Rapid reduction in hospitalizations after an intervention to manage severe asthma. Eur Respir J. 2010;35(3):515–21.

Chapter 11
Global and National Networks and Their Role in Fighting Disparity in Allergic Diseases

Christopher D. Codispoti

Introduction

As defined by the U.S. Department of Health and Human Services Healthy People 2020, a health disparity is a "particular type of health difference that is closely linked with social or economic disadvantage. Health disparities adversely affect groups of people who have systematically experienced greater social or economic obstacles to health based on their racial or ethnic group, religion, socioeconomic status, gender, mental health, cognitive, sensory, or physical disability, sexual orientation, geographic location, or other characteristics historically linked to discrimination or exclusion" [1]. As discussed in the previous chapter, allergic diseases are also influenced significantly by health disparities [2]. These health disparities are a systematic problem. A systematic problem calls for a systematic answer. Fortunately, there are many networks involved in attempting to answer the problem. Often, the stage of the efforts is in epidemiologic studies that define the problem, such as the prevalence and at-risk groups. Other stages of answering the question are at implementation, such as public health measures, improving access or educational programs. The purpose of this chapter is to identify some of the major networks and their work in fighting health disparities in allergic diseases.

C. D. Codispoti (✉)
Department of Internal Medicine, Rush University Medical Center, Chicago, IL, USA
e-mail: Christopher_D_Codispoti@rush.edu

© Springer Nature Switzerland AG 2020
M. Mahdavinia (ed.), *Health Disparities in Allergic Diseases*,
https://doi.org/10.1007/978-3-030-31222-0_11

Governmental Organizations

Agency for Healthcare Quality Research

One of the governmental agencies that work to reduce disparities is the Agency for Healthcare Research and Quality (AHRQ). The mission of the AHRQ is "to produce evidence to make health care safer, higher quality, more accessible, equitable, and affordable" [3]. Asthma and allergic diseases are disorders targeted by the AHRQ. AHRQ achieves this goal in many ways, including funding research grants and producing tools to improve quality. These funding grants have made advances in our knowledge of allergic diseases in minorities and impoverished populations. A key first step is defining the problem and scope. In 2014, with a R21 grant from AHRQ, Baptist et al. conducted focus groups of African-American young adults with physician-diagnosed asthma [4]. Six categories of responses that included concerns and identified barriers for this at-risk group were recognized. These categories of responses included concerns about their quality of life due to asthma; how life responsibilities were interfering with asthma management; difficulty with asthma medication compliance and medication concerns; how asthma management has changed as they reached young adulthood; belief that their physician does not understand their asthma issues; and motivation to participate in an asthma self-management program. The final category found that this was a group very interested in participating in an asthma self-management program. This led to a trial an electronic asthma self-management program for African-American young adults [5]. Over a 6-week period, the program had good retention rates, with 89% completing the 6-week period and 77% available for 3-month follow-up evaluation. Most (97%) at the 2-week postprogram interview would recommend to others. Participation in the program led to significant improvement in control as measured by Asthma Control Test (from 16.1 to 19.3 ($P < 0.01$)) and in asthma-related quality of life as measured by the Asthma Quality of Life Questionnaire (from 4.0 to 5.1 ($P < 0.01$)). These results show evidence of how AHRQ could serve as a funding source for external investigators to test novel tools in order to reduce disparities.

A second method by which AHRQ helps to reduce disparities is through systematic reviews, often in collaboration with the National Institute of Health. An example would be the ARHQ Comparative Effectiveness Reviews, which have been done in collaboration with the National Heart, Lung, and Blood Institute to review the evidence for indoor allergen reduction on asthma [6, 7]. This systematic review found that no single intervention aimed in reducing indoor allergens improved asthma control or pulmonary physiology (forced expiratory volume in 1 second or peak expiratory flow). Multicomponent interventions improved some of the outcomes, but no multicomponent intervention was superior to another. In summary, how we can reduce indoor allergens in order to improve asthma outcomes is going to take further investigation.

National Institute on Minority Health and Health Disparities (NIMHD)

Another federal agency working to reduce health disparities is the National Institute on Minority Health and Health Disparities (NIMHD) of the National Institute of Health (NIH). The NIH has the mission to "lead scientific research to improve minority health and reduce health disparities" [8]. One of the stated missions NIMHD accomplishes is to "conduct and support research in minority health and health disparities." In an example of how NIMHD-funded research has contributed to asthma, Bayly et al. found that secondhand smoke from electronic nicotine delivery systems, such as electronic cigarettes, among children 11–17 years old, was associated with an adjusted odds ratio of 1.27 for reporting an asthma exacerbation within the last 12 months [9].

This is one of the first studies associating secondhand smoke from electronic nicotine delivery systems to a vulnerable population.

National Institute of Allergy and Infectious Diseases (NIAID)

The NIMHD is not the only institute of the NIH fighting to reduce health disparities in allergic diseases. The National Institute of Allergy and Infectious Disease (NIAID), another institute of the NIH, has been supporting the Inner City Asthma Consortium (ICAC) since 1991 [10]. The mission of the ICAC is "to conduct research focused on understanding how the environment, allergens and genetics interact with the body's immune system to cause asthma and aggravate its symptoms" [11]. A major trial from ICAC was the Asthma Control Evaluation study, whose purpose was to "assess the effectiveness of measurement of fraction of exhaled nitric oxide as an adjunct to guideline-based management of asthma" [12]. Asthma patients within the age range of 12–20 years residing in an urban census tract in which at least 20% of households had incomes below the federal poverty threshold were eligible. This led to a sample population that was enriched with racial and ethnic minority groups, including 64% Black, 22% Hispanic, and 14% other or mixed. All eligible asthma participants underwent a 3-week run-in period on a guideline-based treatment regimen defined by their previous treatment, medication adherence, and control. The participant's adherence was monitored, and if their medication adherence, as monitored by a dose counter, was below 25%, they were excluded from the study and not randomized. The results of this study showed that most of the improvement of symptoms occurred during the 3-week run-in period. While exacerbations did occur during the randomization period, the study demonstrated that if this underserved population is provided with guideline-based medications, asthma control could be achieved [13].

In the ACE study, asthma patients with allergen sensitization were one of the subgroups that in post hoc analysis may have significantly (P = 0.0243) benefited from the addition of exhaled nitric oxide measurements (other groups of note included those with elevated total IgE (>460 kU/L at P = 0.0296)). These findings led to another important NIAID-funded ICAC trial among urban children, the Inner-City Anti-IgE Therapy for Asthma (ICATA) study.

The purpose of this trial was to determine if the addition of omalizumab, a humanized monoclonal anti-IgE antibody, would improve disease control by reducing symptoms and exacerbations among inner city children and young adults with persistent asthma [14].

These eligibility criteria again led to an enriched sample of patients from racial and ethnic groups that experience healthcare disparities. Over both groups, 60% were Black and 37% were Hispanic. The addition of omalizumab significantly reduced the number of symptoms (P < 0.001) and the number of exacerbations (P < 0.001). The ACE and the ICATA trials demonstrate the commitment of the NIAID in addressing the asthma epidemic in urban youth who shoulder a disproportionate burden.

Patient-Centered Outcomes Research Institute (PCORI)

Patient-Centered Outcomes Research Institute (PCORI) is an organization focused on improving diseases outcomes. PCORI's mission is to "help people make informed healthcare decisions, and improves healthcare delivery and outcomes, by producing and promoting high-integrity, evidence-based information that comes from research guided by patients, caregivers and the broader healthcare community" [15]. Patient-centered research could serve as an important and effective tool in reducing health disparities in African-American patients [16].

PCORI has funded research to support patient-centered care targeted to reduce health disparities. Sleath et al. conducted interview of children with asthma ages 11–17 years old and their caregivers [17]. They found a discrepancy between adherence reported by children and that reported by their caregivers. They also identified that adherence to asthma medications was associated with having a higher expectations for good outcomes. Other factors that affected their adherence were difficulty in using their inhaler (technique) and difficulty remembering to use their inhaler. These were similar to caregiver predictors of child's adherence. These findings identified an educational opportunity for pharmacists to improve adherence in this asthma group that carries a high burden during the transition from childhood to adulthood.

Nongovernmental Organizations

Networks working to fight health disparities in allergic diseases can take many forms.

The aforementioned government organizations fight health disparities in allergic diseases.

There are also many nongovernmental organizations in this struggle.

While a comprehensive listing is beyond the scope of this chapter, the following sections will provide details of a few nongovernmental organizations and their efforts.

Robert Wood Johnson Foundation

One of the major nongovernmental organization fighting health disparities is the Robert Wood Johnson Foundation. The vision of General Robert Wood Johnson II, the founder of the Robert Wood Johnson Foundation, was to "improve health and health care in America, especially for those most in need" [18]. In staying true to their founder's vision, one of the Guiding Principles is to "seek bold and lasting change rooted in the best available evidence, analysis, and science" and to "... cultivate diversity, inclusion and collaboration." These principles are achieved through dissemination of findings to help communities and grants.

Dissemination of the experiences of different organization who are fighting health disparities is one of the principles of the Robert Wood Johnson Foundation. In 2017, a toolkit was published that presented approaches and tools for addressing disparities [19].

Four different organizations presented their experiences, including successes and barriers.

One success detailed was the experience of Blue Cross of California State Sponsored Business who was able to increase pharmacy consultation, by face-to-face outreach to small pharmacies, which led to an increase rate of appropriate controller medication use for African Americans from 68% to 85%. This demonstrated that pharmacies could be a partner with managed care organizations to fight health disparities.

Another role the Robert Wood Johnson Foundation has played is in grant funding research.

The Robert Wood Johnson Foundation has funded focused literature reviews and systematic reviews. In 2012, Press et al. completed a systematic review to characterized intervention with the potential to improve asthma outcomes for minority patients [20].

From the 24 articles that were included in their review from 1950 to 2010, they found that education from healthcare professionals appeared effective in improving asthma outcomes.

This was despite few of the educational material being culturally tailored, which represents an opportunity for further improvement.

RAND Corporation

Another nongovernmental organization worth mentioning is RAND Health Care.

The mission of RAND Health Care is to "promote healthier societies by improving health care systems" [21]. This mission is accomplished by conducting research for clients, or on its own initiative. Within this mission, RAND Health Care is working to reduce health disparities. One such research project by Lara et al. investigated a clinic- and home-based intervention and showed significant reductions in asthma symptoms, asthma-related emergency department visits, asthma-related hospitalizations, and rescue medication use (while increasing controller medication use) [22]. These findings support the idea that a multidimensional health problem like asthma requires a multidimensional intervention.

Urban Institute

Another nongovernmental organization addressing health disparities is the Urban Institute. The purpose of the Urban Institute is to provide "policymakers and practitioners with the evidence-based, nonpartisan research they need to make smart decisions and implement practical solutions" [23]. Examining how housing affects asthma, Ganesh et al. found that the presence of tobacco smoke, mold, or leaks are associated with higher emergency department visits and urgent care visits and that renters are particularly at risk [24]. They identified that current building code and inspection policies may miss asthma triggers. Additionally, though, solutions were offered including proactive rental housing inspections, quality inspections by the Housing and Urban Development department, smoke-free policies, and integrated pest management. These are action items that agencies can implement to address health disparities.

International Study of Asthma and Allergies in Childhood (ISAAC) and the Global Asthma Network (GAN)

The governmental and nongovernmental organizations described above have mostly a national influence in the United States. There are networks that have an international influence in working to reducing health disparities. The International Study of Asthma and Allergies in Childhood (ISAAC) and its successor, the Global Asthma Network (GAN), have worked to define the global problem of asthma and solutions. Expanding the number of countries involved in Phase 3 of the ISAAC survey, Lai et al. determined by surveys the prevalence of current wheeze among 13- to 14-year-old children varied from 0.8% in Tibet, China, to 32.6% in Wellington, New Zealand [25]. There was also wide variation in the prevalence of current wheeze among 6- to 7-year-old children, ranging from 2.4% in Jodhpur, India, to 37.6% in Costa Rica. To improve asthma care, the ISAAC group established, with the International Union

Against Tuberculosis and Lung Disease, in 2012 the Global Asthma Network (GAN) [26, 27]. The GAN has supported research in asthma, especially in low- to middle-income countries. A possible tool to reduce the burden of asthma is a national asthma strategy (program) that is a formal commitment to improve early detection and access to anti-inflammatory treatments. In a GAN-funded study, to identify how widespread these asthma strategies were adopted, Asher et al. found that 25% of 120 countries had developed a national strategy [27]. The GAN has also fought asthma disparities by publishing the Global Asthma Report of 2018 [28]. This publication identified the global disease and economic asthma burden and the unique barriers in specific regions and countries. Not only did it identify the problems, it recognized some of the solutions that can be accomplished and also should be implemented. For example, the Global Asthma Report identified the value of a spacer for delivering medications. It also described how to make (Table 11.1) and use a homemade spacer (Table 11.2 and Figs. 11.1 and 11.2). These homemade answers to asthma health disparity problems could be helpful.

Table 11.1 Global Asthma Network (GAN) instructions on how to make a homemade spacer from a 500-ml plastic bottle [28]

Step	Instructions
1.	Wash the bottle with soap and water and air dry for a minimum of 12 hours to reduce electrostatic charge on the interior plastic
2.	Make a wire mold similar in size and shape to the mouthpiece of the MDI
3.	Heat the mold and hold in position on the outside of the base of the plastic bottle until the plastic begins to melt (~10 seconds) Rotate the mold 180° and reapply to the bottle until the mold melts through to make a hold
4.	While the bottle is still warm, insert the MDI into the hole to ensure a tight fit between the MDI and the bottle spacer
5.	The new bottle spacer should be primed initially with 10 puffs of the medicine to reduce electrostatic charge on the walls

Table 11.2 Global Asthma Network (GAN) instructions on how to use a homemade spacer [28]

Step	Instructions
1.	Insert the MDI into the hole at the base of the bottle spacer
2.	Hold the neck of the bottle spacer in the child's mouth, simulating a mouthpiece and making it easier to direct aerosol into the airways For a young child who cannot form a tight seal with the spacer in their mouth, a small commercially available facemask that fits on the open end of the bottle can be applied
3.	Give the child a single puff of the MDI with the spacer, followed by normal breathing. Repeat until the desired amount of medication is given, which is frequently 2 puffs, but may be up to 6 puffs for relief of bronchoconstriction

Fig. 11.1 Child using
homemade spacer [28]

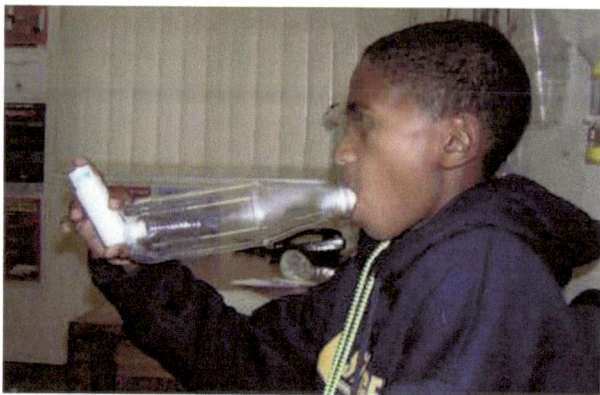

Fig. 11.2 Mother using
homemade spacer for her
infant [28]

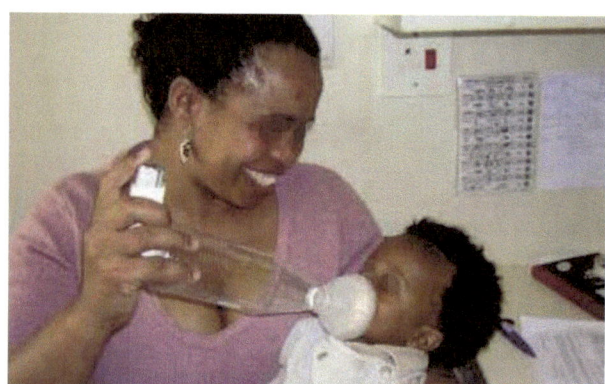

Summary

Health disparities in allergic diseases are increasingly recognized as barriers that need to be eliminated. Many networks are working to eliminate these disparities. These networks include governmental and nongovernmental organizations. These organizations are working at a national and international level, underscoring the prevalence of the problem and trying to provide solutions for it. The efforts of these organizations include identifying the scope of the health disparity problem and its impact on patients and societies, coming up with solutions that are pertinent to high-risk groups, and sharing these solutions broadly for everyone's benefit. Only through constant vigilance can success be measured and, if necessary, new targets acquired. These networks serve as sentinels in the ever-changing fight against health disparities in allergic disease.

References

1. The Secretary's Advisory Committee on National Health Promotion and Disease Prevention Objectives for 2020: Phase I report: recommendations for the framework and format of Healthy People 2020. In: Services USDoHaH, editor, 2008.
2. Forno E, Celedon JC. Health disparities in asthma. Am J Respir Crit Care Med. 2012;185(10):1033–5.
3. Quality AfHRa. About AHRQ: AHRQ; 2017. Available from: https://www.ahrq.gov/cpi/about/index.html.
4. Speck AL, Nelson B, Jefferson SO, Baptist AP. Young, African American adults with asthma: what matters to them? Ann Allergy Asthma Immunol. 2014;112(1):35–9.
5. Speck AL, Hess M, Baptist AP. An electronic asthma self-management intervention for young African American adults. J Allergy Clin Immunol Pract. 2016;4(1):89–95 e2.
6. Leas BF, D'Anci KE, Apter AJ, Bryant-Stephens T, Lynch MP, Kaczmarek JL, et al. Effectiveness of indoor allergen reduction in asthma management: a systematic review. J Allergy Clin Immunol. 2018;141(5):1854–69.
7. Leas BF, D'Anci KE, Apter AJ, Bryant-Stephens T, Schoelles K, Umscheid CA. Effectiveness of indoor allergen reduction in management of asthma. Quality AfHRa, editor. Rockville: Agency for Healthcare Research and Quality; 2018 February.
8. Mission and Vision: National Institute of Health; 2019. Available from: https://www.nimhd.nih.gov/about/overview/mission-vision.html.
9. Bayly JE, Bernat D, Porter L, Choi K. Secondhand exposure to aerosols from electronic nicotine delivery systems and asthma exacerbations among youth with asthma. Chest. 2019;155(1):88–93.
10. Gergen PJ, Teach SJ, Togias A, Busse WW. Reducing exacerbations in the Inner City: lessons from the Inner-City Asthma Consortium (ICAC). J Allergy Clin Immunol Pract. 2016;4(1):22–6.
11. Clinical Studies: National Institute of Health; 2018 [updated September 10], 2018. Available from: https://www.niaid.nih.gov/clinical-trials/inner-city-asthma-consortium.
12. Szefler SJ, Mitchell H, Sorkness CA, Gergen PJ, O'Connor GT, Morgan WJ, et al. Management of asthma based on exhaled nitric oxide in addition to guideline-based treatment for inner-city adolescents and young adults: a randomised controlled trial. Lancet. 2008;372(9643):1065–72.
13. Szefler SJ, Gergen PJ, Mitchell H, Morgan W. Achieving asthma control in the inner city: do the National Institutes of Health Asthma Guidelines really work? J Allergy Clin Immunol. 2010;125(3):521–6; quiz 7-8.
14. Busse WW, Morgan WJ, Gergen PJ, Mitchell HE, Gern JE, Liu AH, et al. Randomized trial of omalizumab (anti-IgE) for asthma in inner-city children. N Engl J Med. 2011;364(11):1005–15.
15. Institute P-COR. Our Vision & Mission https://www.pcori.org/about-us/our-vision-mission. Available from: https://www.pcori.org/about-us/our-vision-mission.
16. Beach MC, Rosner M, Cooper LA, Duggan PS, Shatzer J. Can patient-centered attitudes reduce racial and ethnic disparities in care? Acad Med. 2007;82(2):193–8.
17. Sleath B, Gratie D, Carpenter D, Davis SA, Lee C, Loughlin CE, et al. Reported problems and adherence in using asthma medications among adolescents and their caregivers. Ann Pharmacother. 2018;52(9):855–61.
18. Foundation RWJ. Our guiding principles 2018. Available from: https://www.rwjf.org/en/about-rwjf/our-guiding-principles.html.
19. Martin C, Palmer L. Reducing racial and ethnic disparities: a quality-improvement initiative in Medicaid Managed Care. Martin L, McAndrew M, editors. 200 American Metro Blvd, Suite 119, Hamilton, NJ 08619: Center for Health Care Strategies, Inc; 2007.

20. Press VG, Pappalardo AA, Conwell WD, Pincavage AT, Prochaska MH, Arora VM. Interventions to improve outcomes for minority adults with asthma: a systematic review. J Gen Intern Med. 2012;27(8):1001–15.

21. Care RH. About RAND Health Care 2019 [Available from: https://www.rand.org/health-care/about.html.

22. Lara M, Ramos-Valencia G, Gonzalez-Gavillan JA, Lopez-Malpica F, Morales-Reyes B, Marin H, et al. Reducing quality-of-care disparities in childhood asthma: La Red de Asma Infantil intervention in San Juan, Puerto Rico. Pediatrics. 2013;131(Suppl 1):S26–37.

23. Support Urban Institute: The Urban Institute; 2019. Available from: https://www.urban.org/aboutus/support-urban-institute.

24. Ganesh B, Payton Scally C, Skopec L, Zhu J. The relationship between housing and asthma among school-age children: analysis of the 2015 American Housing Survey. 2100 M Street NW, Washington, DC 20037: The Urban Institute; 2017.

25. Lai CK, Beasley R, Crane J, Foliaki S, Shah J, Weiland S, et al. Global variation in the prevalence and severity of asthma symptoms: phase three of the International Study of Asthma and Allergies in Childhood (ISAAC). Thorax. 2009;64(6):476–83.

26. Pearce N, Asher I, Billo N, Bissell K, Ellwood P, El Sony A, et al. Asthma in the global NCD agenda: a neglected epidemic. Lancet Respir Med. 2013;1(2):96–8.

27. Asher I, Haahtela T, Selroos O, Ellwood P, Ellwood E, Global Asthma Network Study G. Global Asthma Network survey suggests more national asthma strategies could reduce burden of asthma. Allergol Immunopathol (Madr). 2017;45(2):105–14.

28. The global asthma report 2018. Auckland: Global Asthma Network; 2018.

Index